Sexually Transmitted Diseases

Sexually Transmitted Diseases

Edited by

Yehudi M. Felman, M.D., M.A., M.Phil., F.A.C.P.

Clinical Professor of Dermatology
State University of New York, Downstate Medical Center
Brooklyn, New York

Lecturer in Public Health
Columbia University
College of Physicians and Surgeons
School of Public Health
New York, New York

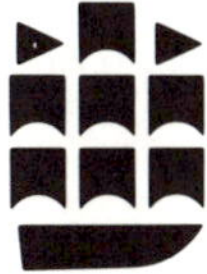

CHURCHILL LIVINGSTONE

New York, Edinburgh, London, Melbourne 1986

Library of Congress Cataloging-in-Publication Data

Sexually transmitted diseases.

   Includes bibliographies and index.
   1. Venereal diseases.   I. Felman, Yehudi M.
[DNLM: 1. Venereal Diseases.   WC 140 S5175]
RC200.S494   1986   616.95′1   86-9710
ISBN 0-443-08331-2

Distributed in the United Kingdom by Churchill Livingstone,
Robert Stevenson House, 1–3 Baxter's Place, Leith Walk, Edinburgh
EH1 3AF, and by associated companies, branches, and representatives
throughout the world.

Accurate indications, adverse reactions, and dosage schedules for
drugs are provided in this book, but it is possible that they
may change. The reader is urged to review the package information
data of the manufacturers of the medications mentioned.

Copy Editor: *Ann Ruzycka*
Production Designer: *Rosalie Marcus*
Production Supervisor: *Jane Grochowski*
Cover Designer: *Gloria Brown Milner*

Printed in the United States of America

First published in 1986

To Brenda, Nahum, and Hillel

Contributors

William R. Bowie, M.D.
Assistant Professor of Medicine, Division of Infectious Diseases, University of British Columbia Faculty of Medicine, Vancouver, British Columbia, Canada

Willard Cates Jr., M.D., M.P.H.
Director, Division of Sexually Transmitted Diseases, Centers for Disease Control, Atlanta, Georgia

John C. Cutler, M.D.
Emeritus Professor of International Health and Health Services Administration, University of Pittsburgh, Graduate School of Public Health, Pittsburgh, Pennsylvania

William W. Darrow, Ph.D.
Research Sociologist, AIDS Program, Division of Viral Diseases, Center for Infectious Diseases, Centers for Disease Control, Atlanta, Georgia

Pierre Dejace, M.D.
Institut Jules Bordet, Centre des Tumeurs de l'Université Libre de Bruxelles, Brussels, Belgium; Former Fellow in Infectious Diseases, Brown University, Providence, Rhode Island

Yehudi M. Felman, M.D., M.A., M.Phil., F.A.C.P.
Clinical Professor of Dermatology, State University of New York, Downstate Medical Center, Brooklyn; Lecturer in Public Health, Columbia University College of Physicians and Surgeons, School of Public Health, New York, New York

Nicholas J. Fiumara, M.D., M.P.H.
Clinical Professor of Dermatology, Boston University School of Medicine; Clinical Professor of Dermatology, Tufts University School of Medicine; Lecturer in Dermatology, Harvard Medical School, Boston, Massachusetts

John D. Frame, M.D.
Adjunct Associate Professor of Public Health (Tropical Medicine), School of Public Health, Columbia University College of Physicians and Surgeons; Director, Associate Mission Medical Office, National Council of Christian Churches, U.S.A., New York, New York

Margaret R. Hammerschlag, M.D.
Assistant Professor of Pediatrics and Medicine, Division of Infectious Diseases, State University of New York, Downstate Medical Center, Brooklyn, New York

William O. Harrison, M.D.
Assistant Clinical Professor of Medicine, University of California, San Diego, School of Medicine; Captain, United States Navy, HTLV3 Screening Project, Naval Hospital, San Diego, California

Axel W. Hoke, M.D.
Clinical Professor of Dermatology, University of California, San Francisco, School of Medicine; Acting Chief, Dermatology Clinics, San Francisco General Hospital, San Francisco, California

Franklyn N. Judson, M.D.
Associate Professor of Medicine and Preventive Medicine, University of Colorado Health Sciences Center; Director, Denver Disease Control Service, Chief, Infectious Diseases, Denver General Hospital, Denver, Colorado

Howard I. Maibach, M.D.
Professor of Dermatology, University of California, San Francisco, School of Medicine, San Francisco, California

James A. Nikitas, M.S.
Former Assistant Director, Bureau of Venereal Disease Control, New York City Health Department, New York, and Clinical Associate Professor of Dermatology, New York Medical College, Valhalla, New York

Robert C. Noble, M.D.
Professor of Medicine, Division of Infectious Disease, University of Kentucky College of Medicine, Lexington, Kentucky

J.D. Oriel, M.D.
Senior Consultant Physician in Genito-urinary Medicine, Senior Lecturer in Medicine, University College Hospital, London, England

Milton Orkin, M.D.
Clinical Professor of Dermatology, University of Minnesota School of Medicine, Minneapolis, Minnesota

David G. Ostrow, M.D., Ph.D.
Associate Professor, Departments of Psychiatry and Community Health and Preventive Medicine, Northwestern University Medical School; Director of Biological Psychiatry Programs, Veterans Administration Lakeside Medical Center and Northwestern Memorial Hospital; Staff Psychiatrist, Veterans Administration Lakeside Medical Center, Chicago, Illinois

Benjamin Raab, M.D.
Assistant Professor of Clinical Dermatology, Northwestern University Medical School, Chicago, Illinois

Ted Rosen, M.D.
Associate Professor of Dermatology, Baylor College of Medicine; Chief, Dermatology Service, Veterans Administration Medical Center, Houston, Texas

Bijan Safai, M.D., D.Sc.
Professor of Medicine, Cornell University School of Medicine; Chief, Dermatology Service, Memorial Sloan–Kettering Cancer Center, New York, New York

Norman Sohn, M.D.
Clinical Assistant Professor of Surgery, New York Medical College, Valhalla; Clinical Assistant Professor of Surgery, New York University School of Medicine, New York; Associate Surgeon, Lenox Hill Hospital, New York, New York

Michael R. Spence, M.D., M.P.H.
Professor and Chairman, Department of Obstetrics and Gynecology, Hahnemann University School of Medicine, Philadelphia, Pennsylvania

Jaime A. Tschen, M.D.
Assistant Professor of Dermatology and Pathology, Baylor College of Medicine; Assistant Chief, Dermatology Service, Veterans Administration Medical Center, Houston, Texas

Nancy Wolfin, M.D.
Dermatology Fellow, Memorial Sloan–Kettering Cancer Center, New York, New York

Stephen H. Zinner, M.D.
Professor of Medicine, Brown University School of Medicine; Director, Division of Infectious Disease, Roger Williams General Hospital, Providence, Rhode Island

Preface

The last few decades have been witness to a veritable explosion of public health problems brought about by sexually transmitted diseases in the United States, in particular, and in the western world in general. Twenty years ago sexually transmitted disease essentially comprised syphilis and gonorrhea. Now the field includes such major public health problems as chlamydial disease, genital herpes simplex, acquired immune deficiency syndrome, and enteric protozoal, bacterial, and viral diseases such as amebiasis, giardiasis, salmonellosis, shigellosis, and hepatitis B, as well as scabies, pediculosis, genital warts, molluscum contagiosum, and a host of other sexually transmitted infections, to all of which are devoted chapters in this book.

Indeed, the problems posed by sexually transmitted diseases cross the boundaries of many specialties, including dermatology, infectious diseases, obstetrics and gynecology, urology, internal medicine, family practice, and adolescent medicine.

This book is designed for practicing clinicians in all the above-mentioned areas. Experts in each disease have written the chapters on that disease. Their views do not necessarily coincide, but represent the gamut of the latest thinking. It is hoped that this book will be of value to all clinicians in the diagnosis and treatment of sexually transmitted diseases.

I would like to acknowledge the gracious help and assistance of the following: Mr. James Nikitas, Mrs. Mildred Marshall, Mrs. Bienveni Arias, Ms. Grace Novick, and Dr. Manuel Scham, without whose assistance this book would not have been possible.

Yehudi M. Felman, M.D.

Contents

Epidemiology and Control of Sexually Transmitted Diseases

Willard Cates, Jr.

A new era of sexually transmitted diseases is upon us.[1] Until recently, the scope of venereal diseases was limited to five classical infections: gonorrhea, syphilis, chancroid, lymphogranuloma venereum, and granuloma inguinale. Through the 1960s, most of the federal emphasis was on syphilis. In 1972 a national gonorrhea control program was initiated; by 1979 gonococcal pelvic inflammatory disease had become a priority.[2] With prevention and control efforts focused on these entities, important advances were made.

During the 1970s, however, a major shift in thinking occurred among those concerned with venereal diseases. Clinicians, public health workers, and policymakers became increasingly aware of the broader spectrum of infection spread from person to person during sexual contact. Just as importantly, public health officials began to understand the magnitude, both in terms of financial cost and human suffering, of the long-term consequences of sexually transmitted infections—primarily infertility, ectopic pregnancy, other types of reproductive loss, and even neoplasia. Thus, as a testimony to the comprehensive nature of this discipline, the term "sexually transmitted diseases" (STDs) has gradually replaced "venereal diseases."

Today, the more expanded list of STDs encompasses *Chlamydia trachomatis* infections, genital herpes, human papillomavirus infections, genital mycoplasmas, cytomegalovirus, hepatitis, vaginitis, enteric infections, and ectoparasite diseases, in addition to the original venereal diseases. Most of these infections have been around for ages, but they have achieved recent prominence as STDs for several reasons. First, laboratory diagnostic techniques improved. New diagnostic approaches facilitated epidemic investigations elucidating the extent, method of transmission, and clinical consequences of STDs. Second, the true incidence of the STDs increased, many at an alarming rate. In the United States, we believe chlamydia infections have become more frequent than gonorrhea; estimates of genital herpes and genital warts range up to one million new cases annually. Third, a higher proportion of systemic diseases are being sexually transmitted. As sexual behavior has changed, hepatitis, cytomegalovirus, group B streptococcal infections,

Organisms	Salpingitis	Infertility	Ectopic Pregnancy	Reproductive Loss	Puerperal Infection	Perinatal Infection	Genital Neoplasms	Male Urethritis	Epididymitis	Vulvovaginitis	Cervicitis/Urethritis	Proctitis	Hepatitis	Dermatitis	Genital Ulceration/Warts
Neisseria gonorrhoeae	X	X	X	X	X	X		X	X		X	X			
Chlamydia trachomatis	X	X	X	X	X	X	X	X	X		X	X			X
Herpes simplex virus				X		X	X			X	X	X			X
Human papilloma virus							X								X
Mycoplasma hominis	X	X	X	X											
Ureaplasma urealyticum				X				X							
Treponema pallidum				X		X							X		X
Cytomegalovirus						X									
Group B streptococcus						X									
Trichomonas vaginalis										X					
Gardnerella vaginalis										X					
Candida albicans										X					
Haemophilus ducreyi															X
Calymmatobacterium granulomatis															X
Campylobacter fetus												X			
Shigella species												X			
Entamoeba histolytica												X			
Hepatitis B virus													X		
Hepatitis A virus													X		
Sarcoptes scabiei														X	
Phthirius pubis														X	

Fig. 1-1 Matrix of sexually transmitted organisms and syndromes.

and some enteric pathogens have become frequent sexually transmitted agents among some subgroups. Fourth, the key impact of STDs on maternal and child health is now apparent. Those interested in improving general reproductive health realize their programs must include activities to prevent and control the STDs.

Thus, during the past decade, the STD field has grown at a logarithmic rate, both in its scope and in its complexity. Over 20 organisms and syndromes are now recognized as being sexually transmitted (Fig. 1-1). Depending on the definition of the illness, more than 50 different pathologic entities can result. Some agents are responsible for many syndromes, while others have been associated with only one. Moreover, the syndromes themselves vary in their incidence, severity, and health care costs.

No longer are the STDs the primary domain of venereologists. The diseases now span the clinical specialties of internal medicine, pediatrics, obstetrics/gynecology, family practice, urology, ophthalmology, and dermatology. However, the supplementary medical disciplines of microbiology, epidemiology, and pathology also contribute to our understanding of the range of STDs. More important from a disease control standpoint, the skills of behavioral scientists, public health managers, and primary field workers can influence the spread of STDs within communities. Thus, the team of health professionals involved with STD is a matrix of medical and public health interests.

EPIDEMIOLOGY OF SEXUALLY TRANSMITTED DISEASES

The Population at Risk

The size of the sexually active population at risk for STDs has never been larger. During the 1970s, various sociosexual changes in the United States have rather dramatically influenced—both quantitatively and qualitatively—those in danger of transmitting or acquiring STDs. By 1985, an estimated 61 million sexually active persons aged 15–34 will inhabit the nation; in 1970, that number was 42 million (Fig. 1-2).

Quantitatively, the factors influencing the population at risk are the coming of sexual age of the baby boom and the increasing percentage of young persons who are sexually active. The baby boom occurred between 1947 and 1964,[3] with the number of births peaking in 1957. The modal age of this uniquely large cohort of the American population increased from 13 in 1970 to 28 in 1985. At the same time, this group became more sexually experienced; by 1979, half of all unmarried teenage women had experienced coitus, compared to 30% in 1971.[4] This increase was found among each year of age from 15 to 19. Because of these two factors, the absolute number of sexually active young persons at greatest risk of STD increased dramatically during the 1970s.

Qualitatively, several other factors also contributed to the increasing population at risk. Those who became sexually active had a greater number of partners than their predecessors of the 1960s. For example, the percentage of sexually experienced unmarried teenage women who had more than one partner increased from 39% in 1971 to 50% in 1976.[5] The number of partners has a multiplier effect on the rate of STD transmission in communities. Also, a greater percentage of the baby boom has remained single—again increasing both the length and likelihood of STD exposure. In 1980 over one quarter of women younger than 25 lived alone; nearly one half of men the same age were in a similar situation.[6]

Trends in Sexually Transmitted Organisms

Gonorrhea has been contained. The implementation of a national program in 1972 to control gonorrhea was eventually followed by a reversal of the spiraling gonorrhea morbidity rate in 1975 (Fig. 1-3). During the previous 10 years, reported gonorrhea had increased at an annual rate of 12% per year. The decline began initially in those aged 20 to 24, but soon spread to other age groups.[7] In 1982 the total number

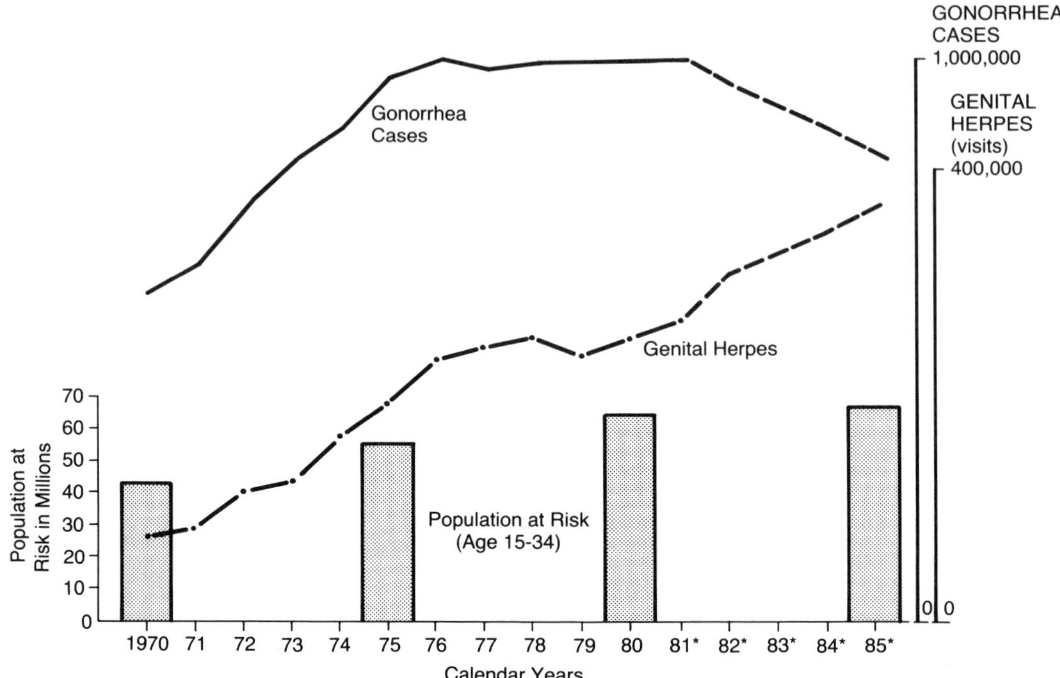

Fig. 1-2 Population at risk (age 15 to 34) and sexually transmitted disease trends in the United States from 1970 to 1985. Numbers for the years 1981 to 1985 were projected. The curve for genital herpes indicates number of visits to private physicians. (From the National Disease Therapeutic Index, IMS, Inc., Ambler, PA.)

of reported cases of gonorrhea fell below 1 million for the first time in 7 years.

This success in the gonorrhea control program was directly correlated with the infusion of federal resources. By 1973, the government expenditures for gonorrhea surpassed those of syphilis for the first time. In constant dollars, the amount committed to gonorrhea control declined gradually during the decade. Because of the increased efficiency of the control strategies—targeted screening, self-referral of sex partners, and more rapid identification of asymptomatic carriers—the number of gonorrhea cases remained level in the 1970s and began to decrease in the 1980s.

Problems with gonococcal antibiotic resistance, however, offset the encouraging trend in reported gonorrhea morbidity. β-Lactamase (or penicillinase)-producing *Neisseria gonorrhoeae* (PPNG) was first isolated in the United States in 1976.[8] Over the next several years, despite prospective surveillance efforts, the reported numbers of PPNG remained quite stable. Most cases were linked to overseas travel or military importation, and immediate intervention by STD caseworkers limited civilian-to-civilian transmission in the United States.

In 1980 things took a turn for the worse. PPNG infections increased dramatically; by 1982, over 4,500 cases had been reported and by 1985 alone there were over 5,000 reported cases. Reasons proposed for these upsurging numbers include continued importation from such high-rate areas as Korea, the Philippines, and Africa, improved laboratory surveillance in recent years, and the entrenchment of PPNG in some communities to produce sustained domestic transmission. Los Angeles, New York City, and Miami were particularly affected. Because of the high cost of treating and controlling PPNG, the increase is of

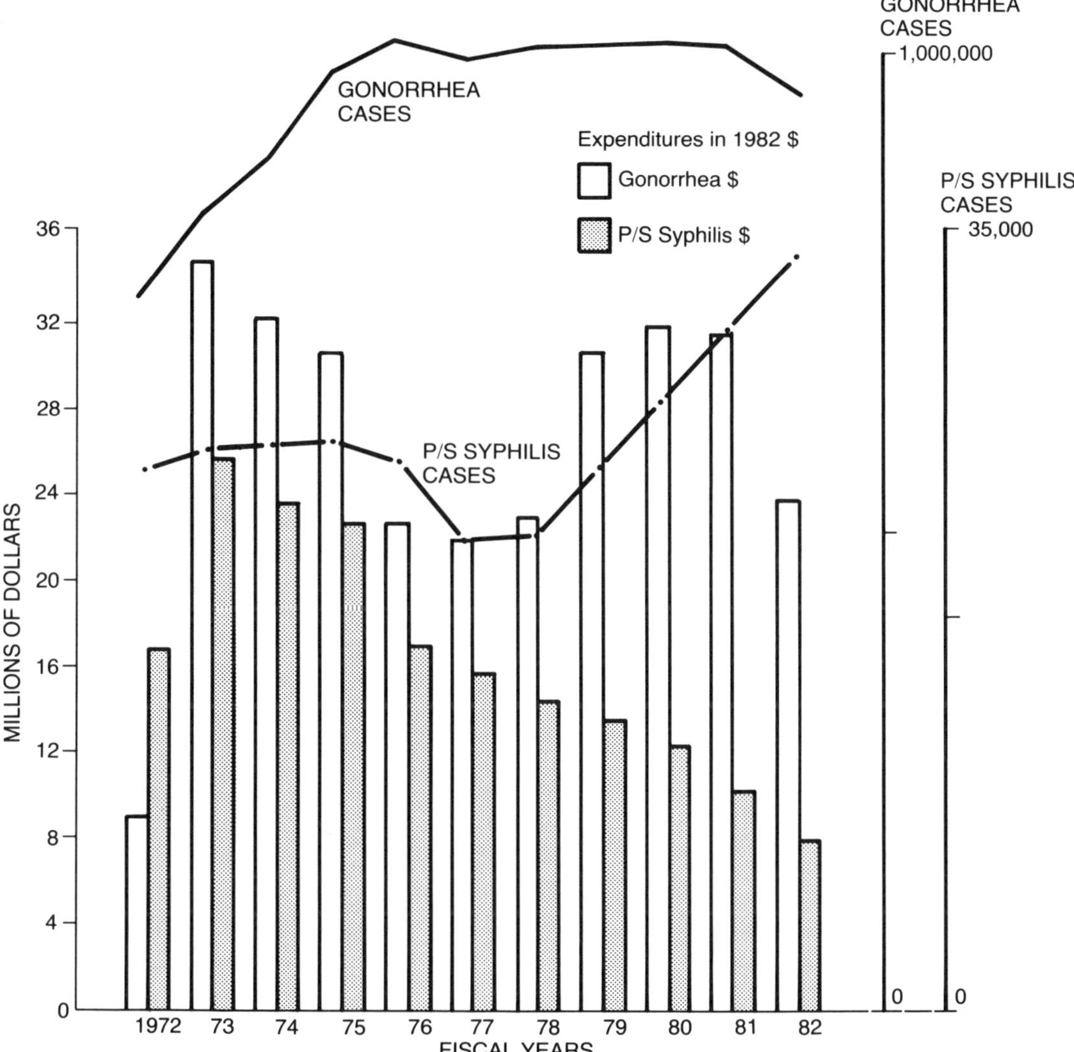

Fig. 1-3 Gonorrhea and primary and secondary syphilis cases versus federal project grants to states in 1982 dollars in the United States in the fiscal years 1972 to 1982. (Adjustments for 1982 dollars were made by Price Deflaters for Federal Government Purchases of Goods and Services.)

great concern to those responsible for STD programs.

In addition, other biological changes of the gonococcal organism created recent outbreaks of resistant strains. In North Carolina, non-PPNG, penicillin-resistant gonorrhea initially appeared in early 1983 and spread throughout the community within a matter of weeks.[9] This was the first instance of the chromosomally mediated, highly resistant organisms in the United States.

In Southeast Asia, more than 20% of gonococcal isolates are non-PPNG strains resistant to penicillin.[10] Even worse, the specter of β-lactamase-producing spectinomycin-resistant gonorrhea appeared in late 1982 and 1983 among Americans stationed in Korea.[11] This doubly resistant strain was shown to be spread among the local civilian and military communities. Thus, although the resistant organisms account for less than 0.5% of reported gonorrhea, they threaten the gains made by the national control program.

Current syphilis trends, while still quite low, warrant consideration. To some extent, the national gains in gonorrhea control were made at the expense of syphilis (Fig. 1-3). As both the relative and absolute amount of federal resources directed to syphilis control decreased, the reported cases of primary and secondary syphilis increased. While the largest portion of the rise occurred among male homosexuals, the number of cases of early syphilis also increased among women.[12] Reported congenital syphilis among infants less than 1 year of age reflected similar trends: in 1982, 159 cases occurred, up 50% from its nadir in 1979. Although the current levels of syphilis morbidity are well below those of the 1940s, when federal control efforts began, its increasing trend through 1982 reflects an acknowledged and necessary tradeoff in the shift of limited STD resources from syphilis to gonorrhea control.

Other sexually transmitted organisms are also apparently increasing, most prominently infections caused by *Chlamydia trachomatis*, herpes simplex virus, and human papillomavirus. *Chlamydia* are among the most common sexually transmitted pathogens in the United States today. Nongonococcal urethritis (NGU) in men is caused by *C. trachomatis* in 30 to 50% of the cases.[13] In 1972 the number of visits to the offices of private physicians was greater for cases of nongonococcal urethritis than for gonorrhea. The gap has widened in recent years. While some of the relative difference is undoubtedly related to more accurate diagnosis of nongonococcal urethritis, the pattern of increasing chlamydia infection compared to gonorrhea is supported by trends in reports from regional STD control programs,[14] as well as national surveillance in other countries.[15]

Chlamydia trachomatis also plays an important role in causing mucopurulent cer-

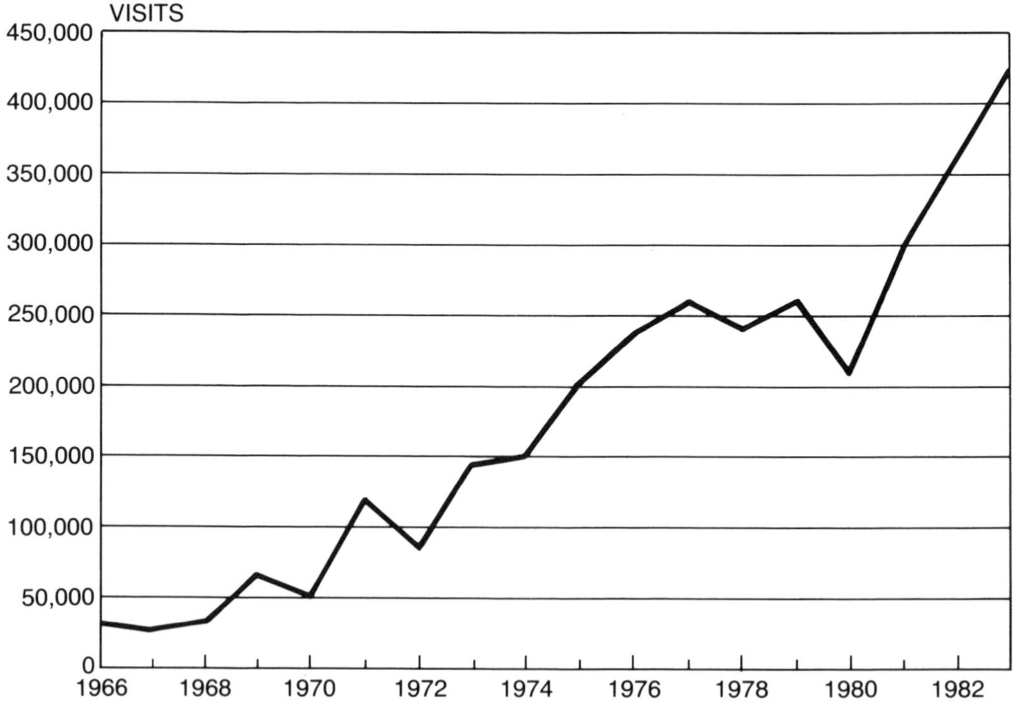

Fig. 1-4 Herpes genitalis: number of visits to private physician's office in the United States from 1966 to 1981. (From National Disease Therapeutic Index, IMS, Inc., Ambler, PA.)

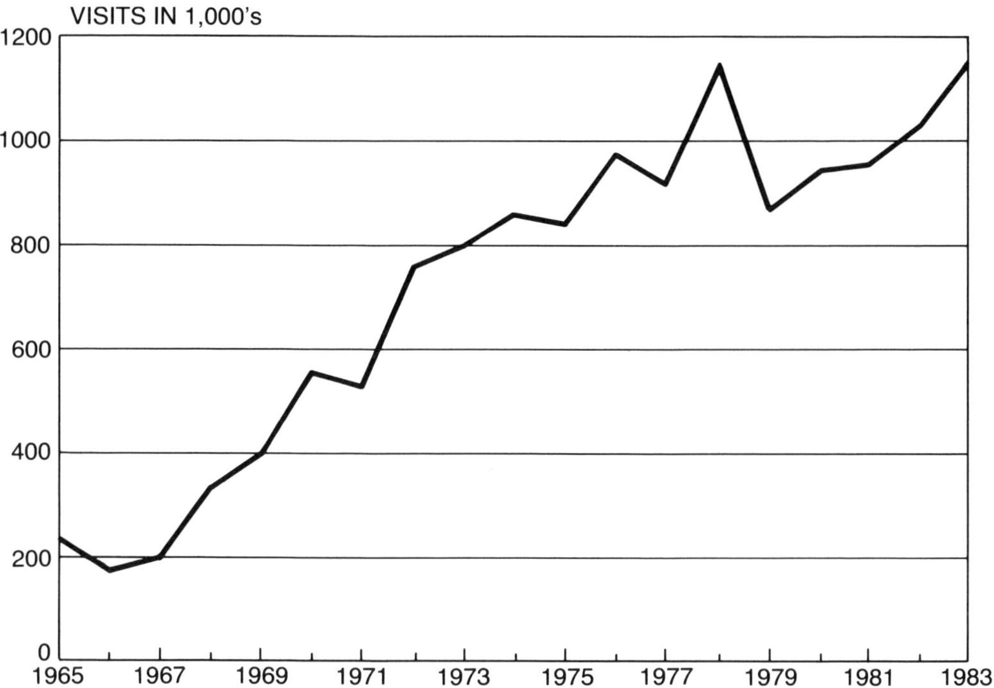

Fig. 1-5 Genital warts: number of visits to private physician's office in the United States from 1966 to 1981. (From National Disease Therapeutic Index, IMS, Inc., Amber, PA.)

vicitis—the female equivalent of nongonococcal urethritis.[13] This condition may predispose to acute pelvic inflammatory disease in nonpregnant women or to infant and maternal infections in pregnant women. Most estimates of the rate of *C. trachomatis* infection in pregnant women have ranged from 7 to 12%; those at highest risk are unwed teenagers living in urban areas,[16] precisely the group at highest risk both for other STDs and for adverse pregnancy outcomes. Finally, the male equivalent of pelvic inflammatory disease, epididymitis, has also been associated with *C. trachomatis,* especially in males aged 19 to 35 years.

Genital herpes infections are also on the rise (Fig. 1-4). The estimated numbers of encounters with private physicians for genital herpes showed a dramatic increase between 1966 and 1981. The *number* of consultations for this condition increased from under 30,000 in 1966 to nearly 300,000 in 1981. The *rate* at which patients consulted

fee-for-service office-based physicians for genital herpes infection increased almost tenfold, from 3.4/100,000 consultations in 1966 to over 33/100,000 in 1981. A similar incidence (and trend) of genital herpes was found in Olmstead County, Minnesota.[17] The current rise of initial genital herpes infections has an effect on the future: clinical manifestations of the infection tend to recur, and infections of the newborn acquired during passage through the birth canal are often life-threatening.

Genital warts caused by the human papillomavirus (HPV) are even more common than genital herpes (Fig. 1-5). In 1981, nearly 950,000 consultations with private physicians were made for condyloma acuminata.[18] Between 1966 and 1981 the increase in the number of visits for genital warts was greater than that of herpes. Moreover, these are minimum estimates of gen ital human papillomavirus infections, since they do not include flat condyloma (cervical intraepithelial neoplasia) caused by the virus. Human papillomavirus is becoming recognized as a serious STD, and its association with precancerous lesions of the cervix, vagina, and vulva is increasingly documented.[19]

Trends in Syndromes Caused by Sexually Transmitted Diseases

Pelvic inflammatory disease (PID) is the most severe complication, with the greatest public health consequences, of lower genital tract infections in women. Trends in PID are more difficult to interpret, however, than those of gonorrhea in women. Results of two databases from physician office visits have demonstrated a remarkably consistent falloff from the peak number of cases of pelvic inflammatory disease in 1973.[20] In the five years between 1973 and 1977, the rate of PID visits fell by about 40%. The decline was greater in women of black and other races than in white women. Since 1978, however, the rate of PID visits has been quite stable.

Hospitalized PID has followed a different course. Overall, rates increased slightly during the decade of the 1970s, with nearly all the increase occurring in young white women.[21] Thus, the outpatient and inpatient data support each other in one event—minority women had more favorable PID trends during the 1970s than white women. Yet they conflict in another—ambulatory visits to private physicians decreased, while hospitalizations increased.

Several factors could account for this apparent conflict: (1) The overall number of visits to physician's offices for all health conditions declined over the decade; trends in PID could reflect this health seeking behavior. (2) The 1973 peak in physician office visits may be an artifact of the national gonorrhea screening program; women with positive cultures may have been diagnosed as PID. (3) Physicians may be more likely to hospitalize patients with PID in recent years as they have become more aware of the long-term consequences. (4) The changing spectrum of sexually transmitted organisms could lead to a form of PID that is less clinically severe at the initial episode, but which eventually produces symptoms requiring direct hospitalization.[13] How many, if any, of these factors are important is unknown.

Involuntary infertility, a portion of which is secondary to STDs, as well as requests for infertility services, apparently increased during the 1970s.[22,23] Between 1965 and 1976, the percentage of couples 29 years of age or younger classified as infertile increased from 5% to 7%; these increases were greater in couples with no children or one child, and in younger black couples. By 1976, an estimated 2 million American families wished to have more children but were unable to conceive. Over 900,000 visits to physicians' offices in 1980 were for infertility counseling and treatment.[23]

The exact proportion of these infertile couples whose status is secondary to the consequences of STDs is unknown; estimates have ranged from 15 to 30%, depending upon the populations involved and the causes of infertility attributed to STDs.[24] Extrapolating from the number of PID cases and the risk of infertility after PID,[25] between 100,000 and 150,000 women would be rendered involuntarily infertile each year because of pelvic infection after STDs. This is probably a minimum estimate of sexually transmitted infertility, since it does not include that portion directly or indirectly related to male factors involving such STDs as *Mycoplasma hominis, Ureaplasma urealyticum, Chlamydia trachomatis,* and *Neisseria gonorrhoeae.*

Prenatal STDs also produce adverse effects on both pregnancy outcome and maternal infant health. The obstetrical consequences of syphilis and gonorrhea have long been known. Nearly 40% of pregnant women with recently acquired, but undetected, syphilis suffer a spontaneous abortion, a stillbirth, or a perinatal death.[26] About half the infants who survive will be infected with *Treponema pallidum* and develop congenital syphilis. Gonococcal infection during pregnancy increases the risk of chorioamnionitis, premature rupture of membranes, and prematurity.[27]

The reproductive sequelae from the other "second generation" STDs are being increasingly documented and may have even more severe impact on pregnancy. Cervical *C. trachomatis* has a complex interaction with the mycoplasmas in contributing to reproductive loss.[13,16,28] Genital mycoplasmas have been implicated in a variety of abnormal outcomes; *U. ureaplasma* is primarily associated with low birth weight infants, and *M. hominis* with postpartum fever.[29] Genital herpes infections influence both pregnancy management and outcome; in women actively shedding virus, cesarean deliveries are recommended to reduce the risk of neonatal herpes.[30] Moreover, parallel to the trend in genital herpes, neonatal herpes has also been increasing in certain regions of the United States.[31]

Ectopic pregnancy has increased dramatically during the last 15 years. Since 1965 the number of ectopic pregnancies quadrupled in the United States, rising to over 60,000 cases in 1981[32,33]; the incidence has tripled, increasing from 38/100,000 women aged 15 to 44 in 1965 to 113/100,000 in 1981. The exact cause of this alarming rise is unknown; however, the data are consistent with a cumulative effect of PID-induced tubal scarring, which eventually causes an ectopic implantation should conception occur. Women with a history of PID are over ten times more likely to suffer ectopic pregnancy than those without such a history.[34] Moreover, careful examination of the role of the intrauterine device in producing an increase in ectopic pregnancy has failed to demonstrate any association.[33] Therefore, experts generally agree that PID

has made the largest contribution to the increase of ectopic pregnancy in the United States.

At least four cancers have been associated with different STDs: cervical intraepithelial neoplasia, vulvar carcinoma, anal carcinoma, and hepatocellular carcinoma. Also, to the extent that the acquired immunodeficiency syndrome (AIDS) and its opportunistic tumors are considered malignant conditions, these are neoplasms apparently associated with a sexually transmissible agent. STDs probably play a complex role in oncogenesis; possible interactions among infectious agents may even potentiate the development of genital malignancies.[35] While the etiology of cervical cancer is probably multifactorial, human papillomavirus and herpes simplex virus remain the strongest infectious candidates.[19,36,37] Other organisms such as *Trichomonas vaginalis, C. trachomatis,* and *T. pallidum* have also been independently linked to cervical cancer. Vulvar carcinoma in situ has likewise been correlated with papilloma- and herpesviruses.[35] Anal carcinoma has been associated with homosexual males[38]; the increased risk of homosexuals having multiple STDs is the hypothesized link between their sexual preference and the anal neoplasm. While these epidemiologic associations do not prove causality, consistency among the studies to date is persuasive in the STD-cancer link.

CONTROL OF SEXUALLY TRANSMITTED DISEASES

These recent trends in STD agents and syndromes have stimulated new directions in STD control programs. Because of the complexity of the United States health care system, our past STD control efforts have generally required timely responses to changes in intervention technology, antibiotic resistance, public funding, and media interest.

History of STD Control

National programs to control STD were established in the United States during the early days of World War I.[39] For the next half-century, the focus was almost exclusively on the control of syphilis and its complications. Federal grants to support venereal disease control initiatives were begun in 1939. Rapid treatment centers for syphilis and gonorrhea were the World War II responses to a perceived venereal disease (VD) problem. Widespread availability of penicillin led to a dismantling of the rapid treatment centers and a dissolution of the clinical specialty of venereology, which had largely been syphilology. Nevertheless, during the 1950s and 1960s, federal assistance continued to support sex partner tracing, serologic screening, and patient education services. The STD "epidemiologist" emerged as a central figure in syphilis control efforts. By the late 1960s, officials became concerned with the rapidly escalating number of gonorrhea cases. Selective culture media stimulated the development of a national gonorrhea control strategy.[40] Pilot projects were undertaken in six cities, both to heighten case-finding of infected women and also to identify sex partners of infected men. These projects demonstrated the feasibility of such an approach. In 1972 the Federal Government dramatically increased its financial assistance to STD control. At the expense of syphilis, gonorrhea gradually received a larger portion of the STD federal dollar during the remainder of the decade. By 1982, expenditures for gonorrhea control accounted for almost 75% of federal STD grant dollars.

The national gonorrhea control efforts evolved through three overlapping phases during the 1970s.[2] Initial program objectives sought to lower disease incidence and arrest the resistance of *N. gonorrhoeae* to antibiotics (Table 1-1). Asymptomatic women were targeted, and ineffective treatments were discouraged. By 1975, the control program had entered a middle phase, emphasizing more focused screening of high-risk patients and more intensive follow-up of treatment failures. The emergence of penicillinase (β-lactamase)-producing *Neisseria gonorrhoeae* (PPNG) warranted highest program concern. Targeted outreach was especially important, since the larger numbers of gonorrhea patients precluded the intensive follow-up of each infected case, which had been a relative luxury of the syphilis era.[39]

By 1979, the gonorrhea control strategies entered into a third phase.[2] Analyses of national data, as well as program experiences, identified the public health importance of pelvic inflammatory disease (PID). Then program objectives expanded to reduce the incidence of, and also limit the consequences from, PID.[41] Asymptomatic men who were partners of women with PID were actively sought. Hospital emergency rooms became additional facilities in which to uncover gonorrhea.

Coincidentally, as emphasized earlier, the importance of sexually transmitted organisms other than syphilis and gonorrhea became recognized not only for their etiologic role in PID, but also for their contribution to a variety of other syndromes causing patients to seek care at STD clinics.[42] Increasingly, control strategies sought to upgrade clinical skills, clinic services, and physical facilities in order to encourage more effective patient recruitment and to provide additional resources for diagnosis of the broad array of STD. Thus, during the 1970s, we saw the concerns evolve from their firm base of "venereal" diseases to consideration of the vast spectrum of the STDs.

Table 1-1. Evolution of National Gonorrhea Control Program in the United States, 1972 to 1983

	Initial Phase	Second Phase	Third Phase
Objectives	Reduce incidence Reduce resistance	Reduce incidence Reduce resistance Limit PPNG	Reduce incidence Reduce PID Reduce resistance Limit PPNG
Approaches	Identify asymptomatic women Use effective therapy	Identify asymptomatic women Identify transmitters Use effective therapy Identify resistant organisms	Identify all infected women Recognize and manage PID Identify transmitters Identify untreated men Use effective therapy Identify resistant organisms
Elements			
Education/training	General public Adolescents Providers	Infected clinic patients Repeaters High-risk groups Providers General public	Clinic staff All clinic patients Women with PID Providers High-risk groups General public
Disease detection	Screen women Quality cultures	Priority screening Test of cure (TOC) Rescreening Quality cultures and followup	Priority screening Hospital emergency room Rescreening of women Quality cultures and followup
Partner referral	Interview infected men	Counsel for infection Interview repeaters Interview men	Counsel for infection Interview patients with gonococcal PID Interview repeaters Interview others
Clinic services	Expand hours Perform smears	Manage genital problems Patient sensitivity Support control	Performance standards Evaluate for PID Collaborate with others

Adapted from Brown ST, Wiesner PJ: Problems and approaches to the control and surveillance of sexually transmitted agents associated with pelvic inflammatory disease in the United States. Am J Obstet Gynecol 138:1096, 1980.

PID = pelvic inflammatory disease; PPNG = penicillinase (or β-lactamase)-producing *Neisseria gonorrhoeae*.

CURRENT SEXUALLY TRANSMITTED DISEASE CONTROL STRATEGIES

A recent World Health Organization/Pan American Health Organization Scientific Group has addressed the key activities necessary to reduce STD.[43] These components of STD intervention strategies provide a framework for describing the current national program in the United States. These components are as follows:

1. Health education and promotion
2. Disease detection
3. Appropriate treatment
4. Partner tracing/patient counseling
5. Clinical service evaluation
6. Training
7. Research

Health Education and Promotion

Health education messages are, in general, an integral part of each of the other six STD intervention activities. Specific community health education efforts, if presented properly, can supplement other strategies by encouraging *primary* preventive behavior *before* infection occurs in healthy persons at risk. Traditionally, "scare tactics" based on judgmental messages have not been a popular or effective method of changing behavior.[44] In fact, stigmatizing infected individuals by widespread social disapproval may even hinder disease control through delaying care.

To have any chance of success, health education must stress the benefits of preventive action and promote individual decision-making. For example, in today's more permissive society, messages emphasizing *discriminative* sexual intercourse among unmarried persons, rather than proscribing coital activity altogether, may have already had an impact. In the United States, in response to increasing concerns with genital herpes, over half of unmarried persons who believed themselves at risk reported changing their sexual behavior to avoid this disease.[45] Similar practices may have occurred in the gay community concordant with CDC's AIDS prevention recommendations.[46]

Other health promotion messages have emphasized appropriate use of contraceptives as prophylaxis against both STD and unintended pregnancy. For example, the condom or other barrier methods can be employed in specific high-risk settings. Such messages could be aired in contraceptive commercials on radio and television, since the National Association of Broadcasters have now lifted their ban against advertising nonprescription contraceptives.[47] Broadcasting this information would be especially useful for getting messages to teenagers.

Health education interventions also have a major role in secondary prevention, namely, in infected persons *after* symptoms appear. Messages to these individuals are directed at encouraging the following behaviors:

1. Prompt attendance for examination after exposure to high-risk situations

2. Early medical examination when symptomatic

3. Compliance with treatment

4. Facilitation of other interventions such as referral of sexual partners

Education strategies to increase the knowledge of STDs in the general public have been emphasized in recent years. Prototype school curriculum materials for grades 6 to 12, based on a self-instructional format, have been field-tested; these will facilitate systematic STD education throughout the country. A VD National Hotline has been implemented to provide both general and referral information to persons at high risk for STD. Thus, health education plays a fundamental role in STD control strategies for the 1980s.

Disease Detection

Early disease detection is an essential component of STD intervention strategies. This intervention takes place at two levels: the STD clinic and the community. At STD clinics, identification of infected individuals through sensitive diagnostic methods, combined with rapid treatment, will reduce disease complications and minimize further transmission. In the community, specific screening activities form the basis for early disease detection in asymptomatic persons and also permit determination of the highest risk groups on which to focus further program efforts.

Accurate diagnosis is the intervention cornerstone for the early detection strategies of STD control. Whether for making specific diagnoses in those with symptoms, or for screening of persons without symptoms, diagnostic tests for STD should ideally be rapid, inexpensive, simple, and accurate.

The usual parameters for assessing diagnostic techniques, sensitivity and specificity have a slightly different interpretation for STD control than for screening of chronic conditions,[48] largely because STD treatment is generally shorter and safer than therapy for other conditions. Consequently, sensitivity, that is, reducing false negatives, takes on an increased importance because missed cases place the infected person at continued risk of more serious complications, and result in further disease dissemination. Specificity, that is, reducing false positives, is less important because treatment of a small percentage of unaffected persons is associated with minimal morbidity, cost, and inconvenience. With the STD, however, the human and emotional costs of erroneously stigmatizing any individual means specificity cannot be neglected. Also, the public health costs of interviewing and tracing large numbers of false positive patients drain limited STD resources.

Advances in laboratory techniques have heralded the major initiatives in STD control. Serologic capabilities improved syphilis case-finding, and selective culture media allowed gonorrhea screening. Breakthroughs for rapid diagnosis of chlamydia will allow a national control program. The decision to initiate or abandon a new diagnostic test should be dictated both by the prevalence of the disease in the population being tested and by the accuracy of the test being considered. The predictive value of test results are crucial to clinical and public health decisions. Deficiencies in sensitivity can cause difficulties, particularly in the testing of populations with a high prevalence of disease. A new test with a sensitivity of 80% when used in an STD clinic would fail to identify 20% of women infected with *N. gonorrhoeae*. If disease prevalence in a clinic is 30%, then 6 women out of 100 tested would not be identified, and some proportion of these infected women would not receive therapy. The risks of those women developing salpingitis and its sequelae are obvious.

Deficiencies in specificity can also have immediate adverse repercussions, especially in low prevalence populations. For example, a new test with a specificity of 95%, when used in a very low prevalence population (2%), produces almost three times as many "false" positive tests unsupported by the "gold standard." In a clinical sense, treating 3 of every 4 patients unnecessarily adds risks and costs. In a case-finding sense, referring and evaluating four individuals to identify just a single diseased individual would tax STD personnel. In a public health sense, screening 20,000 women using the theoretical new test we have just described would increase the follow-up burden from 400 to 1,600 individuals. Such an increase could overwhelm STD resources.

Even with very specific tests (specificity ≥99%), screening for STDs of very low prevalence (<1%) creates many false positives. In the United States, for instance, the prevalence of syphilis has become so low that the cost-effectiveness of serologic screening (e.g., in premarital examinations, prenatal services, and new admissions to hospitals) is being debated.[49,50] Yield and cost considerations may be particularly important in screening activities; selection of the target population may greatly influence these factors. In the United States' gonorrhea program, the cost per case detected varied from a low of $25.00 in metropolitan STD clinics to as high as $350.00 in low prevalence areas.[51] When more selective screening was instituted in one location in 1976, the proportion of positive tests went from 4.5% to 8.1% in 1 year, and the cost per case detected was considerably reduced.[52]

Targeted screening has been implemented in some high-risk groups such as homosexuals, prostitutes, and pregnant women. For example, in some countries, Gram stains for gonorrhea are used in compulsory screening of legalized or semilegalized prostitutes. The yields are usually low, and the impact is severely limited by the insensitivity of the Gram stain. However, screening of prostitutes for PPNG has proved useful in the United States for stemming some specific outbreaks.[53]

Appropriate Treatment

Once the diagnosis is suspected or determined, treatment should be inexpensive, simple, safe, and effective. Early and adequate treatment of patients and their sexual partners is an effective means of preventing both a trend of increasing antimicrobial resistance of STD organisms, and also the spread of STD.[44] Barriers to implementing this strategy include the inability of treatment providers to identify infected persons, the selection of ineffective treatment regimens, and the unavailability of treatment for many patients and their sexual partners. To improve the likelihood of physicians prescribing effective treatment, two approaches have been used in the United States: laboratory monitoring of STD isolates for antimicrobial susceptibilities,[54] and consensus groups to develop standard treatment recommendations.[55]

Studies correlating antibiotic resistance with increasing treatment failure rates for a given antibiotic dose continue to be reported.[54] Widespread use of suboptimal doses of antibiotics for treating gonococcal infection has led to selection of resistant chromosomal mutants in developing countries throughout the world.[10,56] Thus, penicillin had to be used either in higher doses[57] or with a second drug.[10] The recent outbreak in the United States caused by a non-PPNG strain of *N. gonorrhoeae* that is highly resistant to penicillin[9] raises the possibility that such organisms may be widely distributed, but unrecognized, even in developed countries.

The emergence of a plasmid-mediated β-lactamase-producing *N. gonorrhoeae* has posed a much greater problem for STD control strategies.[8] Although disk testing allows relatively rapid laboratory identification of these strains, the sharp increase since 1980 in the reported number of PPNG cases, and the greater expense of treating and tracing individuals infected with these strains, has taxed limited resources of local STD control programs.

To increase the likelihood of successful treatment regimens for specific diagnoses, the United States Public Health Service has established treatment recommendations as a standard part of its control strategy. Initially, these recommendations covered syphilis and gonorrhea, but have been recently expanded to include 18 other sexually transmitted organisms and syndromes.[1,55] The process of achieving consensus among a group of clinicians expert in STD has proved to be a useful approach to establishing treatment guidelines that are applicable to diverse communties and also flexible enough to accommodate alternative treatment regimens.

Selective prophylactic (epidemiologic) treatment also has a major role in STD control strategies. In certain instances, waiting to confirm the specific diagnosis prior to initiating therapy is inappropriate. Rather, based on epidemiologic indications, antibiotics should be administered to some individuals when the diagnosis is considered likely, even before proof of infection by laboratory methods. Thus, selected groups of patients with a high risk of infection are identified by epidemiologic analyses and treated before confirmation of their infection status. This affects STD control in three ways: it interrupts the chain of transmission between the time of testing and treatment; it ensures treatment for infected women with false negative endocervical cultures; and it guarantees treatment for those who might not return when notified of positive tests.

Although this approach results in treating a percentage of uninfected persons, it increases the chances for disrupting transmission, a crucial aspect of STD control. Most recently, this approach of selective prophylactic treatment has effectively limited outbreaks of PPNG and chancroid in metropolitan areas.[53,58] Moreover, an adaptation of the same philosophy was recently used to recommend giving tetracycline concurrently with penicillin to patients with confirmed gonococcal infection,[55] since a relatively high proportion are liable to be harboring coexistent chlamydia organisms.

Partner Tracing and Patient Counseling

Traditionally, STD control programs in the United States have assumed that patients play relatively passive roles in disease control and prevention. Efforts to identify and ensure treatment of sexual partners of infected patients, therefore, emphasized active intervention by the health providers to interview the patient, to locate the named individuals, and to assure that these individuals are evaluated and treated.[39,40] However, during the past several years, this process of active intervention has been modified in some settings to include a more simplified approach. Instead of relying solely on the health worker, the patient may also be encouraged to assume responsibility for locating and referring his or her sexual partners.

Formal sex partner referral by health department personnel is generally unproductive in settings where sound diagnostic procedures are not employed. Furthermore, partner tracing is not indicated either for patients without disease or for those with noninfectious conditions (e.g., late syphilis). Sex partner referral is also less productive with patients whose consorts are anonymous, for example, prostitutes and some homosexuals. Likewise, the process will fail to achieve its objectives if long time delays occur before the sexual partners can be located. Such settings may include interstate or international travelers.

More simplified partner tracing, such as the self-referral method, overcomes some of the serious deficiencies of formal sex partner referral methods.[59] It actively involves patients in the disease control effort, is inexpensive, is normally acceptable to patients, and reserves scarce staff time for other activities. Potential shortcomings of patient referral methods include limited effectiveness, difficulty in evaluating outcomes, and nonproductivity with unreliable patients.

The costs and benefits of partner tracing must be weighed carefully in STD control programs. Under most circumstances, some form of simplified tracing will be cost-beneficial because it will lead to a sizable number of infected individuals being treated for relatively little effort. Only if a high proportion of "contacts" were actually uninfected would this method prove to be excessively costly.

Formal tracing using staff is more expensive; therefore, this activity is worthwhile primarily if those cases located are worth the cost of this activity and no cheaper means exist of achieving the same outcome. For these reasons, we are increasingly restricting active intervention to high-yield cases or to high-risk "core" environments.[60] Special situations where this more costly strategy has been useful include the following: (1) introduction of a serious disease (e.g., syphilis or PPNG infection) into a community previously unaffected[9,61]; (2) all PPNG infections where control of this disease remains feasible[53]; (3) gonococcal pelvic inflammatory disease where a large proportion of male partners are free of symptoms[62]; (4) females and males with repeated STD infections[62]; (5) female consorts of infectious syphilis cases; and (6) STD infections in children.

A further shift in this disease control strategy focuses on the counseling (i.e., educating) of patients to facilitate changes in their behavior.[63] The traditional focus of partner tracing, the assurance that sexual partners are brought to treatment, has been expanded to encourage changing patient behaviors. The following behaviors are advocated:

1. Respond to disease suspicion by promptly seeking appropriate medical evaluation
2. Take medications as directed
3. Return for follow-up tests
4. Assure examination of sexual partners
5. Reduce transmission by avoiding exposure until a follow-up test is completed
6. Prevent exposure by using protection in high-risk settings

Clinical Service Evaluation

Adequate clinical management of patients and their partners is the final common pathway of STD control. In the United States clinical services vary widely in different settings and are often inadequate to provide appropriate care for STD patients. Whether patient care is provided by experts at special STD clinics with sophisticated laboratory support, or by primary clinicians with limited laboratory facilities, the objectives of clinical management are the same[63]:

1. Determine the most likely etiology of the patient's complaint
2. Provide appropriate treatment for that condition
3. Detect other STD
4. Ensure patient follow-up for test of cure after treatment
5. Manage properly those patients who failed treatment
6. Educate patients to reduce their risks of further disease acquisition and to return if symptoms recur
7. Encourage identifiable sexual partners to attend for appropriate evaluation and treatment

In this way, all key STD control strategies are contained in the microcosm of providing clinical services.

For many years in the United States, the public STD facilities were relegated to a lower class status.[40] Recent control efforts have sought both to upgrade the physical appearance and capacity and to improve patient flow within these clinics. For example, a patient flow analysis may lead to more efficient use of existing resources.[64] A redistribution of room use may provide greater privacy for patients during interviews and examinations; working hours can be changed to improve services for employed patients during evening or early morning hours; assignment of specific tasks to existing personnel may increase their efficiency and decrease staff friction.

The content of clinical care is an important determinant of outcome. To assist clinicians in making diagnoses and in providing adequate treatment, use of simplified patient management protocols have been widely encouraged in the United States.[65] Designed as wall charts, these practical summaries describe typical clinical presentations, criteria for diagnosis, appropriate treatment recommendations, and practical prevention points. They are useful in both public and private health care settings. The Quality Assurance Guidelines (QAG)[66] have expanded on these STD summary medical protocols to cover subjects of clinic structure, clinic management, and patient education.

Training

Medical school curricula in the United States have not kept pace with the increasing incidence of STD over the past decade.[67] This has created a dearth of clinicians with the necessary skills to diagnose, treat, and prevent STDs. Both the public and private sectors have suffered from this neglect. Thus, an integral part of STD control strategies in the United States has been to develop a coordinated system for training health care providers in the rapidly changing field of STD. This training involves all specialties affecting STD control: clinicians, laboratory workers, managers, field investigators, and health educators. For each group, both formal education systems and ongoing in-service training opportunities are essential.

The training initiatives have taken several approaches. To respond to acute needs, the Quality Assurance Guidelines[66] were developed to assist STD facilities to improve patient management. The STD treatment recommendations are regularly updated[55] to reflect changing diagnostic capabilities, antibiotic susceptibilities, and pharmacologic breakthroughs. These documents are rapidly distributed to the field and provide public health professionals with access to standardized guidelines that can be adapted to their local needs.

Another training initiative has involved creating regional STD Prevention/Treatment Centers.[68] Each center is based on integration of a university medical school with a model public STD clinic for purposes of providing training for midcareer health care providers, as well as medical, nursing, and paramedical students. By 1983, ten such multidisciplinary centers were in operation, and over 6,500 students have been cumulatively trained since 1979. Further development of these centers will allow them to serve as a focus for testing new disease detection methods, for evaluating recent treatment recommendations, and for expanding patient management protocols.

Research

Both basic and applied research are crucial to STD control. Major changes in intervention strategy have accompanied the introduction of new antibiotics (e.g., penicillin), the development of better detection methods (e.g., Thayer-Martin media), the identification of resistant organisms (e.g., PPNG), and the recognition of high-risk groups (e.g., homosexuals, patients with repeat infections, women with PID). Presently, quantum leaps in STD control programs await such developments as rapid diagnostic techniques for chlamydia and effective vaccines against herpes or gonorrhea.

Most STD research in the United States is supported by the National Institutes of Health and the Centers for Disease Control,[69] although an increasing amount is funded either by voluntary organizations concerned with the magnitude of the STD problem or by pharmaceutical firms or medical diagnostic companies aware of the potential market. The objectives of this research are to characterize the pathophysiology, host response, and epidemiology of STDs to allow further development of improved diagnosis, treatment, prevention, and control strategies.

The National Institutes of Health (NIH), through the National Institute of Allergy and Infectious Disease, supports a variety of basic science and clinical projects. These include development of gonococcal and herpes vaccines, experimental clinical trials with antiviral agents, establishment of herpes transmission patterns within communities, and determination of host responses to chlamydia infections. NIH also sponsors training of postdoctoral fellows in clinical and microbiologic STD research and has undertaken periodic workshops to update the most rapidly advancing areas of STD knowledge. The private sphere has supported both basic and applied research in diagnosis (e.g., nonculture methods for detecting gonorrhea), treatment (e.g., new antibiotics for resistant organisms), and prevention (e.g., vaccines).

The Centers for Disease Control (CDC), through the Division of Venereal Disease Control, and the Sexually Transmitted Disease Laboratory Program, conducts applied research directed toward monitoring practical results and evaluating control strategies. This involves (1) clinical research, including field evaluation of recommended therapies for efficacy and safety, as well as field evaluation of diagnostic tests for their sensitivity and specificity; (2) epidemiologic studies of the etiology, natural history, clinical characteristics, demographic correlates, and geographic distribution of STDs; (3) programmatic investigations to develop and apply new methods of STD control; and (4) related social science studies of STD behavior patterns and motivations.

STD control strategies require close cooperation between those public and private groups conducting research. The limited resources available to study the expanding list of sexually transmitted organisms and syndromes require both a focusing on those areas most likely to influence STD control and an avoiding of wasteful duplication of research efforts on the same topic. Moreover, only through close liaison among researchers will we determine if results gained under controlled laboratory settings or in experimental clinical facilities can be transferred to real-life field operations. The rapid transfer of the latest control technology from research circles to medical practice will depend on harmony among the team of STD professionals.

THE FUTURE

After several decades of apathy and neglect, the STDs are finally becoming recognized for the magnitude of illnesses they cause, the intensity of human suffering they generate, and the amount of health resources they consume. To emphasize how the STDs have emerged as a primary health concern in the United States, the Surgeon General has designated them as one of 15 health priority areas for national prevention and control efforts.[70] To achieve the broad

Table 1-2. 1990 Objectives for Sexually Transmitted Diseases (STD)

Objectives	Rate	
	1990 Objective	1982 Data
Measurable Objectives		
Gonorrhea	280*	418
Gonococcal pelvic inflammatory disease	60*	117 (estimated)
Primary and secondary syphilis	7*	15
Congenital syphilis	1.5**	4.3
Other Objectives		
Neonatal herpes	8.5**	—
Chlamydial pneumonia	360**	—
Nongonococcal urethritis	770*	—
Condom use	25%	—
STD education in high school	100%	—
STD knowledge in clinicians	95%	—

* Per 100,000 population.
** Per 100,000 live births.

national goal of reducing overall death rates and days of disability, specific national prevention objectives were systematically established for the STDs (Table 1-2).

Measurable targets for 1990 prevention objectives include the gonorrhea rate, the gonorrhea pelvic inflammatory disease rate, the primary and secondary syphilis rate, and the congenital syphilis rate; these targets could be tracked relatively easily (Table 1-2). Other 1990 objectives were based on estimated rates and include the neonatal herpes rate, the nongonococcal urethritis rate, the percentage of couples using condom/barrier methods for primary protection, the percentage of high-school students receiving accurate STD education, and the percentage of providers able to diagnose and treat STDs. While some progress has been made in achieving these objectives, far more must be done if the 1990 goals are to be reached.

Future strategies for STD control must build on the successful foundation of the past and must evaluate innovative approaches that are cost-effective. To do this, in the face of the expanded matrix of STDs

Table 1-3. Future Directions for Sexually Transmitted Disease (STD) Control, United States

Components	Future Directions
Health education and promotion	Reproductive life plan Individual decision-making
Disease detection	Nonculture techniques Diagnostic algorithms
Appropriate treatment	Efficacy risks and costs of antiviral treatments Indications for prophylactic treatment
Partner tracing and patient counseling	Factors associated with highest patient yields Role of patient compliance with oral medications
Clinical services	Automatic data systems for record linkage and disease surveillance Integrated Reproductive Health Services
Training	Pilot medical school curricula Model STD academic centers
Research	STD role in pregnancy outcome and human neoplasia Vaccine field testing

and the limited pool of resources, the health consumer—especially the STD patient—will have to play an expanded role in the intervention process. Both primary and secondary prevention must be emphasized.

Refinements to the seven time-honored control measures may make them even more effective (Table 1-3). For example, health education in high schools could stress development of simplified reproductive life plans[71] that would dramatize the role of individual choice to decrease STD risks. Availability of nonculture diagnostic techniques for chlamydia will undoubtedly facilitate a national control program.[72] Effective oral antiviral agents for herpes simplex virus will promote control efforts against this organism. Determination of the variables affecting cost-effectiveness of different gonorrhea interview/investigation approaches will allow managers to conserve future resources.

We must stay abreast of technologic advances by expanding STD information systems to bring the STD control programs technologically into the computer age.[73] To successfully carry out STD control responsibilities, programs must collect, collate, and utilize data from patient medical records, case investigative documents, records of laboratory analyses, and case reports. Most current record systems are manually maintained; such systems are cumbersome, often inefficient, and difficult to link. During the remainder of the decade, state and local health departments should aim to install computer systems that improve the management and operational capabilities of STD control programs. Obviously, plans for the hardware and software components of any data system require that STD program personnel be "computer-literate."

Another priority is the development and evaluation of pilot STD curricula in medical schools. I have previously mentioned the lack of clinical training in STDs in medical schools.[67] While the STD Prevention/Training Centers have been a very important first step in training midlevel practitioners, we still need to reach clinicians during their initial formal training. In this way, we could create a cadre of STD specialists, that is, medically qualified clinicians who have an initial knowledge of, and a career commitment to, the STD field. If we developed such individuals, they would be capable of establishing their own training programs, thus multiplying the effect of the training efforts. In this way, we could meet the 1990 objective of the Department of Health and Human Services that "at least 95 percent of health care providers seeing suspected cases should be capable of diagnosing and treating all currently recognized STD."[70]

Finally, vaccination to provide active immunity against STDs represents the ideal control strategy. Hepatitis B vaccine is already available for high-risk groups. Current research in the United States includes experimental vaccines for gonorrhea, genital herpes, group B streptococcal infection and cytomegalovirus infection.[69] Field trials of gonorrhea vaccine are being conducted by the United States military in Korea, and results may be available by the end of 1984. Integration of effective vaccines into existing control programs will be a major challenge for future managers.

CONCLUSION

What can we say about the outlook for STD prevention and control in the United States? The increased attention shown in STD by patients and health care providers alike is stimulating. The expanded spectrum of organisms and syndromes makes the field especially ripe for innovative approaches. The emphasis on reproductive health consequences of STD has demonstrated how these infections have far-reaching effects on innocent victims. Progress toward effective control of STD will not occur overnight. The population at risk may continue to rise, the availability of new vaccines is still far away, and public health resources are not expanding as fast as the STD. Yet, the opportunity to make further advances has never been better.

REFERENCES

1. Centers for Disease Control: Sexually Transmitted Diseases: Treatment Guidelines, 1982. MMWR 31(Suppl 2):730, 1982
2. Brown ST, Wiesner PJ: Problems and approaches to the control and surveillance of sexually transmitted agents associated with pelvic inflammatory disease in the United States. Am J Obstet Gynecol 138:1096, 1980
3. Department of Commerce: Bureau of the Census population estimates and projections; projections of the population of the United States, 1977 to 2050. Series P-25, No. 704, 1977
4. Zelnik M, Kanter JF: Sexual activity, contraceptive use and pregnancy among metropolitan-area teenagers: 1971–1979. Fam Plann Perspect 12:230, 1980
5. Zelnik M, Kanter JF: Sexual and contraceptive experience of young unmarried women in the United States, 1976 and 1971. Fam Plann Perspect 9:55, 1977
6. Bureau of the Census: Marital Status and Living Arrangements: March 1980. Current Population Reports, Series P-20, No. 365, 1981
7. Zaidi AA, Aral SO, Reynolds GH, et al: Gonorrhea in the United States: 1967–1979. Sex Transm Dis 10:72, 1983
8. Jaffe HJ, Biddle JW, Johnson SP, Wiesner PJ: Infections due to penicillinase-producing Neisseria gonorrhoeae in the United States: 1976–1980. J Infect Dis 144:191, 1981
9. Fletcher JD, Stratton JD, Chandler CS, et al: Penicillin-resistant gonorrhea—North Carolina. MMWR 32:273, 1983
10. Brown S, Warnnissor T, Biddle J, et al: Antimicrobial resistance of Neisseria gonorrhoeae in Bangkok: Is single-drug treatment passé? Lancet 2:1366, 1982
11. Jones O, Strohmeyer G, Brockett J, et al: Spectinomycin-resistant penicillinase-producing Neisseria gonorrhoeae. MMWR 32:51, 1983
12. Fichtner RR, Aral SO, Blount JH, et al: Syphilis in the United States, 1967–1979. Sex Transm Dis 10:77, 1983
13. Thompson SE, Washington AE: Epidemiology of sexually transmitted Chlamydia trachomatis infections. Epidemiol Rev 5:96, 1983
14. Judson FN: Epidemiology and control of nongonococcal urethritis and genital chlamydial infections: A review. Sex Transm Dis 8(Suppl):117, 1981
15. Ripa T, Forslin L, Danielsson D, Falk V: Frequency of gonococcal and chlamydial infections in patients with laparoscopically verified acute salpingitis in 1970 and 1980. p 179. Epidemiologic considerations. In Mardh P-A, et al (eds): Chlamydial Infections. Elsevier Biomedical Press, Amsterdam, 1982
16. Alexander ER, Harrison HR: Role of Chlamydia trachomatis in perinatal infection. Rev Infect Dis 5:713, 1983
17. Chuang T-Y, Daniel Su WP, Perry HO, et al: Incidence and trend of herpes progeni-

talis. A 15-year population study. Mayo Clin Proc 58:436, 1983

18. Centers for Disease Control: Condyloma acuminatum—United States 1966–1981. MMWR 32:306, 1983

19. Reid R, Stanhope CR, Herschman BR, et al: Genital warts and cervical cancer. Cancer 50:377, 1982

20. Centers for Disease Control: Pelvic inflammatory disease—United States. MMWR 28:605, 1980

21. Washington AE, Cates W Jr, Zaidi AA: Hospitalizations for pelvic inflammatory disease: Epidemiology and trends in the United States, 1975–1981. JAMA 251:2529, 1984

22. Mosher WD, Pratt WF: Reproductive impairments among married couples: United States. Vital and Health Statistics. Public Health Service. U.S. Government Printing Office, Washington DC, 1982

23. Aral SO, Cates W Jr: The increasing concern with infertility: Why now? JAMA 250:2327, 1983

24. Moore DE, Spadoni LR: Infertility in women. In Holmes KK, Mardh PA, Sparling PF, Wiesner PJ (eds): Sexually Transmitted Diseases. McGraw-Hill, New York, 1984

25. Westrom L: Effect of acute pelvic inflammatory disease on fertility. Am J Obstet Gynecol 121:707, 1975

26. Ingraham NR Jr: The value of penicillin alone in the prevention and treatment of congenital syphilis. Acta Derm Venereol (Stockh) 31(Suppl 24):60, 1951

27. Amstey MS, Stedman KT: Asymptomatic gonorrhea in pregnancy. Am J Venereol Dis Assoc 3:14, 1976

28. Harrison HR, Alexander ER, Weinstein L, et al: Cervical Chlamydia trachomatis and mycoplasmal infections in pregnancy: Epidemiology and outcomes. JAMA 250:1721, 1983

29. Taylor-Robinson D, McCormack WM: The genital mycoplasmas. N Engl J Med 302:1003, 1063, 1980

30. Committee on Fetus and Newborn, Committee on Infectious Diseases: Perinatal herpes simplex virus infection. Pediatrics 66:147, 1980

31. Sullivan-Bolyai J, Hull HF, Wilson C, Corey L: Neonatal herpes simplex virus in-

fection in Seattle: Trends and clinical correlates. JAMA 250:3059, 1983

32. Rubin GL, Peterson HP, Dorfman SF, et al: Ectopic pregnancy in the United States, 1970–1978. JAMA 249:1725, 1983

33. Sivin I: IUD's and ectopic pregnancy. Stud Fam Plann 14:57, 1983

34. Westrom L, Bengtsson LPH, Mardh P-A: Incidence, trends, and risks of ectopic pregnancy in a population of women. Br Med J 282:15, 1981

35. zur Hausen H: Human genital cancer: Synergism between two virus infections or synergism between a virus infection and initiating events? Lancet 2:1370, 1982

36. Cramer DW: Uterine cervix. p 881. In Schottenfeld D, Fraumeni JF Jr (eds): Cancer Epidemiology and Prevention. Saunders, Philadelphia, 1982

37. Thomas DB, Rawls WE: Relationship of herpes simplex virus type 2 antibodies and squamous dysplasia to cervical carcinoma in situ. Cancer 42:2716, 1978

38. Daling JR, Weiss NS, Klopfenstein LL, et al: Correlates of homosexual behavior and the incidence of anal cancer. JAMA 247:1988, 1982

39. Anderson OW: Syphilis and Society—Problems of Control in the United States, 1912–1964. p 10. University of Chicago Press, Chicago, 1965

40. Henderson RH: Control of sexually transmitted diseases in the United States—A federal perspective. Br J Vener Dis 53:211, 1977

41. Curran JW: Economic consequences of pelvic inflammatory disease in the United States. Am J Obstet Gynecol 138:848, 1980

42. World Health Organization: Nongonococcal urethritis and other selected sexually transmitted diseases of public health importance. WHO Tech Rep Ser 660, 1981

43. World Health Organization: Control of Sexually Transmitted Diseases. WHO, Geneva, Switzerland, 1985

44. Cates W Jr, Wiesner PJ: National strategies for STD control: United States perspective. In Holmes KK, Mardh P-A, Sparling PF, Wiesner PJ (eds): Sexually Transmitted Diseases. McGraw-Hill, New York, 1984

45. Alderman JD: Washington Post/ABC News poll on genital herpes. September 1982 (mimeographed)

46. Judson FN: Fear of Aids and gonorrhea rates in homosexual men. Lancet 2:159, 1983

47. Donovan P: Airing contraceptive commercials. Fam Plann Perspect 14:321, 1982

48. Hart G: Epidemiologic treatment for syphilis and gonorrhea. Sex Transm Dis 7:149, 1980

49. Felman YM: Repeal of mandated premarital tests for syphilis: A survey of state health officers. Am J Public Health 71:155, 1981

50. Kingon RJ, Wiesner PJ: Premarital syphilis screening: Weighing the benefits. Am J Public Health 71:160, 1981

51. St John RK, Curran JW: Epidemiology of gonorrhea. Sex Transm Dis 6:81, 1978

52. Felman YM, Snyder RR, Giordano R, Griffin J: Gonorrhea screening. Experience of a large municipal program. NY State J Med 78:1267, 1978

53. Sidhu S, Barnes R: Penicillinase-producing Neisseria gonorrhoeae—Los Angeles. MMWR 32:181, 1983

54. Jaffe HW, Biddle JW, Thornsberry C, et al: National gonorrhea therapy monitoring study. In vitro antibiotic susceptibility and its correlation with treatment results. N Engl J Med 294:5, 1976

55. Washington AE, Mandell GL, Wiesner PJ: Treatment of sexually transmitted diseases: New additions to an old tradition. Rev Infect Dis 4(Suppl 2):S727, 1982

56. Seth AD, Johnston NA: Penicillin-resistant gonococci. Lancet 2:531, 1980

57. Centers for Disease Control: Current trends: Gonorrhea—CDC recommended treatment schedules, 1978. MMWR 28:13, 1979

58. Greenwood JR, Prendergast T, Ehling LR, et al: Chancroid—California. MMWR 31:173, 1982

59. Potterat JJ, Rothenberg RB: The case finding effectiveness of a self-referral system for gonorrhea: A preliminary report. Am J Public Health 67:174, 1977

60. Rothenberg RB: The geography of gonorrhea: Empirical demonstration of core group transmission. Am J Epidemiol 117:688, 1983

61. Handsfield HH, Sandstrom EG, Knapp JS, et al: Epidemiology of penicillinase-producing Neisseria gonorrhoeae infections: Analysis by auxotyping and serotyping. N Engl J Med 306:950, 1982

62. Potterat JJ, King RD: A new approach to gonorrhea control: The asymptomatic man and incidence reduction. JAMA 245:578, 1981

63. Parra WC, Wiesner PJ, Drotman DP: Patient counseling. In Holmes KK, Mardh P-A, Sparling PF, Wiesner PJ (eds): Sexually Transmitted Diseases. McGraw-Hill, New York, 1984

64. Graves JL, Hudgins AA, DeLung J, et al: Computerized patient flow analysis of local family planning clinics. Fam Plann Perspect 13:164, 1981

65. Centers for Disease Control: Sexually Transmitted Diseases Summary, 1982. Centers for Disease Control, Atlanta, 1982

66. Centers for Disease Control: Quality Assurance Guidelines for STD Clinics, 1982. Centers for Disease Control, Atlanta, 1982

67. Stamm WE, Kaetz S, Holmes KK: Clinical training in venereology in the United States and Canada. JAMA 248:2020, 1982

68. Margolis S: Initiation of the sexually transmitted diseases prevention/training clinic program. Sex Transm Dis 8:87, 1981

69. National Institute of Allergy and Infectious Disease Study Group: Sexually Transmitted Diseases: 1980 Status Report (NIH Publication No. 81-2213). U.S. Government Printing Office, Washington, DC, 1981

70. Department of Health and Human Services: Promoting Health/Preventing Disease: Objectives for the Nation. p 25. U.S. Government Printing Office, Washington, DC, 1980

71. Hatcher RA, Stewart GK, Stewart F, et al: Contraceptive Technology, 1982–1983. 11th Ed. p 9. Irvington Publishers, New York, 1982

72. Wiesner PJ: Developing a national strategy for the control of chlamydial infections—U.S.A. p 437. In Mardh P-A, et al (eds): Chlamydia Infections. Elsevier Biomedical Press, Amsterdam, 1982

73. Fichtner RR, Blount JH, Spencer JN: A statewide management information system for the control of sexually transmitted diseases. In Proceedings of the Seventh Annual Symposium on Computer Applications in Medical Care. Institute of Electrical and Electronics Engineers, New York, 1984

2

Infectious Syphilis: Primary, Secondary, and Early Latent

Franklyn N. Judson

This chapter reviews current concepts of the infectious stages of syphilis: primary, secondary, and early latent infection. Those aspects of epidemiology, clinical manifestations, laboratory diagnosis, and treatment in which there have been changes during the past thirty years or about which there is common misunderstanding are emphasized. The many conflicting theories pertaining to the origins of syphilis and the natural history, pathogenesis, and treatment of late syphilis are discussed in Chapter 3.

EPIDEMIOLOGY

The epidemiology of syphilis and the efficacy of current control programs are best monitored by following the incidence of primary and secondary disease (Fig. 2-1). This is because these stages are of recent onset, highly infectious, and relatively easy to diagnose. Early latent syphilis (i.e., asymptomatic infection under 1 year's duration) is, to a lesser extent, also infectious, but many cases escape diagnosis owing both to the absence of symptoms and the inability to establish duration of infection.

With the widespread use of modern syphilotherapy in the late 1940s and early 1950s, cases of primary and secondary syphilis in the United States dropped from over 35,000 cases per year to a low of approximately 6,500 cases in 1956. An extrapolation of this decline for another 5 to 10 years was used to argue that syphilis might soon be eradicated in much of the developed world. Unfortunately by 1958 (Fig. 2-1) incidence had begun to accelerate upward again for both men and women. This reversal has been attributed to reductions in funds for syphilis treatment and contact tracing. However, probably more important was a major demographic shift toward a much larger and younger at-risk population, along with complex and difficult to measure changes in sexual behavior. The obvious behavioral changes included more numerous casual and anonymous sexual partners, a younger age at first intercourse, and the increasing unpopularity of contraceptive measures—short-term sexual abstinence, withdrawal prior to ejaculation, and condoms—which served to reduce exposure to infectious lesions. Although never adequately monitored, increasing resistance of

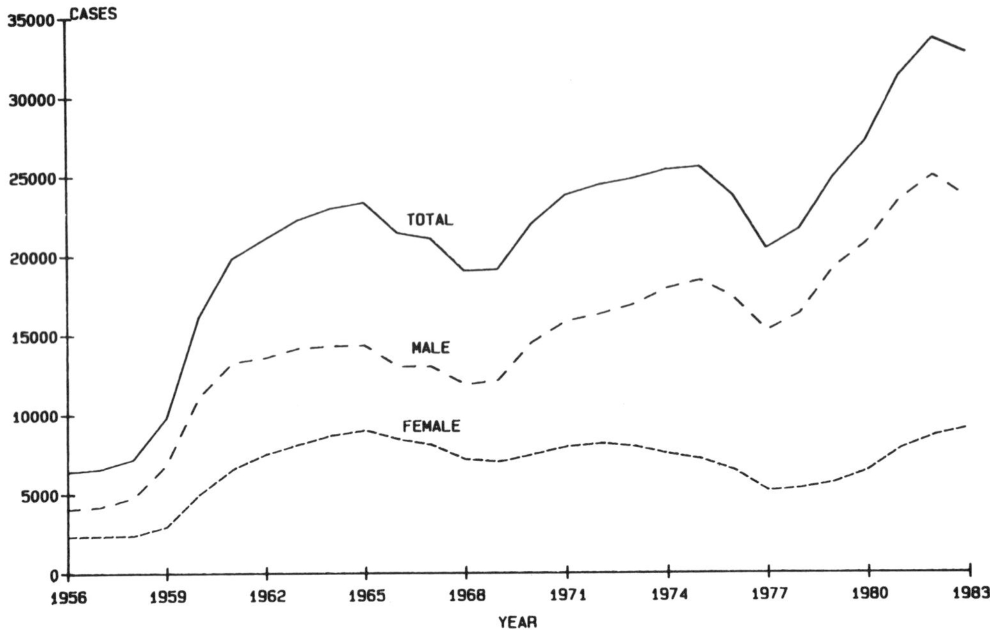

Fig. 2-1 Reported cases of primary and secondary syphilis by sex—United States 1956–1983. (From Centers for Disease Control: Syphilis—United States, 1983. MMWR 33:433, 1984.)

Treponema pallidum to penicillin and tetracycline did not seem to be a contributing factor.

There was another downward trend in incidence of syphilis in 1967, which continued modestly for women until 1977 but was short-lived for men. As a result, a striking change in the sex ratio (males:females) among primary and secondary syphilis cases was noted, increasing from 1.5:1 in 1967 to 3.2:1 in 1980.[1] The percentage of all infected men with early syphilis who named other men as sex partners increased from 23% in 1969 to 42% in 1982, while the percentage of white infected men who reported at least one male sex partner increased from 38% in 1969 to 70% in 1979.[2] Similar statistics have been reported from other developed countries.

Because the reporting system for sexually transmitted diseases in the United States often may fail to correctly identify male homosexual preference, these data underestimate the risk of homosexual men acquiring syphilis. As an example, in 1979 I estimated that the relative risk of early syphilis infection for homosexual men was 28.3 times that for heterosexual men living in the Denver metropolitan area.[3] This was calculated using actual reporting data, which showed that 60% of all early syphilis cases in the metropolitan area occurred in homosexual men, and the assumption that 10% of men are homosexual. The following exemplifies recent secular trends in the United States: In 1953 a "typical" case of early syphilis was more likely to be a poor, rural, heterosexual black man, whereas thirty years later it was more likely to be a middle-class, urban, homosexual white man.

During the past few years syphilis incidence patterns appear to be shifting once again. Overall incidence in the United States is down from its 1982 peak of 14.6 cases per 100,000 population, mainly as a result of fewer cases in homosexual men. This, in turn, may reflect changes in sexual behavior resulting from fear of contracting the acquired immunodeficiency syndrome

(AIDS). Unfortunately, the same trend has not been noted in women, in whom 5 years of increasing syphilis incidence probably accounts for a parallel increase in cases of congenital syphilis, from 104 in 1978 to 158 in 1983.[1]

CLINICAL MANIFESTATIONS

Certain clinical aspects of syphilis relating to its incubation period, infectiousness, and staging are inherently confusing to practitioners who seldom see this infection. The incubation period, or time from exposure to the onset of symptoms, is generally stated to be 10 to 90 days, an admittedly wide range. Actually, the vast majority of incubation periods fall between 3 and 5 weeks. Ninety days is extraordinarily rare, and clearly errs on the side of caution to protect syphilis contact tracers (e.g., public health advisers) who want to be all-inclusive, regardless of cost-yield.

Ten days is the minimum time required by the slowly growing *Treponema pallidum* (i.e., a cell-doubling rate of every 30 to 40 hours) to reach numbers sufficient to cause clinical disease. Short incubation periods are usually associated with large infectious inocula. Finally, incubation period has little meaning for the many patients whose infection is not detected during the first year.

Early syphilis is highly infectious and is transmitted to 10 to 30% of sexual contacts. For example, Schroeter and coworkers[4] reported that 30% of 57 sexual contacts exposed to infectious syphilis within the preceding 30 days, and observed untreated for another 90 days, developed syphilis. Calculated infection rates would be even higher if a study were restricted to patients with proven lengthy and intense exposure to large weeping chancres, mucous patches, or condylomata lata.

The division of early syphilis into primary, secondary, and early latent stages is clinically useful, but somewhat arbitrary. Frequently there is not an orderly progression through these stages. Stages may overlap or be missed altogether. Not uncommonly, chancres may be found in the presence of a secondary rash. Conversely, many patients, particularly homosexual men who are diagnosed as having syphilis because a rash is present, can recall no antecedent chancre. All syphilis is latent at some time. Most late latent syphilis is diagnosed by serologic screening in asymptomatic patients who give no history of chancres or rashes.

Primary Syphilis

The chancre is the first physical manifestation of syphilis infection and develops at the site of inoculation. *T. pallidum* is able to penetrate intact mucous membranes, but may depend upon a small break in cornified epithelium to invade skin. The chancre begins as a minute papule, which breaks down into an ulcer within 3 to 7 days. The ulcer characteristically is described as painless, indurated, smooth, and weeping (Plate 2-1, Fig. 2-2A). It does not tend to bleed or crack when compressed. Regional lymph nodes will enlarge during the first week that the chancre is apparent and sometimes earlier. In the inguinal area adenopathy begins unilaterally, but in the absence of treatment it will become bilateral. The affected nodes are firm, discrete, and nontender. Without treatment the chancre will resolve spontaneously in 1 to 6 weeks. The spirochetes have probably disseminated through the blood long before this time.

More clinical difficulty arises with cases that are not "classical." Although it is often thought that chancres are unitary, at least 25%, and perhaps 47%,[5] of primary patients have two or more lesions. About 20 to 30% of chancres will go unnoticed by the patient. Chancres should be looked for in any sexually active man who develops phimosis; an

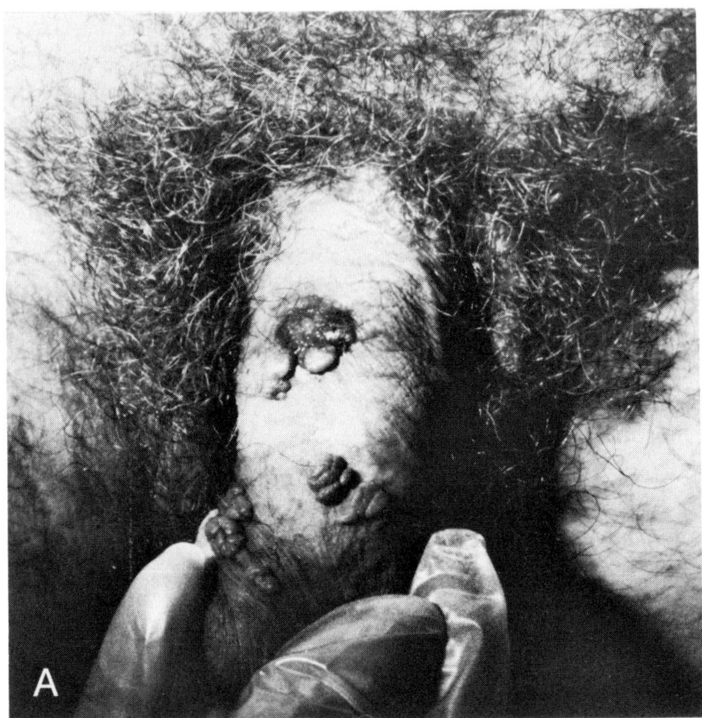

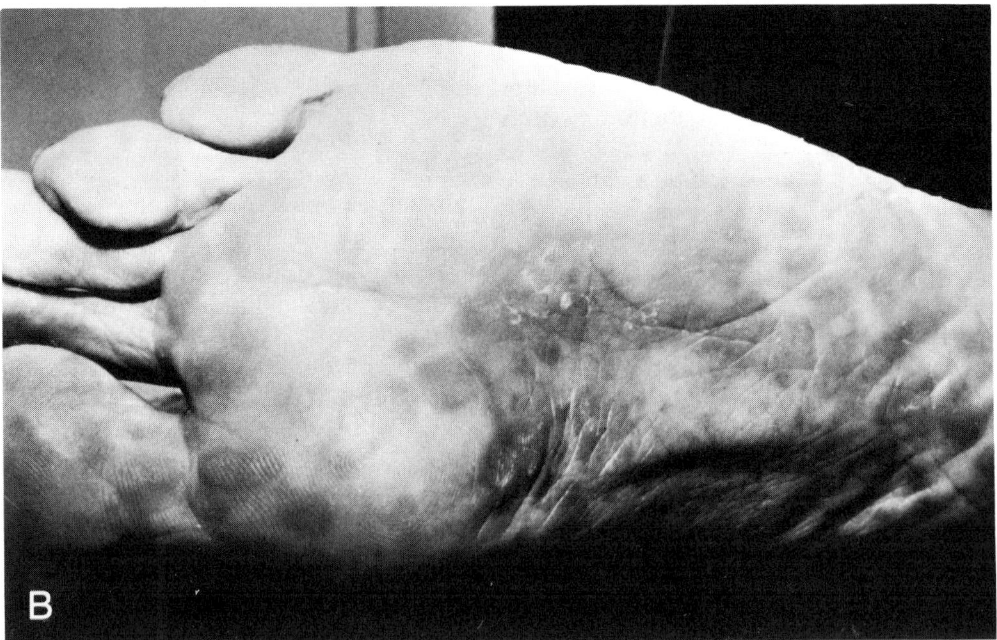

Fig. 2-2(*A*) Primary syphilis: Large midshaft chancre in association with numerous condylomata acuminata. (*B*) Secondary syphilis: Large macular syphilids of foot.

inciting chancre may be found in covered foreskin.

In homosexual men a large percentage of chancres will also go unnoticed by the clinician, particularly if proctoscopy and inspection of the oral cavity have not been performed. About half of all primary lesions in homosexual men will be found in these areas. Plate 2-2 demonstrates the importance of both perianal location and multiple lesions.

Less commonly, chancres have been noted on the breasts of women, axillae, lips, and fingers, and could be expected to occur at any point of effective contact. Reinfection syphilis may bypass the primary stage as a result of preexisting suppressive immunity.

Secondary Syphilis

Secondary syphilis develops 6 weeks to 6 months after the onset of primary syphilis. It is a systemic disease in which spirochetes circulate in the blood and in which there is a generalized endarteritis with the potential to affect all organs. Patients experience malaise, low-grade fever, headache, muscular aches and pains, and sometimes a sore throat. Collectively this manifests as a protracted influenzalike syndrome.

The rash of secondary syphilis usually begins subtly as discrete "copper"- or "ham"-colored macules, which soon become generalized and, unlike pityriasis rosea, involve the face, palms, and soles (Fig. 2-2B). There is a tendency for the rash to evolve sequentially into papules, squamous papules, and occasionally pustules. Highly squamous eruptions are referred to as psoriasiform because this rash clearly can mimic psoriasis. Vesicles and bullae are almost never seen in adults. Condylomata lata are moist, flat, confluent plaques most often found in intertriginous and anogenital areas. They are highly infectious. Chapel[6] has reported that 44 of 105 patients with sec-

ondary syphilis had pruritis, but this is not the usual experience. Marked pruritis should be considered as evidence against uncomplicated syphilis. Mucous patches are syphilitic enanthema (Plate 2-3). They can occur on any mucous membrane and are teeming with spirochetes.

The secondary-stage rash will spontaneously disappear in 4 to 12 weeks, but 25% of patients will have relapses. Two thirds of relapses occur within 6 months, 90% within a year, 95% within two years, and 100% within five years.[7]

The systemic nature of secondary syphilis and its multiple organ involvement is frequently overlooked, leading to misdiagnosis. Inflammatory endarteritis can affect all tissues, including large blood vessels through the vasa vasorum and nerves through the vasa nervorum. Meningeal inflammation causes abnormal cerebrospinal fluid findings in a majority of patients. Uveitis was once reported in 4.6% of patients with early syphilis,[8] but this is now rare. Low level hepatitis remains common.[9,10] An immune-complex glomerulonephritis has been well described,[11] and there have been sporadic reports of syphilitic enteritis and gastritis. Muscle, joint, and bone aches and pains are commonplace and result, respectively, from myositis, synovitis, and periostitis.

Generalized painless lymphadenopathy is a usual concomitant of early syphilis. Including syphilis in the differential diagnosis of lymphadenopathy in homosexual men is particularly important because syphilis is easily treated, whereas some lymphomas, the generalized lymphadenopathy syndrome, and the acquired immunodeficiency syndrome are not.

Early Latent Syphilis

Early latent syphilis is a subclinical stage that may be interrupted one or more times by secondary disease. The World Health

Organization defines "early" syphilis as less than four years of infection; however, the Centers for Disease Control, for epidemiologic purposes, that is, propensity to transmit *T. pallidum,* limits duration of infection to one year. Technically, the diagnosis of latent syphilis requires the results of a negative spinal fluid examination, including a VDRL test, to rule out asymptomatic neurosyphilis. Practically, this is rarely done for syphilis of less than one year's duration, especially when the recommended regimen of benzathine penicillin is used. Early latent syphilis should be considered potentially infectious via spirochetemia to the fetus, to drug addicts who share needles, and to recipients of certain transfused blood products. Finally, some patients with inapparent mucous patches or condylomata lata are misclassified as having latent infections.

LABORATORY DIAGNOSIS

Because so many other diseases can mimic the primary and secondary stages and because latent disease, by definition, has no physical findings at all, laboratory tests are especially important to the diagnosis of syphilis. However, cost-effective use of diagnostic tests requires that the health care provider apply them judiciously by carefully considering the epidemiologic (Is the patient a contact to syphilis? How long ago did contact occur? Is the patient from a known high-risk group?) and clinical circumstances (Is the lesion and/or rash at least compatible with syphilis? Are the results of prior serologic tests available?). In particular, the positive predictive value and cost-yield of any serologic test will be poor if used indiscriminately to screen populations with a low prevalence of infection.

Cultures

Despite an obvious need for *Treponema pallidum* cultures and a great array of efforts over the past 80 years, successful cultivation of *T. pallidum* in vitro has not yet been accomplished. Nutritional requirements for true growth in cell-free medium have never been defined. Recently, attention has been directed at in vitro cultivation using tissue culture methods. Transient but significant multiplication has been achieved by a few investigators, but practical clinical laboratory applications still seem to be a long way off.[12] Currently, the only reliable way to grow pathogenic *T. pallidum* from human clinical specimens is by intratesticular injection into rabbits, a technique practiced by only a few research centers and antigen production facilities.

Darkfield Microscopy

T. pallidum cannot be stained by ordinary laboratory methods and is too narrow to be visualized with a standard light microscope. These problems are circumvented by a darkfield microscope, which uses a condenser that blocks out central rays of light, thereby creating a dark field in which spirochetes are brightly illuminated by peripheral light reflected upward to the objective.

Proper specimen collection technique is essential for success with this method. Diagnostic sensitivity is greatest for specimens taken from active, weeping chancres, mucous patches, and condylomata lata. If the surface is clean, simply apply slow steady pressure to the lesion with gloved fingers until clear serum begins to exude. This should be dabbed directly onto a glass slide. If the specimen is small, a drop or two of room-temperature physiologic saline that contains no bacteriostatic additives can be used to provide sufficient volume to just float the coverslip on the slide.

Lesions that are dirty or have a thick exudate should be wiped clean and abraded slightly with gauze moistened with physiologic saline. Lesions that are difficult to reach, such as those within the anal canal or vagina, often can be adequately sampled with a needle-less tuberculin syringe. Place the syringe tip against the lesion and apply suction with the plunger for about a minute or until a drop of serum collects. Then hold the tip perpendicularly to several drops of physiologic saline on a glass slide, pump the plunger up and down to mix saline and serum, and transfer most of the specimen to the slide. Specimens from abraded dry rash lesions of secondary syphilis are suitable for darkfield microscopy, but in my experience these are positive in less than 30% of cases. It has frequently been said that specimens from a lesion within the oral cavity are not suitable for darkfield examination owing to the presence of resident spiral organisms morphologically similar to *T. pallidum*. In my opinion, if the lesion is compatible with syphilis, is not on the gum-teeth margins, and can be adequately cleaned and sampled, darkfield microscopy should be performed.

Even when petroleum jelly is used to seal the edges of the coverslip, treponemes will exhaust their limited supply of nutrients and lose motility. For this reason, darkfield examination should be carried out immediately after the specimen is collected. The sensitivity of a darkfield examination also is reduced in older lesions that are resolving and by topical or systemic antimicrobials active against *T. pallidum*. The traditional approach is to perform three negative darkfield examinations before giving up; however, it is probably better to do one very careful and thorough examination than to do three suboptimal ones aimed at satisfying an arbitrary recommendation.

The specificity of the test depends very much on the training and experience of the microscopist. The most common error is the failure to observe the strictest criteria for *T. pallidum* morphologic characteristics and motions. *T. pallidum* is tightly coiled, and the important movement is a corkscrew-type rotation about the long axis with slight side to side bending and undulation. In particular, false positive darkfield ex-

aminations are common when *Fusobacterium* spp. from multiple shallow, tender ulcers of fusospirochetal (also known as anaerobic) balanoposthitis[13] are misidentified as *T. pallidum. Fusobacterium* are wide and not so tightly coiled.

Many of the undesirable apsects of darkfield microscopy are problematic. To circumvent some of them, direct fluorescent *T. pallidum* antibody tests for wet mounts or fixed dried smears of clinical specimens have been developed.[14] They have not achieved wide usage, even though they should be more specific and the smears conveniently could be mailed to a central laboratory for later processing.

Serologic Tests

Infection with *T. pallidum* evokes a complex humoral antibody response which can be measured by a variety of serologic tests. These tests are classified as "treponemal" or "nontreponemal" according to the antigen they employ. This section will compare the performance characteristics of the different tests as to sensitivity, specificity, clinical utility, and response after treatment.

HOW THE TESTS WORK

Almost all modern nontreponemal tests use a cardiolipin-lecithin antigen stabilized with cholesterol. This antigen can be obtained from many mammalian tissues, is inexpensive, has a long shelf-life, and can be adapted to a variety of macro- and microflocculation technologies, some of which are readily automated and quantified. The titer is the greatest dilution of serum that can be made while maintaining a fully reactive flocculation reading.

Anticardiolipin antibodies produced during syphilis have been given the confusing name "reagin." It has been assumed that the antibodies are being produced in response to lipid materials in blood vessel endothelium, which are made antigenic by the infectious endarteritis, the fundamental disease process in early syphilis. It has never been determined whether or not the spirorochete itself is required for antigenicity. Given the rather nonspecific nature of the antigen and antibody, it is not surprising that cardiolipin tests suffer from false positive reactions.

The two types of treponemal tests most commonly used today are the fluorescent treponemal antibody-absorption (FTA-ABS) and the microhemagglutination-*T. pallidum* (MHA-TP). The antigen for each is the Nichol's strain of *T. pallidum* grown in rabbit testes. The first specific treponemal test, the *T. pallidum* immobilization test or TPI, was introduced in 1949 and is now only of historic interest. Because it utilized living treponemes, it was very cumbersome, expensive, and even dangerous.

The FTA-ABS test came into wide usage in 1968. Patient's serum is first diluted 1:5 in a diluent called "sorbent," which is prepared from the cultivatable, nonpathogenic Reiter's treponeme and is intended to absorb out cross-reacting antibodies to human commensal nonpathogenic treponemes. Without this step about 30–40% of sera would be false positives by the FTA technique.[15] The diluted serum is then layered on a slide coated with dried *T. pallidum*, incubated, and fluorescein-labeled antibody to human gamma-globulin added. Linear fluorescence along the treponemes indicates that specific antibodies are present. However, the FTA-ABS suffers from some inherent technological disadvantages. The test is labor-intensive, therefore expensive, and it cannot be readily automated or quantified. The test is read qualitatively by subtle gradations of fluorescence (i.e., "borderline," 1+, 2+, 3+, and 4+). Conventional interpretation classifies "borderline" reactions as negative and 1+ to

4+ reactions as positive. Because interpretation is qualitative and reagent quality (sorbent and conjugate) may vary, there have been reports[16,17] of laboratory false positive results, mostly in the 1+ and 2+ range.

The MHA-TP was developed in 1966 but not used widely until a decade later. It employs sheep or turkey erythrocytes coated with particles of *T. pallidum*. Antitreponemal antibody in the serum specimen is indicated by erythrocyte agglutination. The test is highly specific and can be readily automated and quantified. After front-end costs for automated microtiter equipment are borne, unit cost-per-test is very low.

SENSITIVITY

The comparative sensitivity of cardiolipin (e.g., VDRL slide test), FTA-ABS, and MHA-TP tests during different stages of syphilis are compared in Figure 2-3. The following points need to be made:

1. It takes 10–14 days after infection for a detectable primary antibody response to develop.

2. The FTA-ABS test is the most sensitive in early primary disease, and the MHA-TP test is the least sensitive.

3. The diagnosis of primary or secondary stages rarely requires a specific treponemal test if epidemiologic history, physical findings, and results of darkfield examinations and serial quantitative cardiolipin tests are carefully integrated.

4. Secondary and early latent stages are associated with maximal antibody production and all serologic tests should be strongly positive, the sole exception being a rare prozone reaction in which a cardiolipin test is falsely negative due to antibody excess. Prozone reactions can be resolved by further serum dilutions.

5. In the late latent stage, up to 50% of cardiolipin tests may be negative or weakly

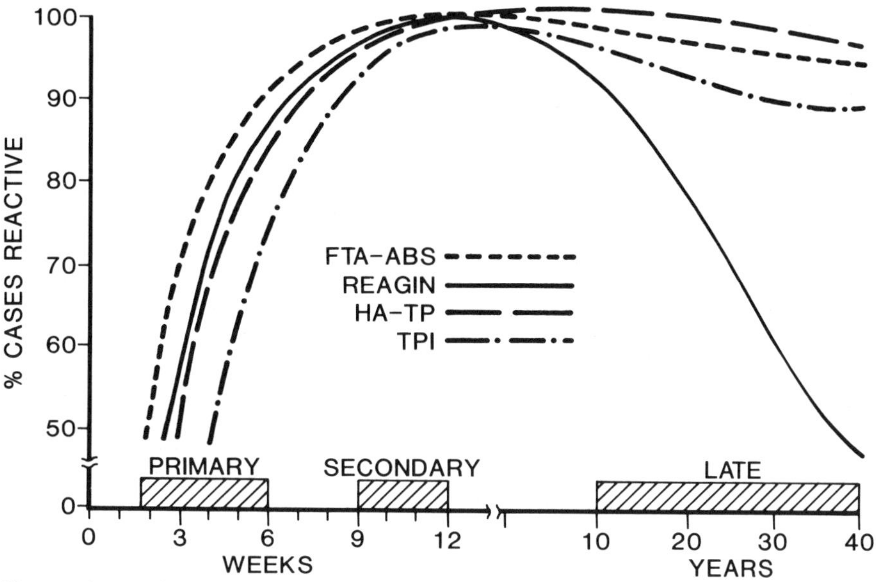

Fig. 2-3 Comparison of reactivity rates of FTA-ABS, reagin, MHA-TP, and TPI tests performed on sera from patients with untreated syphilis, by duration of disease. (From the Laboratory Program Office, Centers for Disease Control.)

reactive; however, both the FTA-ABS and MHA-TP tests should remain reactive for life (see Chapter 1).

Table 2-1 presents the comparative sensitivities of the cardiolipin (VDRL), FTA-ABS, and MHA-TP tests as the approximate percentages that each test will be positive in each stage of disease. Because primary infection lasts a number of weeks, it is not surprising that the VDRL will be positive in less than 50% of patients on the first day of the chancre, but will be positive in more than 90% if the chancre has been present for two to three weeks.

Table 2-1. Comparative Sensitivity of the VDRL, FTA-ABS, and MHA-TP Tests in the Different Stages of Untreated Syphilis

		Test	
Disease Stage	VDRL	FTA-ABS	MHA-TP
Primary	70	85	50–60
Secondary	99	100	100
Late latent or late	50–70	98	98

SPECIFICITY

None of the serologic tests has a specificity of 100%, that is, is negative in all individuals who are not infected with *T. pallidum*. Unfortunately, the comparative rates at which the tests are falsely positive in various other states of disease and health have never been determined for the same large populations. Biologic false positive reactions are, by convention, either "acute," that is, spontaneously revert to negative within 6 months, or "chronic," that is, remain reactive for more than 6 months.

CARDIOLIPIN TESTS. False positive reactions to cardiolipin tests are common even in sexually transmitted diseases clinics and usually fall within three general categories of patients. Many of these reports have been reviewed by Sparling.[18]

1. *Intravenous drug abusers.* As many as 25–30% of chronic intravenous drug abusers will have positive cardiolipin tests,[19]

the majority of which are chronic false positives. Unlike most biologic false positives that have titers of 1:8, the antigenic stimulation from intravenous drug abuse may be so great as to induce titers as high as 1:64, or even 1:128. Moreover cardiolipin tests may remain falsely positive for more than a year after substance abuse has been discontinued.

2. *Autoimmune diseases.* Approximately 10% of patients with systemic lupus erythematosis (SLE) will have falsely positive cardiolipin tests.[20] This may be confusing in sexually transmitted disease clinics because SLE most often afflicts sexually active women who are 25–35 years old. Since the disease is chronic, most false positive reactions are also chronic.

3. *Systemic viral infections and drug reactions.* It is likely that almost any systemic viral infection or drug reaction that lasts a week or more and affects numerous organs and/or causes a rash is capable of inducing anticardiolipin antibodies in a small proportion of patients. It is not clinically important whether the actual rate of false positives in a given viral infection is 1% or 3%. It is only important that this association be considered.

The common pathogenic denominator for each of the above conditions and syphilis is an underlying vasculitis. In this regard, I know of no similar immunopathologic mechanism to explain biologic false positive cardiolipin tests in pregnancy. Consequently, positive reactions should be interpreted as evidence for current or prior infection with *T. pallidum* until proven otherwise.

FTA-ABS TEST. The greatest FTA-ABS specificity problem has not been with biologic false positives, but rather with laboratory false positives in the 1+ and 2+ reactivity range. It is my experience that the FTA-ABS test is only rarely falsely positive in chronic intravenous drug abusers. Rates

in most systemic viral infections have not been adequately studied; however, there have been a few reports of falsely positive reactions in association with genital herpes.[21] The most common cause of chronic biologic false positive reactions in young women is an autoimmune disease. About 10% of women with SLE will have a falsely positive FTA-ABS test, of which about half produce linear fluorescence of the treponeme that is indistinguishable from syphilis, and about half will have an atypical beaded pattern.[20] In the absence of disease the presence of this atypical beaded pattern should serve as a warning that autoimmune disease may be present.

MHA-TP TEST. The MHA-TP test does not seem to be as prone to either laboratory or biologic false positive reactions; however, it has not been adequately studied in many disease states.

RESPONSE TO TREATMENT

One of the least understood aspects of serologic tests for syphilis is their response to treatment. Here are some important concepts that can help with most interpretation problems.

1. *FTA-ABS and MHA-TP tests.* Despite curative antibiotic treatment, once these tests have become fully reactive they will probably remain reactive for years,[22] and perhaps for the life of the patient. The only predictable exceptions occur when treatment has been initiated very early in primary disease (e.g., cardiolipin test negative primary syphilis), in which case the FTA-ABS test may become nonreactive within a year. It is therefore a mistake to offer additional treatment solely on the basis of a persistently reactive FTA-ABS test. The MHA-TP test has not been as extensively studied.

2. *Cardiolipin tests (e.g., VDRL).* Ade-

quacy of treatment of early syphilis should be followed with a quantitative cardiolipin test. Given the 25- to 30-day serum half-life of human immune globulin, one would anticipate the titer decreasing at a maximum rate of a little more than one tube dilution per month. This rate assumes that all anticardiolipin antibody production is shut off after treatment, which does not always occur.

In general, the longer the duration of disease, the slower will be the serologic responses to curative treatment. In primary syphilis the cardiolipin test should become seronegative in 6 to 12 months, while in secondary and early latent stages seronegativity may not be achieved until 12 to 18 months and occasionally longer. Tests will become nonreactive earlier after treatment of macular rashes than after the more established papular and pustular rashes.[23] In late latent and late stages, the cardiolipin test will commonly remain fixed (i.e., serofast) at a low titer.

A fourfold or greater rise in titer (e.g., 1:2 to 1:8) following treatment of any stage indicates that relapse or reinfection may have occurred. Fiumara[24] has demonstrated that the serologic response in men reinfected with primary, secondary, or latent syphilis within 36 months of adequate treatment is brisk and quickly achieves titers severalfold higher than with the initial infection. Because immunologic response is strongly boosted, the duration to seronegativity after treatment of reinfections is greatly increased.

SCREENING

To maximize the cost-effectiveness of any screening program it is important to follow an adaptation of Sutton's law, that is, screen where the disease is and not where it is not. In most communities, mandated premarital tests violate this law because men and women planning to become married are not often homosexual, they tend to be monogamous, and they are more likely to receive appropriate prenatal serologic screening when pregnancy occurs. This assertion is supported by Felman's[25] review of 44 states with mandated tests for syphilis, in which only 1 test in 8,461 was found to be positive for infectious syphilis. Likewise, the screening for syphilis of all patients admitted to general hospitals regardless of epidemiologic and/or clinical risk factors is not productive. These scarce resources should be redirected at screening high-risk homosexual men more frequently, particularly in bath houses and bars.

TREATMENT/PREVENTION

In contrast to treatment of late syphilis (Chapter 3), treatment of early syphilis is relatively uncontroversial. A number of different penicillin and tetracycline regimens have been well studied.[26,27] In addition, the clinical and serologic end points of cure are straightforward, making it possible to continuously monitor therapeutic efficacy of recommended regimens. It is therefore unlikely that increasing treatment failure rates caused by emerging *T. pallidum* resistance to antibiotics would go long unnoticed.

Following are the 1982 recommended regimens of the Centers for Disease Control.[28]

Recommended Regimens

Early syphilis (primary, secondary, latent syphilis of less than 1 year's duration) should be treated with benzathine penicillin G: 2.4 million units total, intramuscularly, at a single session. Patients who are allergic to penicillin should be treated with tetracycline HCl: 500 mg, by mouth, 4 times a day for 15 days. Tetracycline appears to be effective, but has been evaluated less extensively than penicillin. Patient compliance with this regimen may be difficult, so care should be taken to encourage optimal compliance.

Penicillin-allergic patients who cannot tolerate tetracycline should have their allergy confirmed. For these patients there are two options:

1. If compliance and serologic follow-up can be assured, administer erythromycin 500 mg by mouth, 4 times a day for 15 days.
2. If compliance and serologic follow-up cannot be assured, the patient should be managed in consultation with an expert.

The benzathine penicillin regimen is the treatment of choice because penicillin is the most active antibiotic against *T. pallidum* and because it can be administered as a single dose, thereby achieving 100% patient compliance. Intramuscular benzathine penicillin forms a repository that breaks down slowly over 15 to 20 days, releasing penicillin G (benzylpenicillin) into the blood. Serum levels of penicillin are usually maintained at 0.5–1.5 μg/ml, or above the 0.1 μg/ml needed for maximal treponemicidal affect in an animal model.[29]

Although tetracyclines widely are believed to be the drugs of choice in penicillin-allergic patients with early syphilis, there have been few adequate comparative studies.[26] Tetracyclines are many times less active against *T. pallidum* than is penicillin, but this is compensated for by the much larger total dose of 30 g (0.5 g qid) over 15 days.

Erythromycins traditionally have been considered the backup regimens in penicillin-allergic patients who cannot take tetracyclines consequent to gastrointestinal intolerance, allergy (e.g., fixed drug eruptions), age less than 8 years, or pregnancy. Efficacy has not been well established, but in adults it probably depends on taking the full 30-g regimen of a well-absorbed preparation. Either capsules containing enteric-coated pellets of erythromycin base (e.g., ERYC) or erythromycin estolate (despite higher rates of reversible liver transaminitis) would seem to be the best choice. Infants born to mothers treated with erythromycin during pregnancy should receive penicillin.

JARISCH-HERXHEIMER REACTION. This reaction occurs in over half of patients with early syphilis within 2 to 8 hours of starting treatment with penicillin and probably any other effective antibiotic. It consists of a fairly sudden onset of sweating, malaise, fever, and headache, along with an exacerbation of the symptoms of the disease. In 251 patients studied with a test dose of 100,000 units of aqueous penicillin G, Putkonen and coworkers[30] noted this reaction in 55% of patients with seronegative primary syphilis, and about 95% with seropositive primary or early secondary syphilis. In the landmark studies of penicillin therapy of early syphilis, Mahoney and associates[31] reported that 86 of 100 patients experienced some degree of a Herxheimer reaction or "therapeutic shock." Although this reaction is almost always benign in early syphilis, it is extremely important to warn patients what to expect and to advise them to take aspirin or acetaminophen for symptomatic relief. There are many instances in which uninformed frightened patients have fled to an emergency room only to receive an unnecessary fever workup and/or hospitalization.

Follow-up after Treatment

Treatment failures can occur with any of the recommended regimens and all patients with early syphilis should be encouraged to return for repeat quantitative cardiolipin tests at 3, 6, and 12 months after treatment or until they are nonreactive.[28] Careful follow-up serologic testing is particularly important in patients treated with antibiotics other than penicillin. The possibility of reinfection should also be entertained when patients with early syphilis need to be treated a second time.

Retreatment with schedules recommended for syphilis of more than 1 year's duration should be considered when

1. clinical signs or symptoms of syphilis persist or recur;
2. there is a 4-fold increase in titer with a nontreponemal test;
3. a nontreponemal test showing a higher titer initially fails to show a 4-fold decrease within a year.

Treatment of Incubating Syphilis

Syphilis is said to be incubating when infection is very recent, serologic tests (using a cardiolipin test) are nonreactive, and there are not yet any clinical signs. This type of early, undetectable syphilis becomes therapeutically relevant when treating patients for gonorrhea who are also at risk of coinfection with *T. pallidum,* for example, homosexual men. Of the treatment regimens for gonorrhea recommended by the Centers for Disease Control, aqueous procaine penicillin G (APPG), 4.8×10^6 units, with 1 g of probenecid clearly will abort incubating syphilis. This is based on the studies of Schroeter and coworkers,[4] who showed that, even without probenecid, $2.4–4.8 \times 10^6$ units of APPG were 100% effective in aborting incubating syphilis in 117 patients exposed to infectious syphilis within 30 days before treatment. Reasoning by deduction from pharmacokinetic and therapeutic trials in man and rabbits indicates that the recommended ampicillin, amoxicillin, and 7-day tetracycline regimens would also be effective, while spectinomycin would not be effective.[32] This view generally has been accepted by experts in the field.[28]

However, an inconsistency emerges when these same data are applied to established contacts of syphilis, for whom full treatment for early syphilis is recommended.[28] The only obvious difference between a patient with incubating syphilis and a seronegative contact of syphilis is that for the latter case contact has been documented. Because one would not anticipate different response rates to therapy, I have resolved this contradiction in my clinic by not offering additional treatment to seronegative, asymptomatic contacts of syphilis within 30 days before receiving the recommended APPG regimen for gonorrhea. To my knowledge, none of these patients has ever developed primary syphilis within the following 60 days.

Contact Tracing

While the essentials of contact tracing for gonorrhea,[33] nongonococcal urethritis, trichomoniasis, and so on, usually can be cost-effectively carried out by the clinicians managing the patient, this probably is not the best course for infectious syphilis.[34] Given the long-term consequences of untreated syphilis, the special expertise of professional contact tracers, sometimes known as public health advisers, is needed to deal with the problems of long and variable incubation periods, unrecognized infections, large numbers of anonymous contacts, and difficult-to-locate contacts. This is especially true when contact to syphilis has occurred anonymously in a bath house or bar for homosexual men.[35]

Vaccines

Theoretically, vaccines could be developed and used to control, and eventually eliminate, any infectious disease. In practice, development of a vaccine for syphilis has proved to be exceedingly difficult owing to the complex and incompletely understood immune response to natural infection with *T. pallidum,* and to the lack of an in-vitro *T. pallidum* culture system. It is known that increased resistance to challenge with *T. pallidum* occurs as infection progresses.[36] In rabbits, passive antibody to *T. pallidum* attentuates disease but does not provide complete immunity. Immunization of rabbits with attenuated *T. pallidum* induces good protection but the multiple-dose regimen is impractical for use in humans.[36] Until the protective immunogens that regulate host resistance to infection are identified, progress in vaccine development may be slow.

REFERENCES

1. Centers for Disease Control: Syphilis—United States, 1983. MMWR 33:433, 1984
2. Fichtner RR, Aral SO, Blount JH, et al: Syphilis in the United States: 1967–1979. Sex Transm Dis 10:77, 1983
3. Judson FN: High syphilis rate among homosexual men. Medical Aspects of Human Sexuality May:134, 1978
4. Schroeter AL, Turner RH, Lucas JB, Brown WJ: Therapy for incubating syphilis. Effectiveness of gonorrhea treatment. JAMA 218:711, 1971
5. Chapel TA: The variability of syphilitic chancres. Sex Transm Dis 5:68, 1978
6. Chapel TA: The signs and symptoms of secondary syphilis. Sex Transm Dis 7:161, 1980
7. Clark EG, Danbolt N: The Oslo study of the natural history of untreated syphilis: An epidemiologic investigation based on a restudy of Boeck-Bruusgaard material: A review and appraisal. J Chronic Dis 2:311, 1955
8. Moore JE: Syphilitic iritis: A study of 249 patients. Am J Ophthalmol 14:110, 1931
9. Lee RV, Thornton GF, Conn HO: Liver disease associated with secondary syphilis. N Engl J Med 284:1423, 1971
10. Feher J, Somogyi T, Timmer M, Jozsa L: Early syphilitic hepatitis. Lancet 2:896, 1975
11. Gamble CN, Rearclan JB: Immunopathogenesis of syphilis glomerulonephritis. Elution of antitreponemal antibody from glomerular immune-complex deposits. N Engl J Med 292:449, 1975
12. Fitzgerald T: The future of tissue culture methods for growth of Treponema pallidum in vitro. Sex Transm Dis 7:97, 1980
13. Gewart Cree, Willis AT, Phillips KD, Brazier JS: Anaerobic balanoposthitis. Br Med J 284:859, 1982
14. Kellogg DS: The detection of Treponema pallidum by a rapid direct fluorescent antibody darkfield (DFATP) procedure. Health Lab Sci 7:34, 1970
15. Goldman JN, Lantz MA: FTA-ABS and VDRL slide test reactivity in a population of nuns. JAMA 217:53, 1971
16. Burns RE: Spontaneous reversion of FTA-ABS test reactions. JAMA 234:617, 1975
17. Dans PE, Judson FN, Larson SA, Lantz MA: The FTA-ABS test: A diagnostic help or hindrance. South Med J 70:312, 1977
18. Sparling PF: Diagnosis and treatment of syphilis. N Engl J Med 284:642, 1971
19. Cherubin CE, Millian SJ: Serologic investigations in narcotic addicts. I. Syphilis, lymphoguanuloma venereum, herpes simplex, Q fever. Ann Intern Med 69:739, 1968
20. Kraus SJ, Haserick JR, Lantz MA: Fluorescent treponemal antibody-absorption test reactions in lupus erythematosus: Atypical beading pattern and probable false-positive reactions. N Engl J Med 282:1287, 1970
21. Wright JT, Cremer AW, Ridgway GL: False positive FTA-ABS results in patients with genital herpes. Br J Vener Dis 51:329, 1973
22. Schroeter AL, Lucas JB, Price EB, Falcone VH: Treatment for early syphilis and reactivity of serologic tests. JAMA 221:471, 1972
23. Fiumara NJ: Treatment of primary and secondary syphilis. Serological response. JAMA 243:2500, 1980
24. Fiumara NJ: Reinfection primary, secondary, and latent syphilis: The serologic response after treatment. Sex Transm Dis 7:111, 1980
25. Felman YM: Repeal of mandated tests for syphilis: A survey of state health officers. Am J Public Health 71:155, 1981
26. Elliot WC: Treatment of primary syphilis. J Am Vener Dis Assoc 3(Suppl 2):128, 1976

27. Brown ST: Treatment of secondary syphilis. J Am Vener Dis Assoc 3(Suppl 2):136, 1976

28. Centers for Disease Control: Sexually transmitted diseases treatment guide lines. MMWR 31(Suppl):33, 1982

29. Rein MF: Biopharmacology of syphilotherapy. J Am Vener Dis Assoc 3(Suppl 2):109, 1976

30. Putkonen T, Salo OP, Mustakallio KK: Febrile Herxheimer reaction in different phases of primary and secondary syphilis. Br J Vener Dis 42:181, 1966

31. Mahoney JF, Arnold RC, Sterner BL, et al: Penicillin treatment of early syphilis: II. JAMA 126:63, 1944

32. Judson FN: The importance of coexisting syphilitic, chlamydial, mycoplasmal, and trichomonal infections in the treatment of gonorrhea. Sex Transm Dis 6(Suppl 2):112, 1979

33. Judson FN, Wolf FC: Tracing and treating contacts of patients with gonorrhea in a sexually transmitted diseases clinic. Public Health Rep 93:460, 1978

34. Moore MB, Price EV, Knox JM, Elgin LW: Epidemiologic treatment of contacts to infectious syphilis. Public Health Rep 78:966, 1963

35. Judson FN, Miller KG, Schaffnit TR: Screening for gonorrhea and syphilis in the gay baths—Denver, Colorado. Am J Public Health 67:740, 1977

36. Baseman JB: Summary of the workshop on the biology of Treponema pallidum: Cultivation and vaccine development. J Infect Dis 136:308, 1977

3

Late (Tertiary) Syphilis

Nicholas J. Fiumara

Late (tertiary) syphilis is that stage of acquired or congenital syphilis that occurs four or more years after an untreated primary infection. Tertiary syphilis affects about 35% of untreated patients. The disease may occur in the following forms either singly or in combination: mucocutaneous, osseous, visceral, cardiovascular, and neural. For example, late mucocutaneous syphilis and osseous syphilis often occur together, as in perforation of the hard palate. These two types in turn may coexist with cardiovascular syphilis or asymptomatic neurosyphilis. Late mucocutaneous lesions are seldom concomitant with general paresis, tabes, or chronic meningovascular syphilis. However, patients with cardiovascular syphilis, particularly those with aortic regurgitation, more often than not have concurrent neurosyphilis. Since syphilis may appear anywhere in the body, it is obvious that a serologic test should be a routine part of every medical examination.

LATE MUCOCUTANEOUS SYPHILIS

Late syphilis of the skin occurs in about 10% of untreated syphilis cases and may appear from 5 to 10 years or as long as 20 years after the primary infection. The lesions may be nodular, nonduloulcerative, or gummatous. They are hard and indurated, with sharply demarcated borders. Characteristically, the lesions are chronic, painless, asymptomatic, asymmetrical, indolent, slow-growing, and progressively destructive.

Nodular Lesions

Nodular lesions (Figs. 3-1, 3-2, 3-3, Plate 3-1) may vary in size from a few millimeters to several centimeters. The color is generally a reddish-brown. The lesions appear in clusters and may involve any area of the skin, including the scalp, palms, and soles. There is an asymmetry to the eruption, in that one shoulder may have lesions but not the other; there may be lesions on one part of the back or abdomen, but not on the opposite side. All the lesions, both small and large, are hard and indurated, deeply seated in the dermis, and have a shotty feel. The lesions are flat-topped and rounded in shape. A few may have a slight scale and superficially resemble psoriasis. The presence of scales heralds the onset of an impending ulceration. When the nodular lesions spontaneously involute or heal following treatment, they leave a telltale

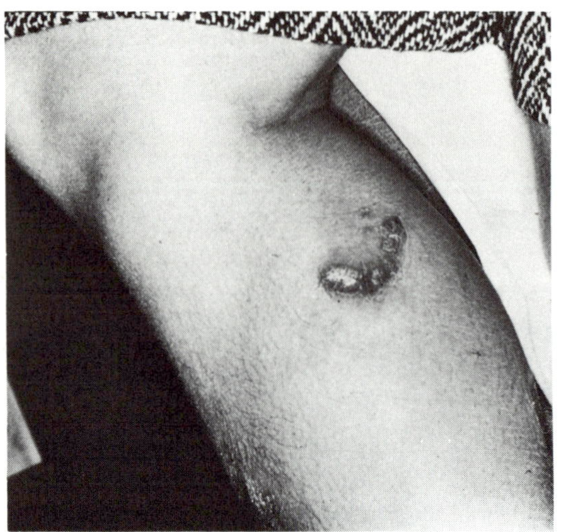

Fig. 3-1 Late nodular syphilis of calf of left leg.

scar. The scar shows some degree of atrophy and spotty pigmentation.

Noduloulcerative Lesions

When some of the nodular lesions ulcerate, the rest may persist without change. Thus, both nodular and nonduloulcerative lesions may coexist. The ulcerations are multiple and usually deep. The destruction is usually in the center of the nodule and is associated with central healing and a scar, followed by progression of the lesions by peripheral extension, ulceration, and scarring. The continuation of the process leads to an arciform or serpiginous contour, which is suspiciously pathognomonic (Fig. 3-4, Plate 3-2).

Gummas

In contrast to the multiple lesions of nodular and nonduloulcerative stages, gummas tend to be solitary lesions. They usually develop at the point of the trauma (Fig. 3-5, Plate 3-3). A gumma arises deep in the dermis, appearing first as a soft tumorlike swelling. The color is first a faint pink, then a dusky red. A softening of the mass occurs, and eventually a central slough develops. With drainage or debridement of the gum-like, clotted, and serous discharge and sponge-adherent slough, an ulcer with a granulomatous base is revealed. The granulomatous ulcer may extend peripherally or may heal spontaneously and forms an atrophic scar with a stippling pigmentation. Only occasionally will involution without breakdown occur. Pain ordinarily is not a prominent factor, but if the gumma is confined within a solid or resistant structure, permitting only limited expansion, pain does occur. In acquired syphilis, the gumma is the least common of the three classified lesions of late mucocutaneous syphilis, but in congenital syphilis, the solitary gumma is the most common.

Late mucocutaneous syphilis must be differentiated from cutaneous tuberculosis, erythema induratum, sarcoidosis, epithelioma,

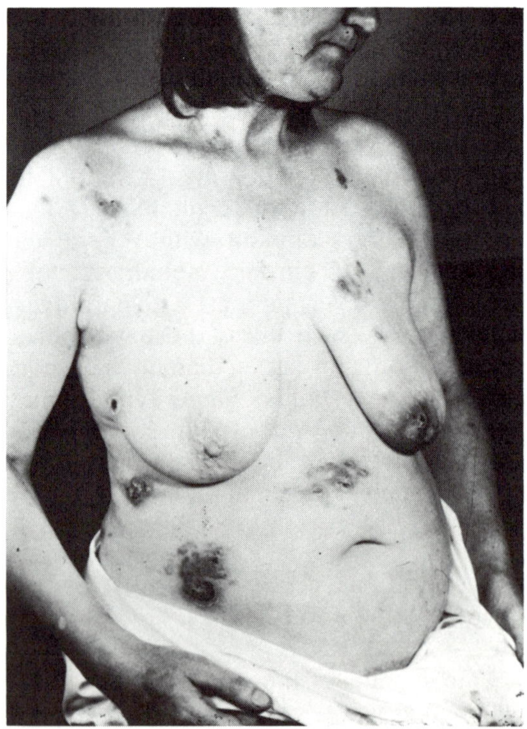

Fig. 3-2 Multiple late nodular syphilis of chest and abdomen.

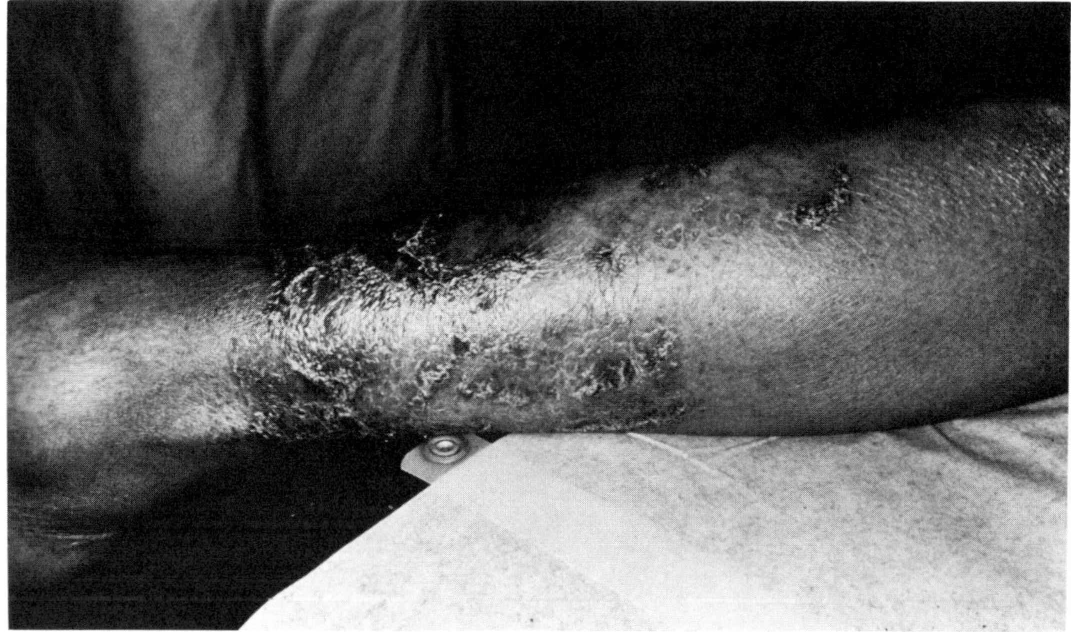

Fig. 3-3 Late nodular syphilis extensor surface of left leg—crusting and ready to ulcerate.

psoriasis, granuloma annulare, stasis ulcer, dermatitis medicamentosa such as bromoderma, leprosy, sporotrochosis, and blastomycosis.

GUMMAS OF THE MUCOUS MEMBRANES. Gummatous lesions may involve the mouth, tongue, soft and hard palate, pharynx, larynx, and the nasal mucous membrane including the septum (Plate 3-4).

The palate is a common site of gummatous infiltration leading to painless ulceration and perforation into the nasal cavity (Plate 3-5). The tongue is a frequent target of late syphilis. The gummatous infiltration compromises the blood supply of the tongue, leading to a vasculitis, then to an obliterative enarteritis. The resulting ischemia causes an atrophy of the tongue with the loss of papillae. The bald tongue of late syphilis appears. At the same time, the endoarteritis causes an atrophy of the musculature of the tongue and the tongue shrinks. Thus the diagnostic features are a bald tongue, a wrinkled tongue (Plate 3-6)

The absence of papillae results in a chronic inflammation of the tongue and a leukoplakia occurs. Malignant degeneration follows and a carcinoma of the tongue is the end result (Fig. 3-6). Thus, a syphilitic glos-

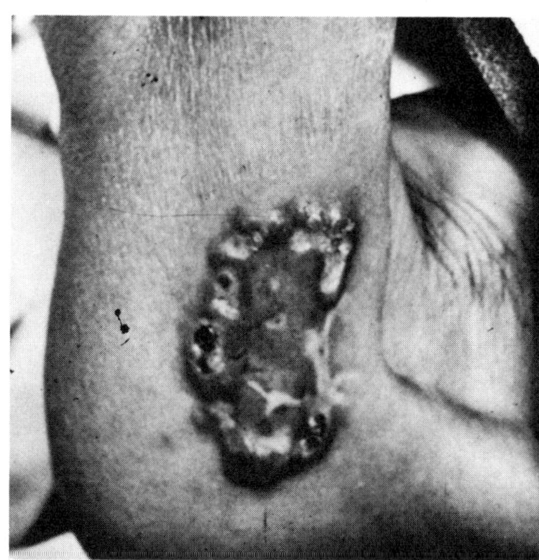

Fig. 3-4 Late noduloulcerative lesion of left upper arm.

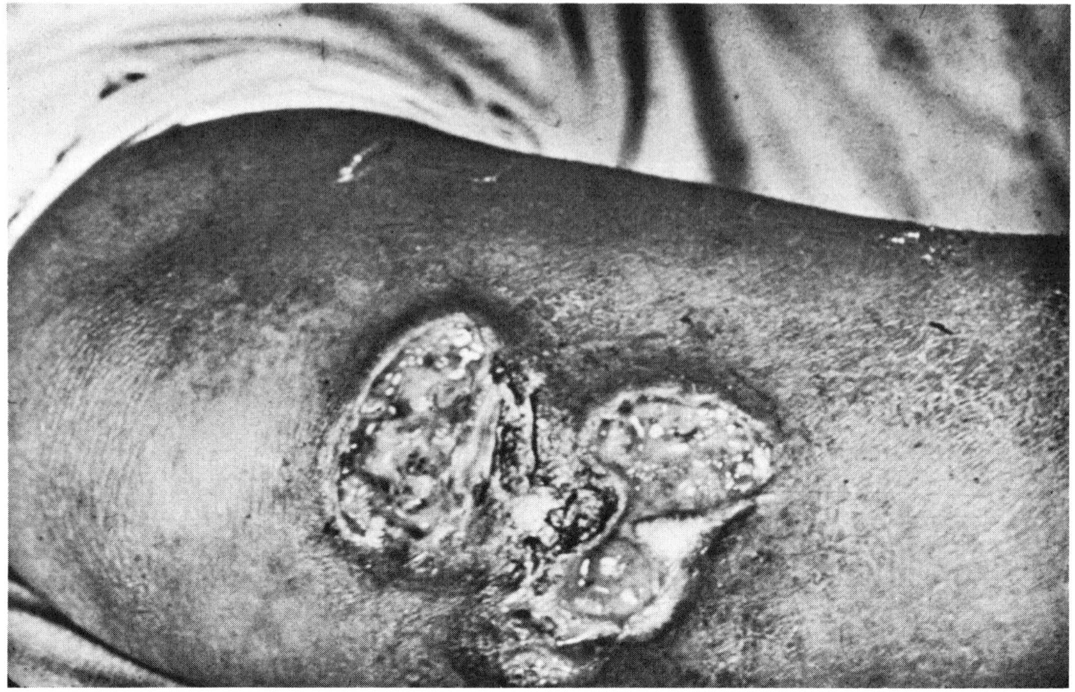

Fig. 3-5 Gumma of the right forearm.

sitis is a precancerous lesion and should be followed throughout the lifetime of the patient. There is no benefit from treatment with antibiotics except to stop the progression of late syphilis elsewhere.

OSSEOUS SYPHILIS

The long bones are more likely to be attacked by syphilis than the flat ones. Of the long bones, the tibia is involved more fre-

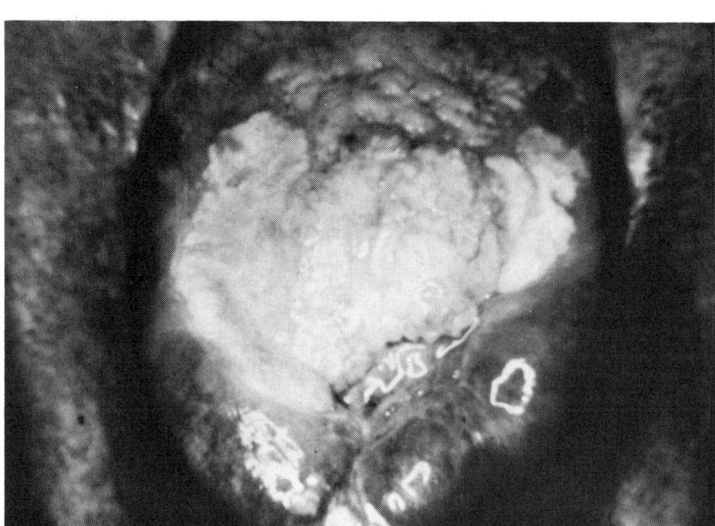

Fig. 3-6 Bald, wrinkled tongue of late syphilis.

quently. The skull and the clavicle, particularly at its sternal end, are the more vulnerable flat bones. In the skull, the syphilitic process first involves the outer table and then may spread to the inner table, with extensive destruction. The process may also penetrate to the meninges and brain, and there may be nodular lesions or localized areas of tenderness over the eroded, "worm-eaten" skull. On the chest, syphilis of the clavicle (Plate 3-7) usually manifests itself as a nodular swelling that is hard and not painful. The nodule sometimes breaks down and ulcerates the overlying skin. The syphilitic process may involve the sternoclavicular joint and the sternum itself. Syphilis of the clavicle is seen in both acquired and congenital syphilis, more often in the latter (Higoumenakis' sign).

The tibia, when involved, manifests a roughened, thickened anterior surface and is shaped like a saber. Sometimes the surface of the tibia is pitted by holes that can be felt.

The joints may be involved in secondary syphilis, and, less so, in primary syphilis. The patient complains of arthralgias, but physical and x-ray examination reveal nothing abnormal. However, in late syphilis, particularly in late congenital syphilis, there may be painless hydrarthrosis (chronic infusion) of the weight-bearing joints, knees (i.e., Clutton's joints, first described in 1886), ankles, elbows, and wrists. These infusions are more often bilateral than unilateral (Plate 3-8). Charcot's disease, or neurogenic arthropathy (first described in 1868), is often seen in tabes dorsalis. It attacks especially the joints of the knees, ankles, hips, shoulders, elbows, wrists, hands, and spine. The disease process is more often unilateral than bilateral and may involve many joints, more often, only one (Plate 3-9).

The pathologic changes are the result of damage to the trophic nerves of the joint. Subsequent damage is due to the lack of sensation in the joint. The onset is gradual, usually with painless swelling. The disease may progress to eventual loss of normal joint contour, enlargement of the joint, hypermobility, and destruction of bone, with small broken pieces producing crepitus and a "bag-of-bones" sensation to the touch. Because of the loss of function of sensory nerves, trophic ulcers may form on pressure areas such as the sole of the foot (mal perforans) (Plate 3-10), particularly at the first or fifth metatarsophalangeal joint.

VISCERAL SYPHILIS

Syphilis of the respiratory tract is rare. The diagnosis usually is established at autopsy or indirectly as the result of a therapeutic test with penicillin. Symptoms, if present, include persistent hoarseness, dysphagia (if the epiglottis is involved), and, sometimes, respiratory stridor. The lesions usually are nodular, noduloulcerative, or gummatous and involve the larynx or bronchi. Gummas of the lungs have the same characteristics on physical examination as any mass in the lungs. The differential diagnosis usually includes pulmonary tuberculosis, neoplasm, fungal infection. The history is one of easy fatigability, gradual and continual loss of weight, cough, and hemoptysis. There often is an afternoon rise in temperature. The x-ray film may suggest a localized neoplasm or a more widespread exudative or fibrotic process. The response to penicillin in gummas of the lungs is dramatic.

Syphilis of the stomach is also rare, and there is no specific finding on physical examination. The history suggest peptic ulcer or gastric neoplasm. Syphilis may be suspected following x-ray study or gastroscopy, but the final test may be either the therapeutic response to penicillin or the pathologic examination after surgery. There may be one or more nodules or a gummatous infiltration in the submucosa, which ulcerates and finally scars and constricts the stomach, particularly at the pre-pyloric end. A series of these infiltrations may result in a "leather-bottle stomach" (linitis plastica).

In secondary syphilis, the liver is occasionally enlarged, and this is often accompanied by jaundice. In late (tertiary) syphilis, a gummatous hepatitis may be seen, characterized by an irregular enlargement of the liver on palpation. The surface may feel pebbly or nodular, and syphilitic hepar lobatum may be suspected. If the gummas are not on the surface, an enlarged and smooth liver is felt. When the liver is enlarged, splenomegaly is also frequent. Because syphilitic hepatitis is rare, other causes of hepatic disease should first be considered, despite a positive blood test. However, patients with positive blood tests should be treated with penicillin if all other procedures are ineffective.

The gallbladder rarely is involved with syphilis. Infrequently, the intestines are affected by gummatous infiltration. The diagnosis is made at operation or autopsy. There are no specific physical findings on palpation of the abdomen. Early symptoms are those associated with an acute enteritis and late symptoms are those of an obstruction.

For some unexplained reason, the ovaries, fallopian tubes, and uterine body are spared.

Unlike the female reproductive organs which are spared, gummatous infiltration of the testes and epididymis do occur. Usually only one testis is involved and if there is an epididymitis, it follows after the testicular involvement. The patient complains of a hard nontender swelling of the testicle—it usually does not ulcerate into the skin. Penile gummas do occur but are much less common than testicular gummas (Plate 3-11).

CARDIOVASCULAR SYPHILIS

Cardiovascular syphilis occurs in 10–15% of untreated patients and becomes evident about 15 to 20 years after contracting the infection. Thus, it is a disease of middle life. It may manifest itself as a syphilitic aortitis, aortic insufficiency, aneurysm of the aorta and great vessels, and stenosis of coronary ostiae.

Uncomplicated aortitis may be suspected in a middle-aged patient, usually a male, with a history of substernal discomfort, who also has an accentuated tambourlike or bell-like second aortic sound. However, hypertension or arteriosclerosis must be ruled out before an x-ray diagnosis of syphilitic aortitis can be made. The electrocardiogram offers no specific diagnostic help.

Aortic regurgitation causes hypertrophy of the left ventricle and eventually congestive heart failure. It is found in rheumatic endocarditis, syphilis, and arteriosclerosis. Syphilitic aortic insufficiency usually occurs in males of middle age; it comes on later than aortic insufficiency of rheumatic endocarditis and earlier than that due to arteriosclerosis. The diastolic aortic murmur usually is quite distinct, soft and blowing. The distribution of the murmur follows the direction of the regurgitant stream, that is, downward and to the left. It may be heard at the second right intercostal space close to the sternum (Erb's point), but in many patients the murmur often is loudest along the left sternal border at the second, third, and fourth ribs or over the sternum itself. In many cases there is a concomitant systolic apical murmur, with or without a diastolic Austin-Flint murmur. The systolic blood pressure is increased, with normal or low diastolic pressures that produce a wide pulse pressure, evidenced by pulsating carotid arteries in the neck and at the suprasternal notch and associated with a jerk of the head that is synchronous with each heartbeat (Musset's sign). The face is pale, in contrast to the flushed cheeks of mitral stenosis. The wrist pulse is of the characteristic Corrigan or water-hammer type (described in 1832). Both Duroziez's murmur and pistol shot sounds may be heard over the large arteries of the extremities. The capillary pulse of Quincke may be disclosed by gentle pressure on the fingernails or by shining a flashlight under the fingertips and observing the alternating flush and pallor of the nailbed synchronous with the pulse. X-ray examination and fluoroscopy will reveal hypertrophy of the left ventricle, dilation of the aorta, and Corrigan's pulsation of the aortic arch. The electrocardiogram is not diagnostic.

Although most of the aneurysms of the thoracic aorta (Plate 3-6) are syphilitic in origin, traumatic, arteriosclerotic, and congenital aneurysms are seen occasionally. The signs and symptoms will depend on the location and size. Aneurysms of the ascending aorta usually are silent. Those in the transverse and descending aorta may produce pressure on the trachea and major bronchi, causing cough, tracheal tug, hoarseness, and aphonia from pressure on the recurrent laryngeal nerve; dysphagia from compression of the esophagus; difference in blood pressure in both arms; pupillary inequality from pressure on the cervical sympathetic nerves; or pain in the chest or back from bone erosion. Because of these possible involvements, x-ray examination of the chest should be done on all patients with late as well as latent syphilis.

Syphilitic coronary artery disease is similar in its manifestations to coronary sclerosis and, therefore, should be suspected in a middle-aged patient with an abnormal electrocardiogram. Patients with cardiovascular syphilis, particularly those with aortic insufficiency, have a concomitant neurosyphilis more often than not.

NEUROSYPHILIS

The invasion of the central nervous system occurs early during the course of infection when there is a generalized dissemination of spirochetes. About 20 to 30% of patients in the secondary stage will manifest abnormalities in the spinal fluid, such as an increase in lymphocytes and total protein and even a reactive VDRL. These will continue during the years when secondary relapses may be expected. Realistically, this will be most frequent during the first year of the disease, less often during the second year, and not at all after the fourth year. Thus, if the spinal fluid VDRL is nonreactive 4 years or more after infection, one can postulate that neurosyphilis would not occur, barring a reinfection.

Symptomatic neurosyphilis, other than acute meningitis, does not appear for at least 2 years after the initial infection. Neurosyphilis may be divided into the following stages: asymptomatic, acute meningitis, chronic meningovascular, general paresis, and tabes dorsalis.

Asymptomatic Neurosyphilis

Asymptomatic neurosyphilis is defined as the presence of syphilis characterized by repeated reactive blood reagin and treponemal tests and a reactive spinal fluid reagin test such as the VDRL. The FTA-ABS test for spinal fluid examination is not recommended at this time. There is also an absence of clinical signs and symptoms of central nervous system disease. In addition to the reactive spinal fluid VDRL test, if infection is active, the spinal fluid will have an increase in lymphocytes (5 cells/mm^3 or more) and total protein (35 mg/dl or more).

Acute Meningitis

Acute meningitis may occur within the first 2 years of infection, usually associated with the secondary stage of syphilis or a relapsing secondary process. Most cases, however, occur during the first 6 months of the disease. Acute syphilitic meningitis presents essentially the clinical picture of any acute meningitis, except that there is a greater variability in the extent and intensity of the symptoms because of the constant absorption and reformation of the exudate. The meningitis is principally a basilar type with headache appearing either continuously or in paroxysms, which are usually worse at night. Attacks of vertigo, nausea, and vomiting are frequent. The convulsions are usually generalized. The patient may become stuporous but may have periods of alertness and greater activity, often merging into delirium. There is cervical rigidity and positive Kernig's and Brudzinski's signs. The fever is irregular and moderately high.

Depending on the location of the exudate, which is usually more intense at the base, various cranial nerves are involved by a perineuritis. The third cranial nerve is most frequently implicated in whole or part. Various ocular palsies and gradations of external and internal ophthalmoplegia may be seen. Nystagmus, facial palsies, deafness, and facial pain are likely to appear.

but, most commonly, the middle and posterior cerebral arteries and their branches are affected. Therefore, the patient may suffer from a weakening of one side of the body, progressing to hemiplegia. However, hemiplegia is rarely complete, and there is rapid recovery with treatment.

The meningeal involvement will cause the patient to complain of headache, tenderness to the head on percussion, irritability, and double vision. With increased intracranial pressure, nausea, and vomiting occur. The cranial nerves may be completely on incompletely involved. Argyll Robertson pupils frequently are found. There may be papilledema and secondary optic atrophy. The third, fourth, and sixth cranial nerves are frequently affected. Less often, there is vertigo and deafness from the eighth cranial nerve impairment. With all of this, the spinal fluid examination will show increased pressure, marked increase in lymphocytes, elevated total protein, and positive serologic findings.

Chronic Meningovascular Neurosyphilis

In 2 to 5 years, but no later than 10 years, after the initial infection, meningovascular syphilis occurs as a result of no treatment, inadequate treatment, or a reinfection. The signs and symptoms will vary, according to the degree of involvement of the cerebral blood vessels and cranial nerves. There is a proliferative endarteritis and a perivascular infiltration with lymphocytes and plasma cells.

Perivascular cuffing is particularly marked around the blood vessels of the pia-arachnoid. Because of the swelling of the endothelial cells of the small and middle-sized vessels and diminution of blood supply, vascular thrombosis results in infarction of the nerve tissue. Gradual intellectual and emotional deterioration follows. Any of the cerebral blood vessels may be involved

General Paresis

About 5% of patients with untreated syphilis develop general paresis. This condition usually appears 20 or more years after the original infection. In general paresis, both the blood and spinal fluid will have reactive reagin and treponemal tests. Both neurologic and psychiatric symptoms are present in varying proportions. These may be summarized by the following acrostic schema:

P *Personality changes:* Deterioration of social habits, exaggeration of basic personality—neurosis with organic symptoms, euphoria, depression, overactivity, paranoid reactive state, follows crowd, moral offenses.

A *Affect:* Quantitative term to express patient's capacity and degree of reaction. The reaction is not consistent with or appropriate to the problem. Mood encompasses, mood shifts, irritability, and emotional reactions of an "all-out" type, such as those seen in childhood, which are not regulated in intensity to fit the situation.

R *Reflexes:* Hyperactive.
E *Eyes:* Argyll Robertson pupils.
S *Sensorium:* Delusions, illusions, hallucinations, and paranoid ideas.
I *Intellect:* Reduction in mental capacity, orientation, memory, retention and recall, calculations, general information, judgment, and insight.
S *Speech:* Slurred speech, consonants *s* and *l* pronounced slowly, coarse tremors of lips and tongue; patient omits words and phrases, repeats last few words, face often smooth and masklike.

General paresis can be classifed into the following forms.

Early Stage. The early symptoms of general paresis are usually manifested by a change in the personality, irritability, outbursts of temper, and inability to concentrate. Slovenliness of the person or dress may become apparent in individuals previously not showing such characteristics. Insomnia, anxiety states, headache, and fatigibility may offer reasons for the patient's going to a doctor. Loss of weight is often marked. Lack of judgment in a formerly astute businessman may be striking. With progression of the disease, loss of memory becomes prominent, a lowering of ethical and moral standards take place, and loss of the ability to make simple calculations appears. Because of the clouding of consciousness, the patient loses rapport with his environment and, as a result, has difficulty in comprehending the details of business and family life. As this condition increases, the patient becomes more and more disoriented until he is unaware of time, place or person and seems to live in an isolated dreamlike

state. Hallucinations are not common, but delusional states frequently recur.

Simple Dementia. The most common type of paresis is the simple dementing form, in which a simple organic deterioration occurs without excitement or emotional changes. There is a rapid and profound lowering of ethical and moral standards. Patients quickly lose interest in their environment and rapidly pass through a phase of forgetfulness into a state of dullness and apathy, with little insight into their condition. These patients eventually become entirely demented and bedridden. They lose weight, soil themselves, and die in a state of general paralysis.

The Euphoric or Expansive Paretic. The euphoric paretic has delusions of grandeur. The course of this form of the disease is longer and beset with remissions. Aside from the delusions of power, position, and wealth, the patients are cheerful and euphoric. Like the manic individual, they are in a constant state of psychomotor activity. At the same time, mental deterioration gradually progresses.

The Agitated Paretic. The agitated paretic is dangerous, especially since his type of psychosis is so frequently and suddenly precipitated. Mental deterioration may be quickly succeeded by an impulsive manic state in which the patient becomes violently excited and destructive. Homicide is not infrequently the result of such outbursts in the noninstitutionalized patient.

The Depressed Paretic. The depressed paretic is melancholy and has somatic hypochondriacal delusions. There is a marked psychomotor slowing and other physiologic disturbances. Typical depressive guilt feelings with self-condemnation, self-accusation, and self-punishing tendencies are present. At times the negativism and catatonic state of a schizophrenic are present.

TABES DORSALIS

Tabes dorsalis becomes evident 5 to 20 years after the primary or secondary stages. About 5% of patients with untreated syphilis develop tabes. Tabes is divided into three stages of development: preataxic, ataxic, and paralytic. Pain is characteristically the earliest symptom of tabes. The patient thinks that he has had rheumatic or muscular pain for years before other symptoms develop. The pain is often described as like lightning, because of its characteristic sudden appearance, rapid spread, and disappearance. It is often described as radiating from the gluteal region to the heel or foot, although it may be limited to the leg and, less commonly, to the arm. The pain may simulate a constricting band about the trunk and under such circumstances is named girdle pain. In addition to the pain, there may be marked paresthesia and hypesthesia. The paresthesia is most commonly referred to the soles of the feet and is described as a sensation of walking on a thick, soft carpet or walking on wood. The patient develops a loss of sense of position and passive motion. He may be able to recognize imperfectly, if at all, the movement of his toes or feet. As a result, the patient has poor control of his extremities. The vibratory sensibility is usually affected to the same degree as is the position sense.

Because of a deep sensory loss, the patient is ataxic. He at first notices slight difficulty in maintaining his balance. When washing his face and shutting his eyes, he tends to sway back and forth. At night he is less sure of his gait, and has to be observant of even visible landmarks. He gradually unconsciously assumes a broad base while walking, and, when not moving, he tends to take hold of nearby fixed objects. The patient can keep his sense of balance as long as his eyes are open. On closing his eyes, he begins to sway from side to side. Normal equilibrium in humans is maintained by three systems: the somatic afferents, principally from the muscles and joints; the labyrinthine afferents; and the visual system. Any two of these may compensate, even though imperfectly, for the loss of one. The patient uses gravity as a supplemental control of movement. He holds his body stiffly and gropes for his position by continual muscle stimulation. He consciously watches his movements and position in efforts to control them. He attempts to obtain the maximum effect of his proprioceptive sense when while walking, he overflexes his knees to be sure that his feet have cleared the ground and brings his extremities down forcibly to stimulate any remaining deep sensibility. Later, the tabetic must use one or even two canes.

TREATMENT

Once the physician has made the diagnosis of late symptomatic syphilis and has established the systems of the body affected, the next decision is to select the proper antibiotic and dosage schedule. There are many treatment regimens, and the choice of the treatment is the physician's. There is no dispute that the antibiotic of choice is penicillin. Thus, the physician must first determine if the patient is allergic to penicillin. If the answer is yes, obviously the alternate drug will need to be tetracycline or one of its analogs such as doxycycline or minocycline.

Logically, the next step is for the clinician to choose a satisfactory schedule of penicillin or tetracycline. When oral therapy is instituted, the physician must assess the reliability of the patient in following the prescribed course of therapy.

The recommended treatment for late symptomatic syphilis, except neurosyphilis, is benzathine penicillin G 2.4 million units intramuscularly each week for no less than two weeks. Patients with neurosyphilis

receive the benzathine penicillin G 2.4 million units intramuscularly for no less than three weeks. There is no objection to more treatment; it does the patient no harm, but it does no good either. It primarily comforts the physician.

Patients who are allergic to penicillin are prescribed tetracycline hydrochloride orally, 500 mg four times a day for no less than 15 days and no less than 20 days for neurosyphilis.

As with the treatment of any disease, the physician must evaluate the results of therapy. In late symptomatic syphilis both the clinical and serologic results are different from early syphilis.

In early syphilis, there are no destructive changes in the skin, muscles, and other organs, and after treatment the involved areas heal completely with no significant scarring or no scarring at all. Furthermore, effective treatment results in a seroconversion of the reagin tests to negativity.

In contrast, the lesions of late symptomatic syphilis are destructive and when they heal, they do so with fibrosis and tissue damage. Furthermore, in spite of effective therapy, seroreversal of the reagin tests do not usually occur. Thus, the physician must not only treat the syphilis, but also the destructive changes.

Mucocutaneous syphilis, whether nodular, noduloulcerative, or gummatous, will respond dramatically to the recommended treatment. However, the mucocutaneous lesions leave a noncontractible atrophic stippled scar. The reagin blood tests can be expected to remain reactive, that is, Wassermann or reagin-fast.

In the patient with cardiovascular late syphilis, the physician needs the assistance of a cardiologist and a vascular or cardiac surgeon. Uncomplicated aortitis is not a clinical entity. Usually the diagnosis may be made occasionally in an upper middle-aged patient, usually a man with reactive RPR-CT and FTA-ABS blood tests. An x-ray

may then reveal egg shell calcification of the proximal ascending thoracic aorta. However, most often the diagnosis is made at autopsy.

In addition to specific therapy for syphilis, the patient with aortic insufficiency needs digitalis support and equally, if not more importantly, aortic valve replacement. Without this surgery, in a patient who has had one cardiac decompensation, the prognosis is death, usually within two years. The patient with aortic aneurysm needs the same specialized assistance.

Patients with active neurosyphilis will have a normal lymphocyte count in CSF three months after treatment without any marked change in the total protein or in the cerebrospinal fluid VDRL test. One year after treatment, the protein level and the quantitative cerebrospinal fluid VDRL titer will be decreased notably but will not necessarily become normal. Wassermann fastness of the spinal fluid VDRL does occur.

Patients with chronic meningovascular syphilis will be markedly improved, but some patients may have residual neurologic weakness. Patients with general paresis show marked improvement and may be integrated into the general community, although they will have some neurologic and psychiatric residua. For example, most such patients will have difficulty in making important decisions, can be easily persuaded, and are manipulated by the gang.

When one reaches the state of tabetic neurosyphilis, the physician can expect very little, if any, improvement. Progression to a destructive Charcot joint is common. Tabetic crises respond to no presently known therapy. Some patients can anticipate their onset and take preventive measures in an attempt to abort them. The physician now needs the assistance of a good brace man and the advice of an orthopedist for possible joint replacement.

Late syphilis represents a failure to detect and treat early syphilis on the part of clinic and public health medicine. The patient needs every bit of help the physician can muster.

SUGGESTED READINGS

Fiumara NJ: Diagnosis and treatment of latent and late syphilis. Ch. 10, p. 127. In McCormack WM (ed): Diagnosis and Treatment of Sexually Transmissible Diseases. Wright-PSG Publishing, 1983

Gabay EL, et al: Computerized tomographic findings in meningovascular syphilis: A case report: Sex Transm Dis 10(1):39, 1983

Handsfield HH, et al: Demonstration of Treponema pallidum in a cutaneous gumma by indirect immunofluorescence. Arch Dermatol 119(8):677, 1983

Matsuda SS, et al: Nodular late syphilis. J Am Acad Dermatol 9(2):269, 1983

Moskovitz BL, et al: Meningovascular syphilis after "appropriate" treatment of primary syphilis. Arch Intern Med 142(1):139, 1982

Punt J: Multiple cerebral gummata. Case report. J Neurosurg 58(6):959, 1983

Romanowski B, et al: Treatment of neurosyphilis with chloramphenicol. A case report. Br J Vener Dis 59(4):225, 1983

Sacks JG, et al: Progressive visual loss in syphilitic optic atrophy. J Clin Neurol Ophthalmol 3(1):5, 1983

Smith JL: Syphilitic optic atrophy. J Clin Neurol Ophthalmol 3(1):3, 1983

COLOR PLATES

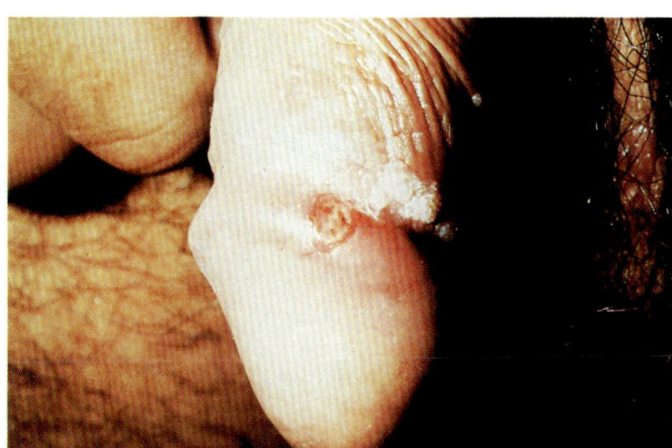

Plate 2-1

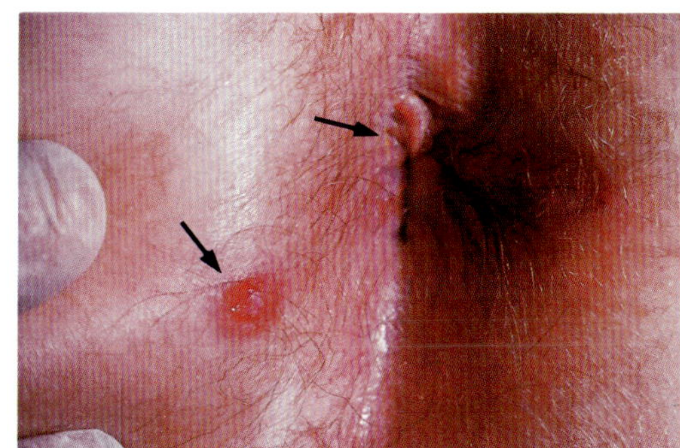

Plate 2-2

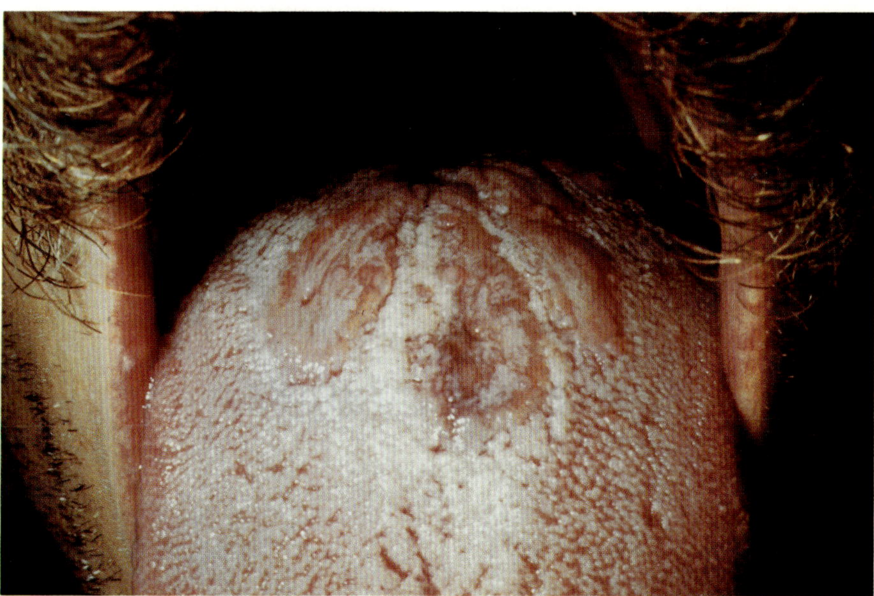

Plate 2-3

Plate 2-1 Primary syphilis: Typical coronal chancre in association with condylomata acuminata.
Plate 2-2 Primary syphilis: Twin perianal primary chancres (arrows) in a homosexual man.
Plate 2-3 Secondary syphilis: Multiple large mucous patches of the tongue.

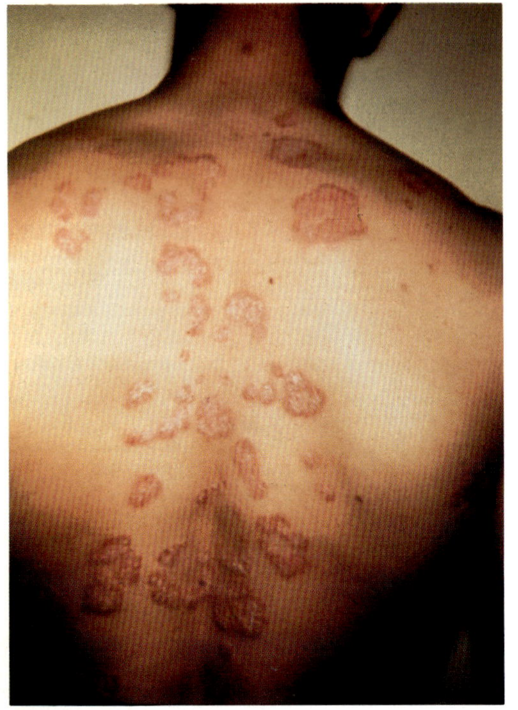

Plate 3-1

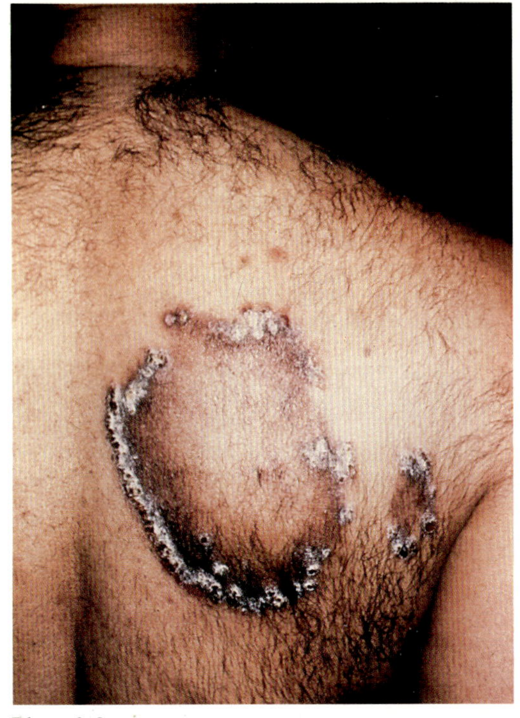

Plate 3-2

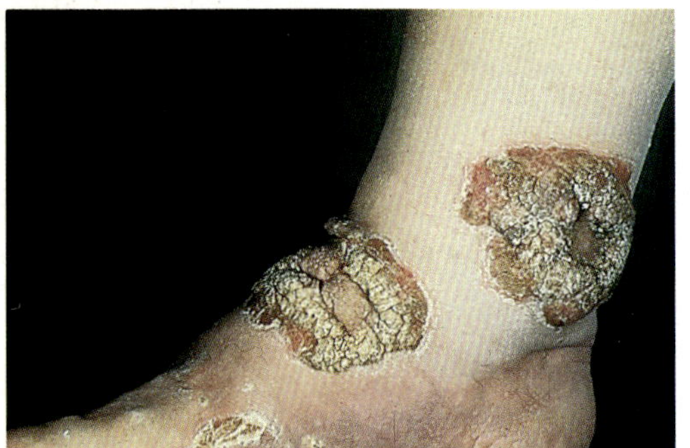

Plate 3-3

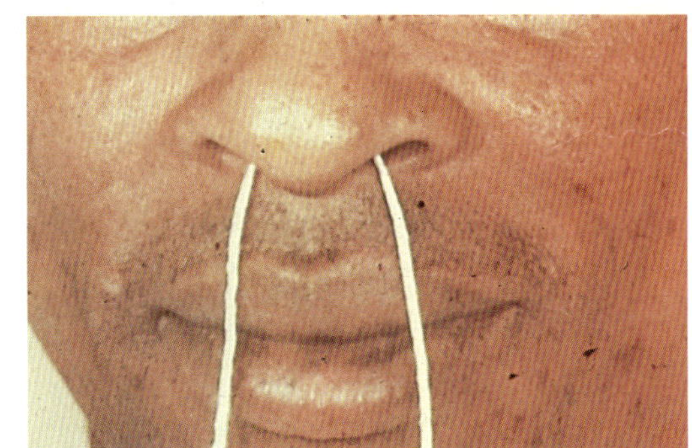

Plate 3-4

Plate 3-1 Late nodular syphilis of the back.
Plate 3-2 Late nodular syphilis of the back: Crusted and early ulceration.
Plate 3-3 Gummas of the right ankle.
Plate 3-4 Gumma of the nasal septum.

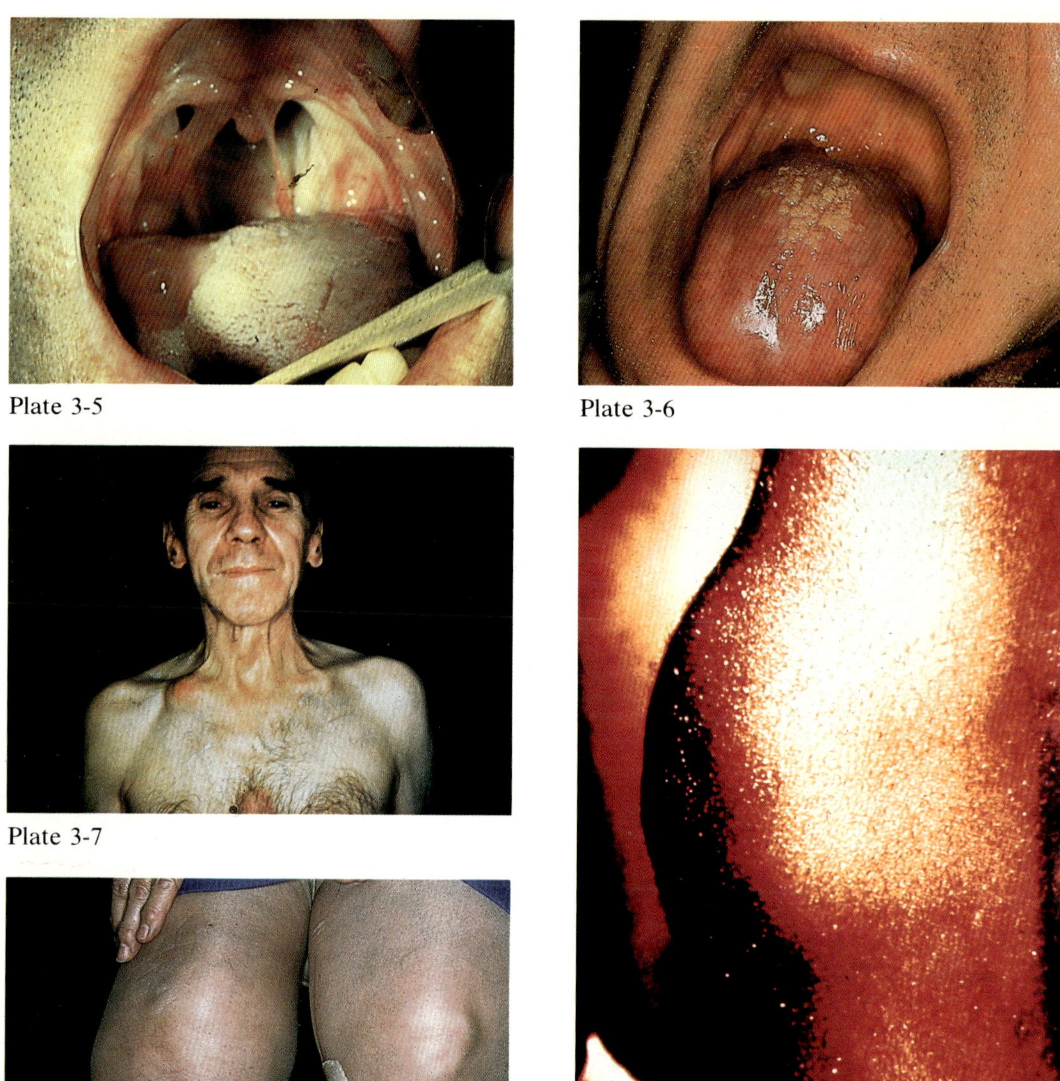

Plate 3-5

Plate 3-6

Plate 3-7

Plate 3-9

Plate 3-8

Plate 3-5 Gumma perforating the hard palate into the nasal cavity.
Plate 3-6 Gummatous infiltration of the tongue.
Plate 3-7 Late mucocutaneous, osseous syphilis of the right clavicle and overlying skin.
Plate 3-8 Late congenital syphilis with Clutton's joints of both knees.
Plate 3-9 Charcot's joint, both knees, more extensive on the right.

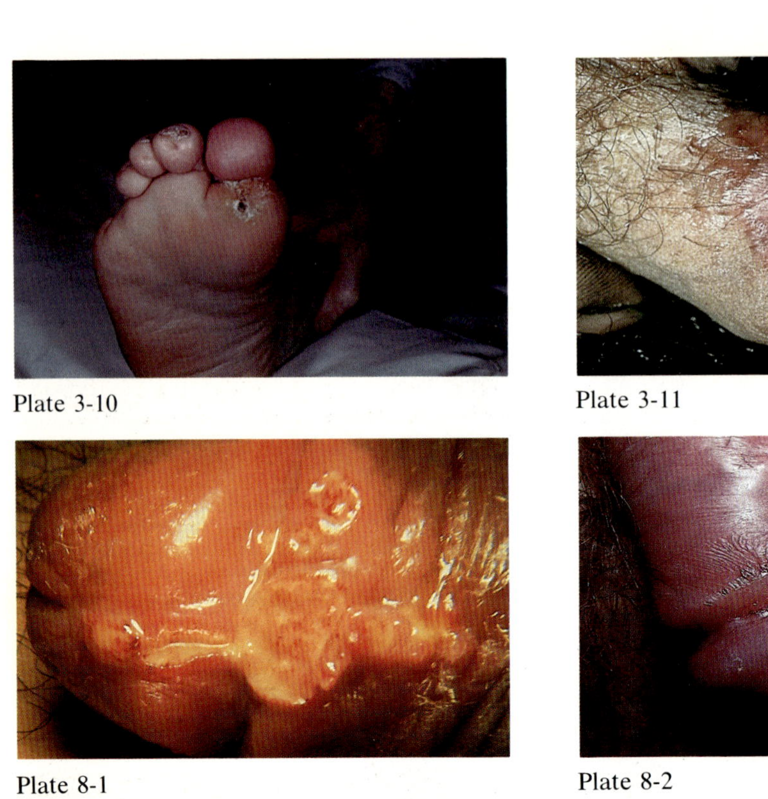

Plate 3-10

Plate 3-11

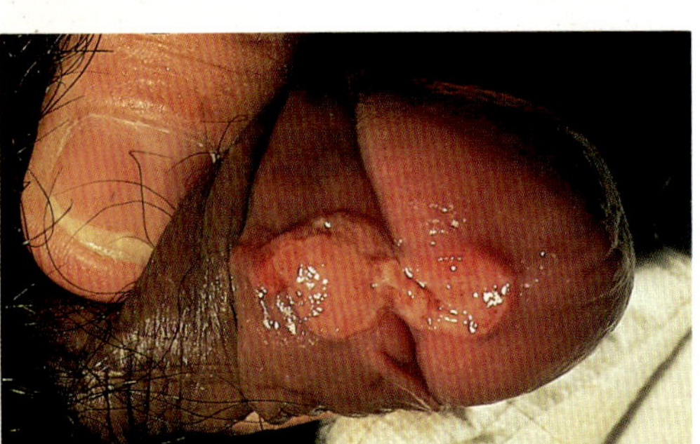

Plate 8-1

Plate 8-2

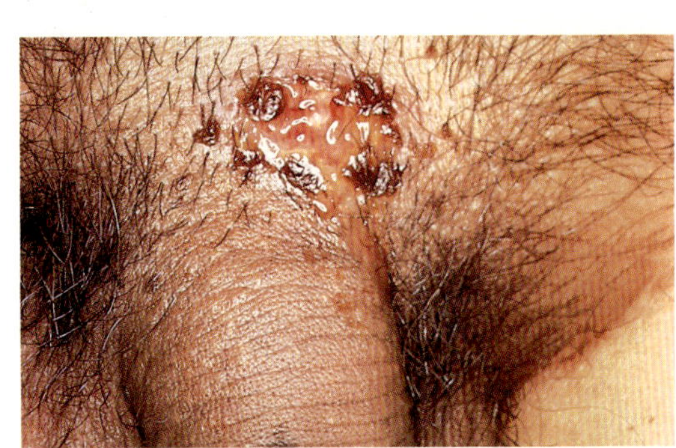

Plate 8-3

Plate 8-4

Plate 3-10 Mal perforans, sole of the right foot.

Plate 3-11 Gumma of the shaft of the penis.

Plate 8-1   Typical presentation of chancroid in a male. Multiple, autoinoculated, "dirty," purulent, painful ulcerations destroying the frenulum.

Plate 8-2   Early "kissing ulcers" of chancroid showing mucopurulent exudate and an erythematous halo.

Plate 8-3   A common site of chancroid ulcerations in males. Note the soft rolled margin and granulating base seen after cleaning the purulent exudate. (Courtesy of John Reeves, M.D.)

Plate 8-4   Chancroid ulcer at site not protected by a condom.

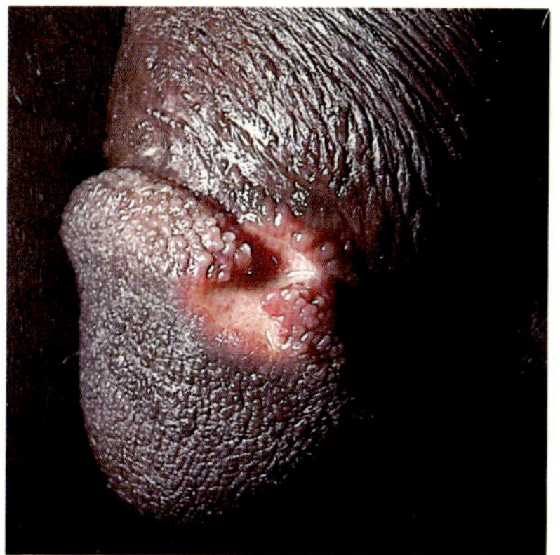

Plate 8-5

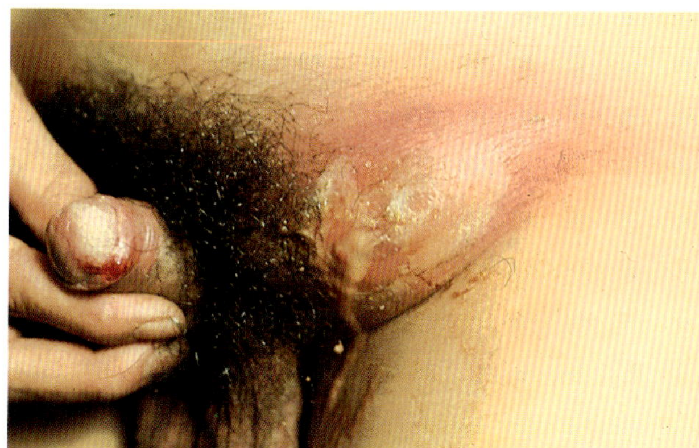

Plate 8-6

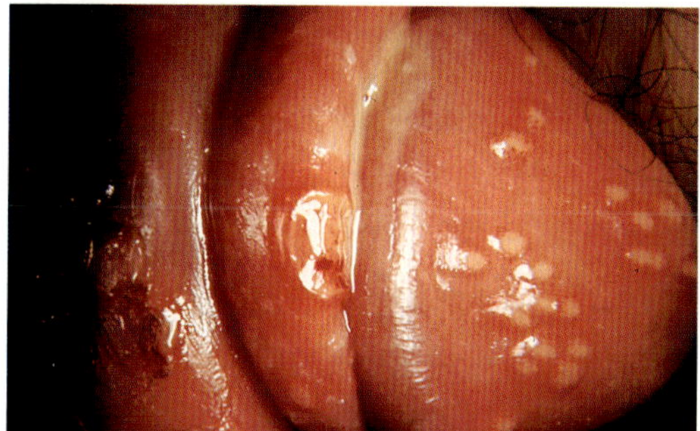

Plate 8-7

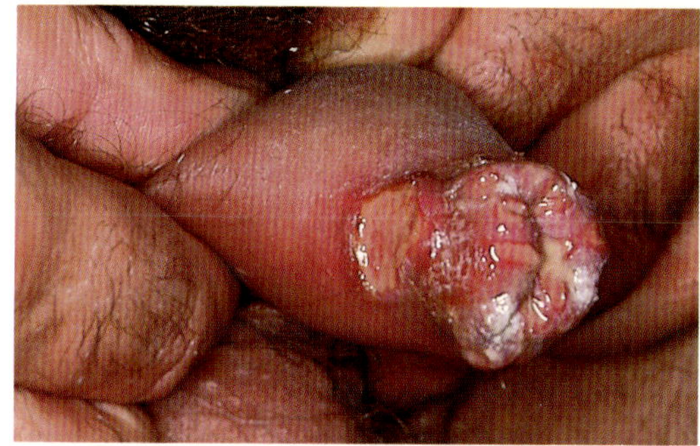

Plate 8-8

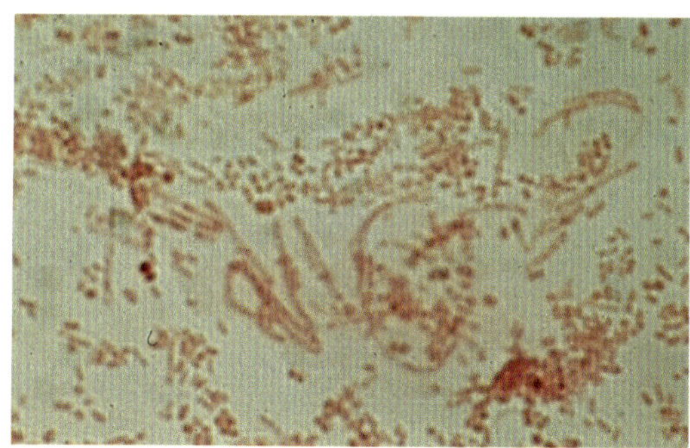

Plate 8-9

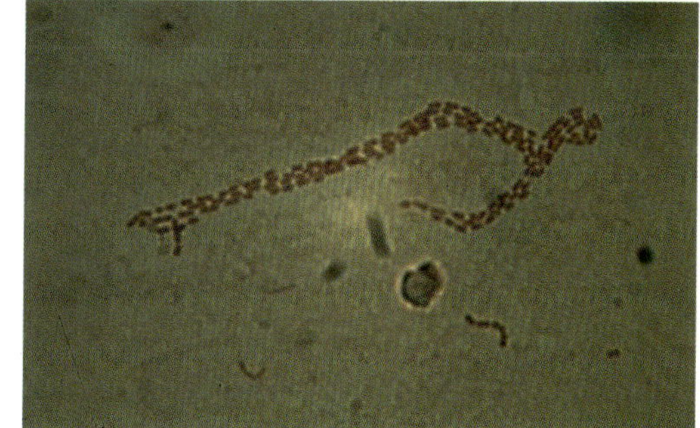

Plate 8-10

Plate 8-5 Phagodermic chancroid. This ulcer is only 3 days old.

Plate 8-6 Ruptured "bubo" of chancroid. This must be differentiated from lympho-granuloma venereum.

Plate 8-7 Balanitis and paraphimosis complicating chancroid.

Plate 8-8 Multiple severe chancroidal ulcerations with phimosis.

Plate 8-9 Smear from a chancroid lesion showing parallel chains of gram-negative streptobacillary organisms in the "school of fish" arrangement.

Plate 8-10 *Haemophilus ducreyi* from culture on patient's blood. Parallel chains of gram-negative bacilli are characteristic.

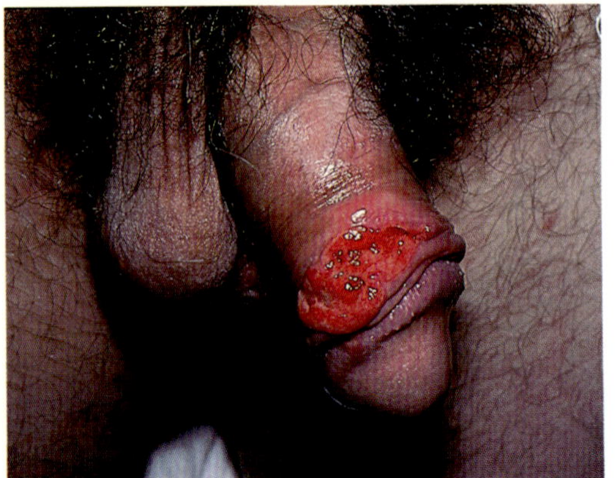
Plate 9-1A

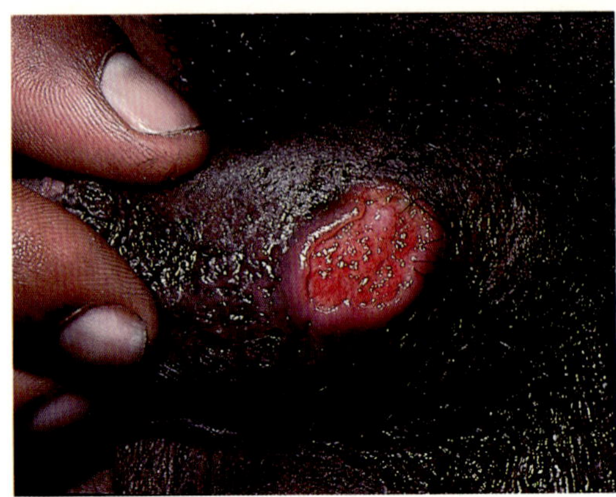
Plate 9-1B

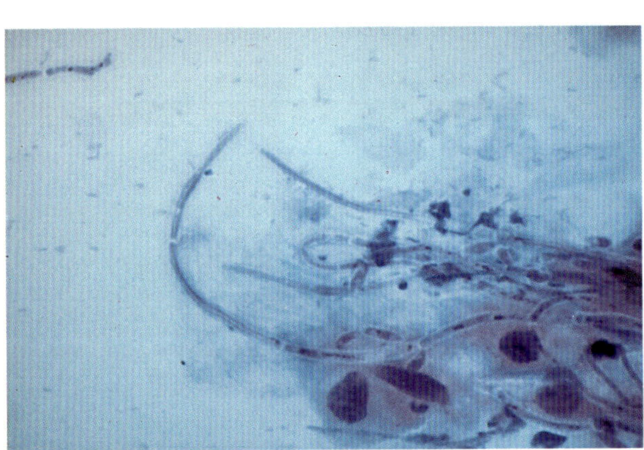
Plate 10-1

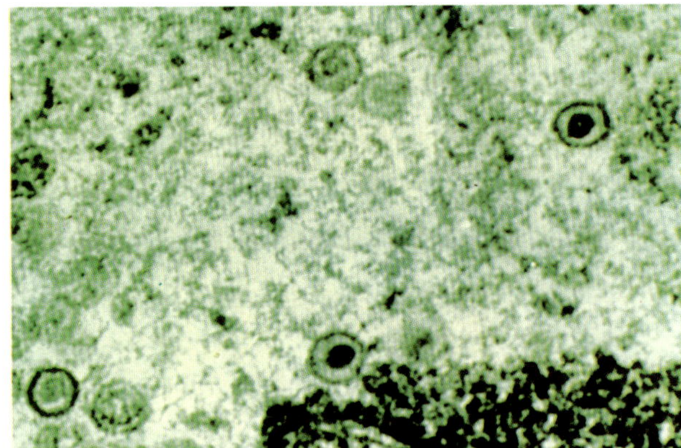
Plate 11-1

Plate 9-1 (A,B) Typical granuloma inguinale presents with a friable ulceration with a rolled border.
Plate 10-1 KOH-methylene blue stain of vaginal fluid showing yeast and pseudohyphae from a
  patient with vaginal candidiasis. (Courtesy of John Evrard, M.D.)
Plate 11-1 Herpes simplex virus as seen using the electron microscope.

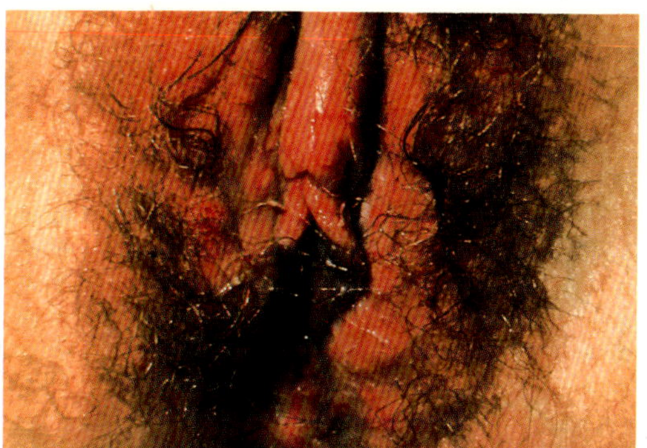

Plate 11-2

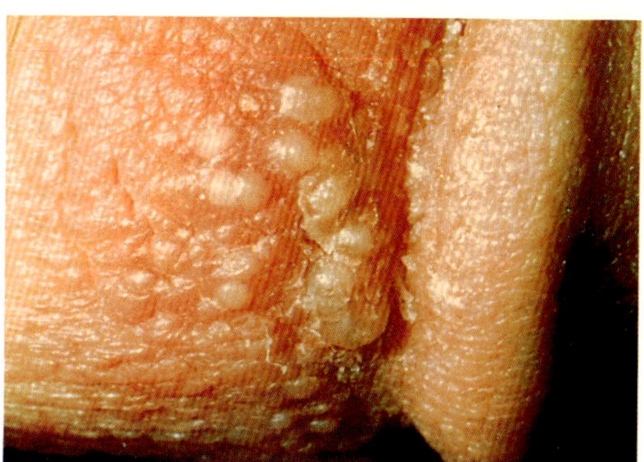

Plate 11-3

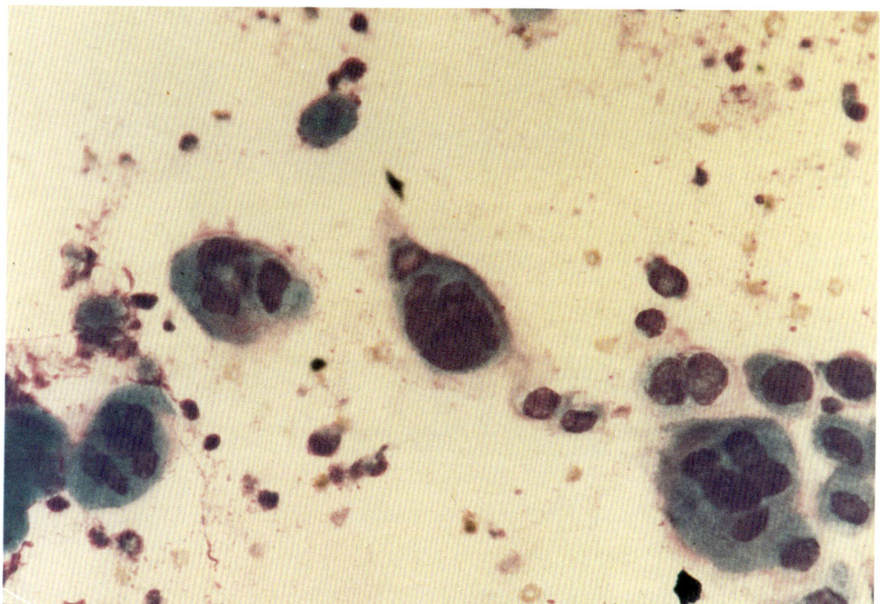

Plate 11-4

Plate 11-2 Primary genital herpes infection in the female.
Plate 11-3 Recurrent genital herpes infection in the male.
Plate 11-4 Multinucleated giant cells as seen in a positive Tzanck smear.

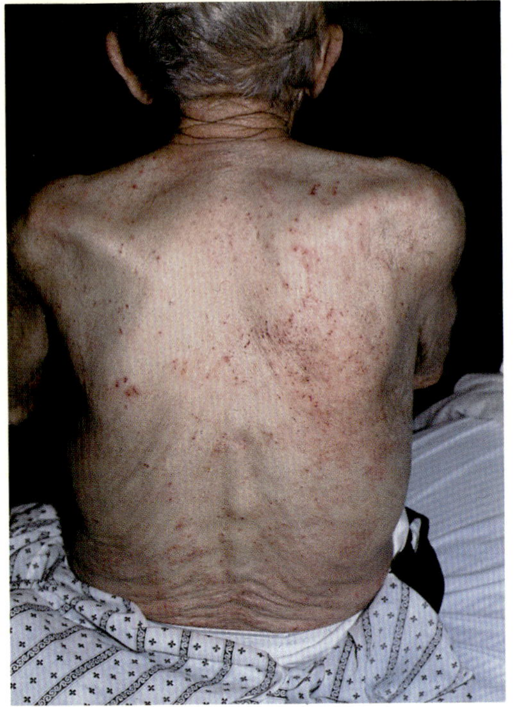

Plate 13-1

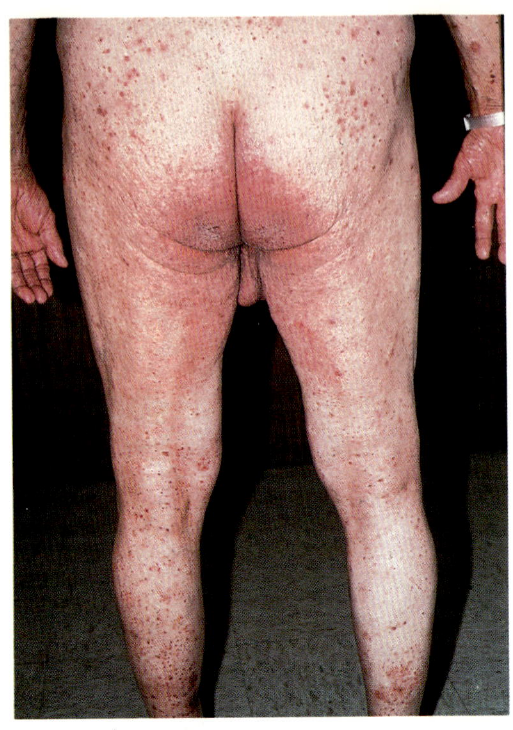

Plate 13-2

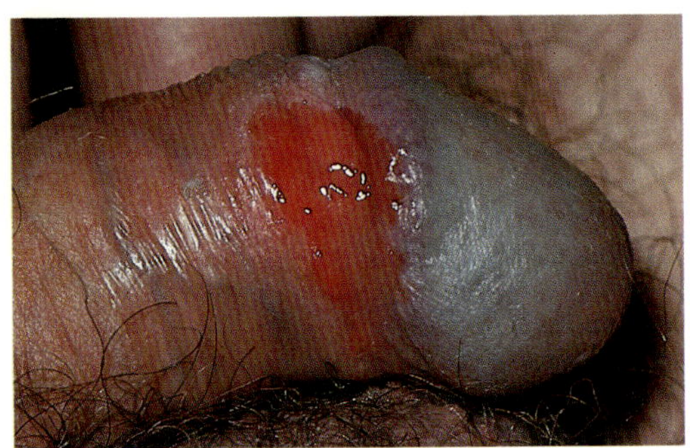

Plate 14-1

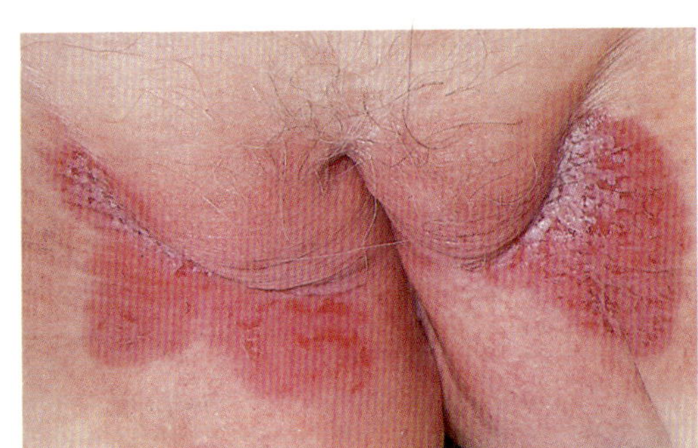

Plate 14-2

Plate 13-1 Scabies in a nursing home patient. Excoriations (no primary lesions) on back. (Courtesy of Russell W. Currier, M.D.)

Plate 13-2 Clinical vasculitis on buttocks and lower extremities, overshadowing the elements of scabies. (Courtesy of Frank Parker, M.D.)

Plate 14-1 Erythroplasia of Queyrat of the penis. (Hall-Smith P, Cairns RJ: Dermatology: Current Concepts and Practice. 3rd Ed. Butterworth, Woburn, Mass., 1981)

Plate 14-2 Paget's disease of the anogenital region.

4

Gonorrhea

William O. Harrison

Gonorrhea is a bacterial infection that primarily affects male and and female genital mucosa but can involve other areas of the body. It has been endemic throughout the world for many centuries. Probably the earliest description of gonococcal urethritis can be found in the Bible, in the Book of Leviticus. The Phoenicians, Persians, and Egyptians were also familiar with the disease, but it remained for Galen, practicing in Rome during the golden age of Greek medicine, to give the disease its present name. He mistakenly believed that the discharge (*Rheos*) was composed of semen (*Gonos*). Thus he named the disease *gonorrhea*, meaning a flowing of seed.

From earliest history until modern days gonorrhea has continued to be a problem of serious impact with sequelae as serious as sterility, blindness, and, in some cases, death. Despite the use of antimicrobials specifically effective against the gonococcus, gonorrhea remains in the unenviable position as the most common reportable infectious disease in the United States. In 1980 there were more than one million reported cases of gonorrhea of all types in the United States,[1] the majority of which were male urethritis.

MICROBIOLOGY

The causal agent of gonorrhea, *Neisseria gonorrhoeae*, is a gram-negative diplococcus closely related to commensal *Neisseria* commonly inhabiting mucous membranes in various parts of the body. It was described by Albert Neisser over 100 years ago as being the etiology of gonorrhea.[2]

Neisseria gonorrhoeae is a capneophilic aerobe and does not survive for long outside the host because of its susceptibility to drying, heat, and low concentrations of anions. Although Fuchs[3] has reported recovering viable organisms from toilet seats for as long as 18 hours after inoculating them there, and Elmros[4] noted gonococcal survival on wet towels for 10 to 24 hours, these are exceptional circumstances.

Gonococci are usually described as "kidney-bean" shaped, but may be oval or spherical as well, and may show arrangements other than the classic diplococcal form. Using light microscopy, they are readily seen under the oil immersion lens, but it is impossible to visually differentiate pathogenic from nonpathogenic *Neisseria*. Specific biochemical or immunologic tests are required to positively identify *N. gonorrhoeae*.

EPIDEMIOLOGY

Despite patient claims to the contrary, gonococcal infections are acquired by sexual contact. Studies done by Hooper and coworkers[5] show that the risk of a white male acquiring gonorrhea during a single episode of intercourse with an infected partner is approximately 17%. The risk increases to 100% as the number of episodes or the number of partners increases. Gonococcal urethritis is most commonly transmitted by either genital or rectal contact, but there is increasing evidence that infection can be transmitted from an infected pharynx to the urethra as well.[6] Complicated gonococcal infections generally begin as genital infections.

Most gonococcal infections are sexually acquired, but there have been cases reported of genital gonorrhea without vaginal penetration, as well as nongenital infections acquired by contamination with infected secretions.[7,8]

The incubation period for gonococcal urethritis varies from 3 to 10 days, but there are exceptions to this generality. For example, strains of gonococci from the western Pacific area will produce symptoms and positive cultures in as short a time as 12 hours after exposure, or may take as long as 3 months to manifest themselves.[9]

Classic symptoms of gonococcal urethritis include dysuria and urethral discharge—"dripping and burning." The dysuria may be only a slight discomfort on urination or may be exquisitely painful. The same variability holds true for the urethral discharge. It may be absent or profuse, with all stages intermediate. Although the classic gonococcal discharge is profuse and purulent, in some cases it may be only mucoid or mucopurulent.[10] Thus to attempt to diagnose gonorrhea only by the qualitative evaluation of discharge is to allow for the probability of missed diagnoses.

The number of men who have asymptomatic gonorrhea is a matter of some debate. Several studies of sexually active men who were voluntarily screened to rule out asymptomatic gonorrhea showed an absolute incidence of from 0.5 to 1.5%,[11,12] but other surveys of men likely to be infected who had not sought treatment spontaneously have reported a prevalence of from 40 to 60% of asymptomatic infection.[13–15]

Infections in Women

Although many women with uncomplicated gonorrhea have no symptoms, the majority are symptomatic.[16] Undue emphasis on the lack of symptoms in women has probably resulted from studies of women identified by tracing them as contacts or by screening. The primary site of infection is usually the endocervix with secondary infection or colonization of the urethra or rectum.

Gonococci may ascend the genital tract in women to infect the fallopian tubes and pelvic peritoneum, causing pelvic inflammatory disease or salpingitis. Acute salpingitis usually begins with diffuse pelvic pain and tenderness, fever, and malaise. Subacute salpiginitis causes prolonged or recurrent attacks of pelvic pain and tenderness usually associated with episodic low-grade fever and menstrual disturbances. Chronic salpingitis causes prolonged or recurrent attacks of pelvic pain and tenderness usually preceded by acute or subacute attacks but may appear de novo with sterility, ectopic pregnancy, or as asymptomatic thickening or abscess formation in the adnexal regions.

Gonococcal infection usually causes inflammation with subsequent signs and symptoms that are useful in diagnosing gonococcal urethritis. Even though such inflammation usually subsides in 2 to 4 weeks without treatment, the host may remain a carrier and potentially infectious.[17] Thus, establishing a definitive diagnosis even in women without symptoms is important.

DIAGNOSIS

The initial differentiation point in evaluating an organism suspected of being gonococcus is to test for the production of oxidase. A gram-negative diplococcus which is oxidase-positive is almost certainly one of the *Neisseria*, and this fact can be used in clinical settings to plan and execute therapy.[18] To fully identify the bacteria as to species, however, a common technique is the carbohydrate utilization test.[19] There are a number of more sophisticated tests that can further delineate the characteristics of the gonococcus, but a full description of them is beyond the purview of this chapter. The interested reader is referred to textbooks such as those of Brooks and colleagues[20] and Morton.[21]

The effectiveness of laboratory diagnosis depends upon meticulous care being paid to the collection and subsequent testing of specimens. Disinfectants should not be used for preparing the patient and the only lubricant used should be sterile water. Specimens must be transferred as rapidly as possible onto suitable culture or transport medium. Because gonococcal infections often occur in areas with extensive normal bacterial flora, or adjacent to such areas, it is extremely important that specimens be obtained in a manner so as to avoid contamination with other bacteria. In the case of gonococcal urethritis or endocervicitis, this means that urethral specimens must be obtained from within the urethra or endocervix, not by simply using a drop of expressed urethral discharge or vaginal pool secretions to inoculate a swab or culture plate.

Urethral specimens should not be collected until at least one hour after the patient has urinated, in order to avoid having viable bacteria swept from the anterior urethra by the stream of urine. A calcium alginate urethrogenital swab (Calgiswab, Inolex) should be carefully inserted into the urethra or endocervix, rotated gently, and inoculated directly onto the culture or transport medium. Cotton swabs should be avoided because of the bactericidal effect of free fatty acids contained within cotton fibers.[19] Specimens from other areas of interest such as pharynx, anal canal, blood, or joint aspirate may be collected as necessary, depending upon symptoms. Some investigators recommend culturing the sediment of a spun-down urine specimen, or prostatic fluid, but these techniques may not be as sensitive as urethral or endocervical cultures and are somewhat more difficult to do correctly.[22]

Except in the case of male gonococcal urethritis, Gram staining of material collected for culture is not necessary because of the significant number of false negative and false positive tests that result. For gonorrhea in women and for all complicated gonococcal infections, adequate cultures are mandatory.

The swab should be inoculated onto culture medium first, and then applied to a clean microscope slide for Gram staining, if this test is to be done. Once the inoculum for culture has been planted, the swab should be carefully rolled across the center of the slide, ensuring that all surfaces of the swab are touched to the slide. It is important to roll, rather than "scrub" the swab onto the slide. Too vigorous an effort can disrupt white blood cells, thus obscuring the classical appearance of "intracellular gram-negative diplococci" by which the initial diagnosis of gonococcal urethritis is made.

Slides should be air-dried and heat-fixed. They should be stained and examined immediately, but if this is not possible, heat-fixation should be done prior to transporting the slides to the laboratory. A variety of simple staining procedures can be used, and there are many different stains and counterstains recommended for the Gram procedure. The technique described in the second edition of the *Manual of Clinical Microbiology* is satisfactory, but any method that gives comparable results may be used routinely. When evaluating specimens from men with urethritis, trained laboratory personnel who prepare and read Gram stains on a regular basis can make the diagnosis of male gonococcal urethritis with approximately 95% sensitivity and 99% specificity.[23]

The transfer of specimens for culture from clinic to laboratory in transport medium should be avoided if at all possible. The best results are obtained when specimens are inoculated directly onto culture plates and immediately incubated. When transfer is necessary, it should be done under full or partial environmental control, or by holding the specimen in a nonnutrient transport medium designed to minimize overgrowth by other bacteria.

The most common transport devices available offer only partial environmental control but when properly utilized can be effective.[24] These include the use of candle jars to transport already-inoculated culture plates; the Transgrow system of Thayer-Martin medium in a small CO_2-containing vial; and the JEMBEC system, which also utilizes modified Thayer-Martin medium but in a flat plate with a CO_2-generating system and self-contained pouch. The efficiency of all of these systems is enhanced by pretransport incubation.

Holding medium is useful for transport of swabs from wards or clinics to the clinical laboratory when they cannot be inoculated onto agar medium with 5 minutes. Holding medium is least successful when there is a prolonged time lapse between collection of the specimen and its inoculation onto culture plates. Amies modified Stuart medium is the most commonly used holding medium.

The use of cultures to confirm the clinical and microscopic diagnosis of gonococcal urethritis is becoming a necessity rather than an option. The major reason for this change is the rapid increase in resistance of the gonococci to many commonly used antibiotics. Whereas in former days it was

necessary only to establish a diagnosis by means of Gram stain and to culture only in the event of treatment failure, the emergence of penicillin- and tetracycline-resistant strains of gonococci have made it mandatory to culture initially. In the case of male gonococcal urethritis, treatment may still be offered on the basis of microscopic diagnosis alone.

The two most effective media to use for initial cultures of gonococci are the modified Thayer-Martin medium[25] and the New York City medium.[26,27] Both of these media are very sensitive when properly prepared and give a very low rate of false negative results. As with any culture technique, quality control and competent laboratory support are mandatory. Further details concerning the culturing of gonococci may be obtained from publications of the American Society for Microbiology.[19]

Although there are a number of serologic and fluorescent antibody tests available commercially, the high level of sensitivity and specificity of the combination of Gram stain and culture of urethral discharge in gonococcal urethritis makes the routine use of any adjunctive test unnecessary. There are few situations where the patient cannot be rapidly and easily diagnosed and properly treated using these two simple and relatively inexpensive procedures.

TREATMENT

Preantibiotic-era treatments for gonorrhea included the application of various salves and ointments to the genitalia or the instillation of various antiseptic solutions into the urethra.[28] In 1936–1937 such remedies were discarded in favor of the newly discovered sulfa drugs.[29] Over the next several years, however, resistance to sulfas developed at an increasingly rapid rate. By 1943 the majority of isolates of gonococcus were resistant to sulfadiazine.[30]

The discovery of penicillin began the current era of treatment of gonorrhea, and in 1943 the first cases of gonorrhea were being successfully treated. During the subsequent 40 years the amount of penicillin needed to eradicate the infecting gonococcus has steadily increased.[31] Treatment has been with several different formulations of penicillin and according to many different treatment regimens. In 1972 the Centers for Disease Control (CDC) issued a set of standard recommendations for the treatment of gonorrhea and other sexually transmitted diseases, and they have updated the recommendations at regular intervals since.[32] Table 4-1 is a resume of the current CDC recommendations.

Penicillin

The current penicillin regimen is 4.8 million units of aqueous procaine pencillin intramuscularly accompanied by 1 gram of oral probenecid. This regimen has both advantages and disadvantages. The major disadvantage is the increasing presence of beta-lactamase-producing strains of gonococcus, which will be discussed in detail in a later section. Other significant problems with the regimen include the fact that procaine penicillin in this dose is a large, painful series of injections which some patients find intolerable; and the additional disadvantage that the recommended amount of procaine penicillin contains a significant level of procaine, which may cause a toxic reaction in some patients.[17]

The major advantage of the regimen is that it can be given in one session while the patient is still under the supervision of the health care provider. This makes it an ideal regimen for the transient, poorly motivated, or otherwise unreliable patient. It is also the most effective regimen for associated pharyngeal or rectal gonococcal infections.

Table 4-1. Recommended Treatment Regimens for Gonococcal Urethritis Infections (The order of presentation does not indicate preference)

Parenteral
  Aqueous procaine penicillin G
    4.8 million units injected intramuscularly (IM) at two sites and accompanied by 1 gram of probenecid by mouth *or*
  Spectinomycin HCl (Trobicin)
    2 grams injected as a single dose intramuscularly (IM)
  Ceftriaxone
    250 mg IM

Oral
  Ampicillin
    3.5 grams as a single dose, accompanied by 1 gram of probenecid by mouth *or*
  Amoxycillin
    3 grams as a single oral dose, accompanied by 1 gram of probenecid by mouth *or*
  Tetracycline HCl
    500 mg by mouth four times daily for 7 days (total dose 14 grams). Doxycycline hyclate 100 mg by mouth, twice daily for 7 days may be substituted, but it is no more effective than tetracycline HCl. All tetracyclines are ineffective as single-dose therapy

Combination therapy
  (This regimen is theoretically effective against both gonorrhea and coexisting chlamydial infections, but it has not been evaluated in a rigorous manner)
  Ampicillin/Amoxycillin
    3.5 grams of ampicillin or 3.0 grams of amoxycillin by mouth in a single oral dose, accompanied by 1 gram of oral probenecid *plus*
  Tetracycline HCl
    500 mg by mouth 4 times daily for 7 days. Doxycycline hyclate 100 mg by mouth twice daily for 7 days may be substituted for tetracycline HCl

Ampicillin

Oral penicillin V and K do not attain adequate serum or urethral levels to be effective against gonococci in a single-dose therapy.[33] The use of ampicillin overcomes this problem and provides a mechanism for single-dose oral therapy. Ampicillin is as effective as procaine penicillin in treating either urethritis or endocervicitis and may be substituted for it if an oral penicillin regimen is desired. This ameliorates two of the three major disadvantages of the parenteral agent, pain on injection and procaine reactions. Unfortunately, beta-lactamase-producing strains of gonorrhea are resistant to ampicillin as well as penicillin.

Amoxicillin

Amoxicillin offers no significant advantage over ampicillin except that it can be given in a slightly lower dose, and the cost of amoxycillin may be lower in some circumstances than that of ampicillin.[34] All three of these penicillin-derivative regimens are 95% effective or better, except against the beta-lactamase-producing strains of gonococci.

Tetracycline

An alternative to penicillin therapy is the tetracycline group. (Table 4-1) Tetracycline hydrochloride has been used successfully in the United States for many years and is a primary drug of choice for uncomplicated gonococcal urethritis in recommendations developed by the CDC. Tetracycline is generally well-absorbed and achieves good urine and urethral levels. It is effective orally as well as parenterally. The oral regimen is quite well accepted by most patients. The delineation of *Chlamydia trachomatis* as the causative agent of many cases of postgonococcal urethritis (PGU) makes the use of tetracycline even more attractive, since this therapy could, at least theoretically, cure gonococcal urethritis and simultaneously abort incubating PGU. Tetracycline is also a very inexpensive drug, making it attractive to facilities with limited budgets. Disadvantages of the tetracycline group include the requirement for multiple doses and contraindications for use in children under the age of eight or pregnant women. The more expensive tetracycline analogs (minocycline, doxycycline) are no

more effective than tetracycline hydrochloride, but may be better tolerated by patients.

Spectinomycin

Spectinomycin hydrochloride is the recommended alternative therapy for patients with penicillin allergy or those in whom penicillin-resistant infections are either proven or suspected. The 2-gram intramuscular dose is effective for most cases of uncomplicated gonorrhea, although there have been reports from Korea and Europe of the emergence of spectinomycin-resistant strains of gonococci.[35,36] There is no rationale for using a higher dose of spectinomycin, since resistance, when it develops, is of a high order of magnitude. Unlike penicillin, spectinomycin will not abort incubating syphilis.

Sulfamethoxazole/Trimethoprim

Since the early development of resistance to sulfas caused these drugs to fall from favor in the treatment of gonorrhea, there has been little experience with their use. The combination antibiotic sulfamethoxazole/trimethoprim has had good success in several studies,[37,38] and could be considered an alternative for a multiple-day/multiple-dose oral regime.

Erythromycin

Erythromycin in a dose of 500 mg 4 times daily for 7 days is also an effective regimen, but no more so than the penicillins or tetracyclines. Its use is primarily restricted to those with multiple drug allergies, children, or pregnant women.

Cephalosporins

Many of the first generation cephalosporins have been used in the treatment of gonococcal infections, but in most cases they offer no advantage over penicillin or tetracycline.[32] The real efficacy of cephalosporins is in the treatment of gonorrhea caused by penicillin-resistant strains of gonococci. These regimens will be discussed below under the separate heading of penicillinase-producing *Neisseria gonorrhoeae* (PPNG).

FOLLOW-UP

Reevaluation of patients treated for gonorrhea is mandatory. All patients should be reevaluated between 3 and 7 days after therapy and repeat cultures obtained. Cultures should be obtained from the same sites as pretreatment cultures; in addition, women should have anal canal cultures taken because of the occasional failure of therapy to eradicate gonococci from that location. If male patients are still symptomatic, a Gram stain of urethral secretions should also be obtained. This will assist in making a preliminary determination as to whether the symptoms are due to recurrent gonorrhea or PGU. If gram-negative diplococci are seen, it can be presumed that the patient has either failed therapy or has been reinfected, and appropriate antigonococcal therapy can be given. If there are no diplococci seen, tetracyclines can be given for presumed PGU.

TREATMENT FAILURES

Patients whose symptoms persist after therapy and who have evidence of persistent or recurrent gonococcal infection (see above) should be given spectinomycin HCl in the standard two-gram dose. If they had been initially treated with spectinomycin, treatment should be with penicillin, tetracycline, or cefoxitin (see Tables 4-1 and 4-2), depending upon the antibiotic sensitivities of the pretreatment cultures. Recurrent gonococcal infections after treatment with recommended regimens frequently are due

Table 4-2. Antibiotics Effective against Penicillinase-Producing *Neisseria gonorrhoeae*

Spectinomycin	2 grams intramuscularly (single dose)
Cefoxitin	2 grams intramuscularly, plus 1 gram of probencid by mouth
Cefotaxime	1 gram intramuscularly
Ceftriaxone	250 mg intramuscularly
Ceftizoxime	1 gram intramuscularly

The following regimens are effective but have not been approved by the FDA

Cefaclor	500 mg orally 4 times daily for 5 days
Sulfamethoxazole/ trimethoprim	9 single-strength tablets in a single daily dose for 3 days total therapy

Other regimens are either not as effective as the above or have not yet been released by the FDA for general use

to reinfection and suggest a need for improved patient education and counseling, as well as better contact tracing. Because an increasing proportion of treatment failures are due to PPNG (see below), all posttreatment gonococcal isolates should be tested for beta-lactamase production.

EPIDEMIOLOGIC TREATMENT

The treatment prior to making a firm diagnosis in asymptomatic contacts of patients with known or suspected gonorrhea is a well-established practice.[32] Such epidemiologic treatment is justified by the frequency of such concurrent infection, the likelihood of further spread of disease while awaiting diagnosis and the frequent failure of patients to return for follow-up. Epidemiologic treatment should be carried out with both the male contacts of men and women with suspected or proven gonorrhea and female contacts of men with proven or suspected gonorrhea, whether symptomatic or not.

COMPLICATIONS

Gonococci may spread by extension beyond the anterior urethra or endocervix to cause significant local complications, or they may disseminate widely via the blood or lymphatics to produce distant disease. Untreated anterior urethritis usually reaches a symptomatic peak in 2 to 3 weeks if not treated, but may persist for months.[17] Local extension to the posterior urethra, seminal vesicles, or epididymis occurs frequently in men with untreated disease and may occur even in promptly treated cases.[39] Posterior urethritis in preantibiotic days commonly led to urethral stricture and sterility,[40] but this complication is rare in developed countries today.

Epididymitis in younger men is frequently caused by gonococci[41] and cultures of epididymal aspirates should be obtained for both gonorrhea and *Chlamydia trachomatis* (if such culture is available). A technique to maximize therapeutic success in such cases is to treat with tetracycline or one of the long-acting analogs in order to eradicate both pathogens. Such treatment should be for at least one or, preferably, two weeks. Epididymitis in men over 40 generally is caused by gram-negative rods and may be associated with nonvenereal urinary tract infections.

Genital abscess may also accompany genital gonorrhea, particularly if there are anatomic abnormalities present or the sexual activity was accompanied by trauma.[42,43] These infections generally respond to simple local care and standard regimens of effective antibiotics.

Gonococcal Proctitis

Gonococci may infect the rectum after anal intercourse in women or male homosexuals or by secondary spread from the vulvar area in women.[44] The stratified squamous epithelium of the anus withstands invasion, but the columnar epithelium of the rectum becomes inflamed and friable. Mucopurulent or bloody discharge may occur, but many patients remain asymptomatic.

Gonococcal proctitis or pharyngitis in homosexual men frequently accompanies symptomatic urethritis. In any patient with gonococcal urethritis, a tactful inquiry into sexual preference and behavior should be a part of the initial history, in order to enable the practitioner to determine exactly what diagnostic measures to take.

Pharyngitis

Gonococcal pharyngitis is a disease of women and homosexual men who practice fellatio. Most carriers are asymptomatic, but pharyngitis, tonsillitis, and gingivitis have been ascribed to the gonococcus. Among patients with gonorrhea in other sites, about 20% of homosexual men and 10% of heterosexual women harbor gonococci in the pharynx. Gonococci disseminate in the blood more frequently from the pharynx than from other sites.

Disseminated Gonococcal Infection

Disseminated gonococcal infection (DGI) is occasionally a concomitant of urethral or cervical gonorrhea, but more often it occurs unaccompanied by genital infections.[45] The diagnosis and the treatment of DGI is well-delineated in other sources.[46]

Conjunctivitis

Conjunctivitis in neonates is most often caused by the gonococcus but also by *Chlamydia*, staphylococci, *Haemophilus*, or *Moraxella*. Neonatal gonorrheal ophthalmia appears 3 to 7 days postpartum, usually as a bilateral, profuse, and purulent conjunctivitis. Adult gonococcal conjunctivitis is caused by autoinoculation, sexual activity, or laboratory accidents.

ANTIBIOTIC-RESISTANT GONOCOCCI

In 1975 the first cases of beta-lactamase-producing *N. gonorrhoeae* were noted in the Philippines,[47] followed soon thereafter by occurrence in England,[48] and the United States.[49] The mechanism by which the gonococcus had become absolutely resistant to penicillin was by the incorporation of a cytoplasmic packet of DNA called a plasmid, or R factor, which coded for the production of TEM beta-lactamase.[50] This enzyme opens the beta-lactam ring and renders penicillin inactive. The strains that produce beta-lactamase have in the intervening ten years become the majority in the Philippines,[51] and have reached an incidence of from 30 to 50% in many other parts of the Far East. In Europe and the United States the strains have not become a significant problem, but they have established endemic foci in London,[36] Rotterdam,[52] Los Angeles,[53] New York, Miami, and Seattle.[54]

More recently gonococci from Korea and the Philippines have been isolated which both produce beta-lactamase and are resistant to spectinomycin.[35] A recent report from North Carolina[55] notes an outbreak of penicillin-resistant gonorrhea which is not caused by beta-lactamase-producing isolates. These developments necessitate a hard look at traditional therapies for gonorrhea, especially in areas where there is likelihood of importation of gonococci from areas with large numbers of resistant organisms.[56]

Except for antibiotic sensitivities, PPNG strains are not different from sensitive gonococci. An evaluation of several hundred men with gonococcal urethritis caused by either PPNG or sensitive strains from southeast Asia showed no difference in incubation period, symptomatology, or complications between the two groups.[9]

The diagnosis of PPNG is also accomplished in a similar manner as with sensitive strains. The single caveat is that if an individual has had sexual exposure in an area known to have a high incidence of PPNG (e.g., the Far East or West Africa), or has been exposed to prostitutes in any of the metropolitan areas mentioned above, a test for beta-lactamase production or for antibiotic sensitivities should be ordered along with the initial culture. In addition, if such strains are suspected, spectinomycin is the treatment of choice.

Until the occurrence of spectinomycin-resistant PPNG in Korea,[35] spectinomycin HCl in a single intramuscular dose of 2 grams was the recommended therapy for PPNG. Although the number of cases of multiply resistant gonorrhea is still small, the availability of alternate regimens for use in these cases should be recognized. Table 4-2 lists regimens which have been proven effective and which are available in the United States.

The most experience has been with cefoxitin in a single dose of 2 grams intramuscularly. In our hands this regimen has a 99% cure rate, which prompted an evaluation of a 1-gram dose.[57] This was also highly effective, and its use would ameliorate both the cost of the drug and some of the pain on injection. Cefotaxime,[58] cefaclor,[59] cefonicid,[60] ceftizoxime,[61] and sulfamethoxazole/trimethoprim[62] are also very effective. The cephalosporin that is even more effective is ceftriaxone.[63] This drug can be given in as small a dose as 250 mg with excellent results, and has recently been approved by the Federal Drug Administration.

COMPLICATED PENICILLINASE-PRODUCING *NEISSERIA GONORRHOEAE* INFECTIONS

Although most infectious caused by resistant strains of gonococci have been uncomplicated urethritis or endocervicitis,

Table 4-3. Complicated Penicillinase-Producing *Neisseria gonorrhoeae* **Infections Seen at the Naval Hospital, San Diego, California 1978–1982**

Disseminated gonococcal infection

Gonococcal bacteremia

Pelvic inflammatory disease

Adult conjunctivitis

Bartholin gland abscess

Penile abscess

Epididymoorchitis

Acute monoarticular arthritis

Proctitis

Pharyngitis

there are increasing reports of the occurrence of complicated infections. Table 4-3 lists various complications that have been seen at the United States Naval Hospital in San Diego, California. Most of these infections have been treated with cefoxitin, either as a single 2-gram intramuscular dose, or given intravenously. Disseminated gonococcal infection or bacteremia has been cured using intravenous cefoxitin given at either a 1-gram or 2-gram dose four times daily. Pelvic inflammatory disease has responded well to intravenous cefoxitin, 1 gram 4 times daily, or to spectinomycin, 2 grams intramuscularly twice daily for 5 to 7 days.[9] Because of the possibility of spectinomycin resistance, this latter regimen probably should no longer be used.

Gonococcal conjunctivitis in adults has responded well to cefoxitin,[64] cefaclor, or ceftriaxone. Abscesses and proctitis have been treated successfully with cefoxitin, but PPNG pharyngitis should be treated with either trimethoprim/sulfamethoxazole for 5 days,[32] or with ceftriaxone.

PREVENTION

The major preventive measure which can be taken to reduce the occurrence of gonococcal urethritis is monogamy or at least limitation of sexual contacts. Although such recommendations are generally not well re-

ceived by most patients, the recent upsurge in herpes genitalis and the occurrence of the acquired immunodeficiency syndrome (AIDS) have caused many people to reconsider the advantages of monogamy.

Gonorrhea can also be prevented by the regular use of condoms, prophylactic or postcontact antibiotics, or the intravaginal application of various chemicals, antiseptics, or antibiotics. While there are no epidemiologic drawbacks to the use of condoms, Hooper and associates[5] noted that in a large group of sexually active men with access to free condoms, fewer than 10% availed themselves of the protection. The use of prophylactic antibiotics selects for resistant strains of gonococci,[65] and so is self-defeating if employed for any length of time in a large population.[66] The impact of intravaginal agents is largely unknown.[67]

Immunization against gonorrhea is an attractive measure that is being aggressively pursued in several areas.[68] Wide use of even a partially effective vaccine could be helpful in reducing the incidence of gonorrhea, if the technical problems in producing and field-testing such a vaccine can be overcome.

CONCLUSION

Despite early optimism that the widespread use of penicillin would rapidly eradicate gonorrhea, the epidemic rise in incidence in the United States during the 1960s and early 1970s showed that such was not to be the case. Although with intensive contact-tracing and improved strategies for control, numbers of cases have not continued to increase during the 1980s, neither have they declined. The occurrence of strains of gonorrhea resistant to penicillin, tetracycline, and spectinomycin suggest that the treatment of gonococcal urethritis will not only become more complicated but may also be more expensive. Even if a vaccine is developed that provides permanent immunity against the gonococcus, events in England and Scandinavia suggest that as the gonococcus is eliminated from its niche, *Chlamydia*-caused nongonococcal urethritis may move to fill the void. Perhaps monogamy is the simplest solution.

REFERENCES

1. Centers for Disease Control: Sexually transmitted disease statistical letter. U. S. Department of Health and Human Services, Atlanta, Georgia 30333
2. Neisser A: Zentralbl Med Wiss 17:497, 1879
3. Gilbaugh JH, Fuchs PC: The gonococcus and the toilet seat. N Engl J Med 301:91, 1979
4. Elmros T, Larrsen PA: Survival of gonococci outside the body. Br Med J ii:403, 1972
5. Hooper RR, Wiesner PJ, Harrison WO, et al: Cohort study of venereal diseases: I. Risk of transmission from infected women to men. Am J Epidemiol 107:235, 1978
6. Soendjojo A: Gonococcal urethritis due to fellatio. Sex Transm Dis 10:41, 1983
7. Frazier JJ, Miller, J, Pickering LK: Orbital cellulitis due to Neisseria gonorrhoeae in an enucleated socket. Arch Ophthalmol 7:2345, 1979
8. Pareek SS: Gonococcal otitis externa. N Engl J Med 300:1490, 1979
9. Harrison WO: Unpublished data
10. Rothenberg R, Judson FN: The clinical diagnosis of urethral discharge. Sex Transm Dis 10:24, 1983
11. Handsfield HH, Lipman TO, Harnisch JP, et al: Asymptomatic gonorrhea in men. N Engl J Med 290:117, 1974
12. Harrison WO, Hooper RR, Weisner PJ, et al: Prevention of gonorrhea: Evaluation of prophylactic antibiotics. Proceedings of the 13th Interscience Conference on Antimicrobial Agents and Chemotherapy. Abstract #64. American Society of Microbiology, Washington, DC, 1973
13. Crawford G, Knapp JS, Hale J, et al: Asymptomatic gonorrhea in men. Science 196:1352, 1937
14. John J, Donald WH: Asymptomatic urethral gonorrhea in men. Br J Vener Dis 54:322, 1978
15. Portnoy J, Mendelson J, Clecner B, et al: Asymptomatic gonorrhea in the male. CMA J 110:169, 1974
16. McCormick WM, Stumacher RJ, Johnson D, Donner D: Clinical spectrum of gonococcal infection in women. Lancet 1:1182, 1977
17. McCutchan JA: Gonorrhea and nongonococcal urethritis. In Braude AI (ed): Medical Microbiology and Infectious Diseases. Saunders, Philadelphia, 1981
18. Miller MA, Millikin P, Griffin PS, et al: Neisseria meningitidis urethritis: A case report. JAMA 242:1656, 1979
19. Kellogg DS, Holmes KK, Hill GA: Cumitech 4: Laboratory Diagnosis of Gonorrhea. American Society of Microbiology, Washington DC, 1976
20. Brooks ST, Thompson SE, Biddle JW, et al: Treatment of uncomplicated gonococcal infection with trimethoprim-sulfamethoxazole. Sex Transm Dis 9:9, 1982
21. Morton RS: The gonococcus. In Morton RS: Gonorrhea. p 25. Saunders, London, 1977
22. Moore G, Pittard WB III, Mosca N, et al: Gonorrhea detection by urine sediment culture. JAMA 224:1499, 1973
23. Judson FN: Gonococcal urethritis—Diagnosis and Treatment. Arch Androl 3:329, 1979
24. James-Holmquest AN, Wende RD, Mudd RL, et al: Comparison of atmospheric conditions for culture of clinical specimens of Neisseria gonorrhoeae. Appl Microbiol 26:466, 1973
25. Thayer JD, Martin JE: Improved medium selective for cultivation of Neisseria gonorrhoeae and Neisseria meningitidis. Public Health Rep 81:559, 1966
26. Granato PA, Schneible-Smith C, Weiner LB: Use of New York medium for improved recovery of N. gonorrhoeae from clinical specimens. J Clin Microbiol 13:317, 1979
27. Riccardi NB, Felman YM: Laboratory diagnosis in the problem of suspected gonococcal infection. JAMA 242:2703, 1979
28. Kampmeier RH: Introduction of sulfonamide therapy for gonorrhea. Sex Transm Dis 10:81, 1983
29. Dees JE, Colston JAC: The use of sulfonilamide in gonococcic infections. JAMA 108:1855, 1937

30. Campbell DJ: Gonorrhea in North Africa and the central Mediterranean. Br Med J 2:44, 1944

31. Halverson CW, Keys TF, Clarke EJ Jr: In vitro susceptibility of Neisseria gonorrhoeae to different antibiotics. Milit Med 134:1427, 1969

32. Centers for Disease Control: Sexually transmitted diseases, treatment guidelines 1982. MMWR 31:35S, 1982

33. Kvale PA, Keys TF, Johnson DW, et al: Single oral dose ampicillin-probenecid treatment of gonorrhea in the male. JAMA 215:1449, 1971

34. Willcox RR: Amoxycillin in the treatment of gonorrhea. Br J Vener Dis 48:504, 1972

35. Centers for Disease Control: Sexually transmitted diseases, treatment guidelines 1982. MMWR 31:35S–60S, 1982

36. McCutchan JA, Adler MW, Berrier JRH: Penicillinase-producing Neisseria gonorrhoeae in Great Britain, 1977–1981. Br Med J 285:337, 1982

37. Austin TW, Brooks GF, Bethel M, et al: Trimethoprim-sulfamethoxazole in the treatment of gonococcal urethritis. J Infect Dis (Suppl) 128:S666, 1973

38. Brown ST, Thompson SE, Biddle JW, et al: Treatment of uncomplicated gonococcal infection with trimethoprim-sulfamethoxazole. Sex Transm Dis 9:9, 1982

39. Greenberg SH: Male reproductive tract sequelae of gonococcal and nongonococcal urethritis. Arch Androl 3:317, 1979

40. Engelbercht HE, Movson IJ, Van den Bulcke C: Urethral stricture in males. S Afr J Radiol 5:28, 1967

41. Watson RA: Gonorrhea and acute epididymitis. Milit Med 144:784, 1979

42. Katsman L: Gonorrheal abscess of the penis. Vestnik Derm I Ven (Moscow) 5:64, 1980

43. Kleibl K: Primary gonococcal abscess on the raphe perinei. Cz Derm 54:9, 1979

44. Klein EJ, Fisher LS, Chow AW, Guze LB: Anorectal gonococcal infection. Ann Inter Med 86:340, 1977

45. Holmes KK, Wiesner PJ, Pederson AHB: The gonococcal arthritis dermatitis syndrome. Ann Intern Med 75:470, 1971

46. Holmes KK, Counts GW, Beaty HN: Disseminated gonococcal infection Ann Intern Med 74:979, 1971

47. Splinter RJ: Personal communication.

48. Phillips I: Beta-lactamase-producing, penicillin-resistant gonococcus. Lancet 2:656, 1976

49. Ashford WA, Golash RG, Hemming VG: Penicillinase-producing Neisseria gonorrhoeae. Lancet 2:657, 1976

50. Sparling PF: Treatment of gonorrhea: What effect will antibiotic resistance have in the future? Sex Transm Dis 6:120, 1979

51. Basaca-Sevilla V, Riel RS, Sevilla JS, et al: The prevalence of Neisseria gonorrhoeae and penicillinase-producing N. gonorrhoeae in the Philippines. Phil J Microbiol Infect Dis 9:45, 1980

52. van Klingeren B, van Wijngaarden LJ, Dessens-Kroon M, et al: Penicillinase-producing gonococci in the Netherlands in 1981. J Antimicrob Chemother 11:15, 1983

53. Centers for Disease Control: Penicillin-resistant gonorrhea—North Carolina. MMWR 32:273, 1983

54. Centers for Disease Control: Global Distribution of the penicillinase producing Neisseria gonorrhoeae (PPNG). MMWR 31:1, 1982

55. Centers for Disease Control: Penicillin-resistant gonorrhea—North Carolina. MMWR 32:273, 1983

56. Berg SW, Harrison WO: Spectinomycin as primary treatment of gonorrhea in areas of high prevalence of penicillinase-producing Neisseria gonorrhoeae. Sex Transm Dis 8:38, 1981

57. Berg SW, Kilpatrick ME, Harrison WO, et al: Cefoxitin as single-dose treatment for urethritis caused by penicillinase-producing Neisseria gonorrhoeae. N Engl J Med 301:509, 1979

58. Lancaster DJ, Berg SW, Harrison WO, et al: Treatment of penicillin-resistant gonorrhea with cefotaxime. Drug Therapy (Suppl) p 87 1981

59. Harrison WO: Cefaclor in the treatment of uncomplicated gonococcal urethritis. Postgrad Med J 55:85, 1979

60. Sanchez PL, Wignall FS, Berg SW, Harrison WO: Two new cephalosporins, cefonicid and FK 749, are effective in the treatment of uncomplicated urethritis due to penicillinase-producing Neisseria gonorrhoeae (PPNG). Proceedings of the 21st In-

terscience Conference on Antimicrobiol Agents and Chemotherapy, 1981

61. Harrison WO, Sanchez PL, Lancaster DJ, et al: Ceftizoxime (FK 749) is effective therapy for urethritis caused by penicillinase-producing Neisseria gonorrhoeae. Sex Transm Dis 11:54, 1984
62. Harrison WO, Hooper RR, Kilpatrick ME, et al: Penicillin-resistant gonorrhea: Alternative therapy. Cur Chemother 1:194, 1978
63. Handsfield HH, Murphy VL, Holmes KK: Dose-ranging study of ceftriaxone for uncomplicated gonorrhea in men. Antimicrob Agents Chemother 20:839, 1981
64. Berg SW, Harrison WO, Baeza CR, et al: Gonoccoccal eye infections in adults—California, Texas, Germany. MMWR 28:341, 1981
65. Harrison WO, Hooper RR, Wiesner PJ, et al: A trial of minocycline given after exposure to prevent gonorrhea. N Engl J Med 300:1074, 1979
66. Babione RW, Hedgecock LE, Ray JP: Navy experience with oral use of penicillin as a prophylaxis. US Armed Forces J 3:973, 1952
67. Cates W Jr, Weisner PJ, Curran JW: Sex and spermicides: Preventing unintended pregnancy and infection. JAMA 148:1636, 1982
68. Marx JL: Vaccinating with bacterial pili. Science 209:1103, 1980

5

Nongonococcal Urethritis

William R. Bowie

Nongonococcal urethritis (NGU) is the most frequent cause of urethritis in heterosexual men, and accounts for a considerable, but smaller proportion of urethritis in homosexual and bisexual men. Although initial management is usually straightforward and physical sequelae are unusual, NGU that does not respond to initial treatment may result in considerable patient and physician frustration. Urethritis has numerous causes. The best-known cause of urethritis is *Neisseria gonorrhoeae*, but, by definition, diagnosis of NGU requires the presence of urethritis and the exclusion of *N. gonorrhoeae* urethral infection. Of the numerous causes of NGU, *Chlamydia trachomatis* and *Ureaplasma urealyticum* are the most frequent and the most important. *C. trachomatis* may be present without symptoms and signs, but, like *N. gonorrhoeae*, it is always considered to be a pathogen requiring treatment. In contrast, *U. urealyticum* is usually not associated with urethritis, but causes urethritis occasionally. Thus its presence, even in a man with urethritis, does not necessarily mean that it is contributing to the urethritis. When NGU arises after treatment of gonococcal urethritis, it is called postgonococcal urethritis (PGU).

Although the syndrome of urethritis occurs in both men and women, NGU is usually only diagnosed in men. When urethritis not due to cystitis arises in women, it is called the urethral syndrome. *C. trachomatis* has been shown to be a major cause of the acute urethral syndrome when pyuria is present concurrently.

EPIDEMIOLOGY

Accurate data on the overall incidence of NGU are very hard to obtain, and, with the possible exception of England and Wales, are greatly compromised by lack of standard diagnostic criteria, and the fact that NGU is not usually reportable. In England and Wales, gonorrhea and NGU have been reportable since 1951, and the number of reported cases of both diseases has risen markedly.[1] Gonorrhea was more frequent until the mid-1960s, but since then NGU has been more frequent, so that over two thirds of reported urethritis in England and Wales is nongonococcal. Although the incidence of gonococcal infections has remained stable since 1972, the incidence of NGU is still rising, although at a slower rate. In the United States it took longer for the reported rate of gonorrhea to stabilize. It is not certain what is happening to the rate of NGU. It is very likely that well in excess of 50% of urethritis is nongonococcal.[2] That generalization has significant implications for overall health care delivery, but has less meaning to individual clinics and physicians because the relative importance of NGU is highly dependent upon the sexual preference and clientele. When the population served is primarily homosexual, or inner city, gonococcal urethritis predominates. In contrast, when primarily heterosexual populations are seen, especially in Student Health Services or private practice, then up to 80–90% of urethritis can be nongonococcal.[1] There are no adequate data on the prevalence of chlamydial or ureaplasma-associated urethritis. It would be a reasonable guess that the incidence of chlamydial urethritis has risen in parallel with the total rise of NGU, since rates of isolation of *C. trachomatis* from men with NGU have been quite stable since the 1960s, when specific chlamydial diagnosis became possible.

Although NGU can arise in a male in a totally monogamous relationship, it is unusual. In most cases, the male or his partner(s) has had one or more new partners in the preceding months. The most frequent incubation period is 2 to 3 weeks, with a range of 1 to 5 weeks. However, it is often difficult to accurately determine the incubation period. Possible explanations for this dilemma include the high frequency of asymptomatic disease, a tendency for symptoms to be missed or ignored, the difficulty in knowing whether a sex partner has had other recent partners, and the probability that the numerous causes of urethritis have different incubation periods. Early studies performed in sexually transmitted disease (STD) clinics indicated that, in contrast to men with gonorrhea, men with NGU were more likely to be Caucasian, better educated, older at the time of first sexual intercourse, and to have had NGU rather than gonorrhea in the past.[3] However, all sexually active groups are at risk for acquiring NGU. The risk factors in general parallel those of gonorrhea. Indeed, the age distribution is almost identical, with the largest number of cases in men aged 20 to 24, and the next highest rates in men aged 15 to 19, and then in those aged 25 to 29.

ETIOLOGY

The major causes of NGU are *C. trachomatis* and *U. urealyticum* (Table 5-1). However, discussion of etiology should be further characterized according to the particular situation being considered. Sexual preference also makes a difference, albeit a smaller one. Thus when a man has not recently received treatment for urethritis (with the exception of single-dose treatment for gonorrhea), and the episode is the first, or arises many months to years after the last, episode, then *C. trachomatis* and/or *U. urealyticum* are recovered in 70 to 80%.[4] Under treatment with tetracyclines or erythromycin, symptoms almost always improve. In the small proportion of men in whom urethritis is still present at the end of treatment, *C. trachomatis* is no longer a problem, but *U. urealyticum* becomes relatively very important. In the more usual unfavorable outcome, when NGU recurs weeks or months later, *C. trachomatis* is still not very important. *U. urealyticum* is a cause in some cases, but in 70 to 80% of cases, neither organism appears to be the cause.

Research studies to evaluate the etiology must be carefully designed and performed. In general, studies require thorough evaluation for at least known causes, using optimal examination procedures, specimen collecting and transport, and laboratory processing. Choice of a control group or groups is critical because there are always organisms in the meatus and urethra, and because culture or serologic evidence of acquisition of many genital organisms is highly correlated with the total number of sex partners, and history of past or present STD. Studies may be further complicated because of inadequate diagnostic tests,

Table 5-1. Etiology of Sexually Transmitted Nongonococcal Urethritis (NGU)

Agent	Acute (%)	Persistent (%)	Recurrent (%)
Chlamydia trachomatis	30–50	0	0–5
Ureaplasma urealyticum	30–40	40–50	10–20
Trichomonas vaginalis	1–2	5–10	1–2
Herpes simplex virus	1–2	10–20	0
Anaerobic gram-negative rod	?	?	?
Unknown	20–30	30–45	80–90

Acute NGU = NGU of less than one month's duration, without prior treatment for that episode.

Persistent NGU = NGU that persists unchanged or only minimally improved at the end of 1 week of a tetracycline or erythromycin.

Recurrent NGU = NGU that recurs within 6 weeks of starting treatment, without intercourse with a new or untreated partner.

even when the organism is known (e.g., diagnosis of *Trichomonas vaginalis* infection in men).

Chlamydia trachomatis

Although it is possible that symptomatic *C. trachomatis* infection sometimes arises after reactivation by some other process or infection, the evidence that *C. trachomatis* is a primary cause of urethritis is convincing.[5] The evidence includes isolation data, development of humoral antibody, development of blood lymphocyte transformation, development of postgonococcal urethritis, production of urethritis in primates, selective antimicrobial treatment studies, and rates of detection of *C. trachomatis* in partners. *C. trachomatis* is recovered from the urethra of 25 to 60% (usually 30–40%) of heterosexual men with untreated NGU, and in some studies a lower proportion of homosexual men with NGU. Among heterosexual men with urethral gonorrhea, 4 to 35% (usually 15–25%) have urethral *C. trachomatis*. In homosexual men with gonorrhea 4 to 5% have urethral *C. trachomatis*, but another 5 to 6% have rectal *C. trachomatis* infection.[6] In contrast to the rates in symptomatic men, *C. trachomatis* is recovered from 0 to 7% of asymptomatic men

in STD clinics. If, in addition, pyuria is excluded, the rate of isolation is only 0 to 3%. Chlamydial infections are characterized by a tendency to long-term persistence, and manifestations are often subtle and certainly are usually less dramatic than with gonorrhea. Consequently, the possibility of high rates of asymptomatic infection was a distinct consideration. This has, in fact, turned out to be true. In a recent study *C. trachomatis* was isolated from the urethra of 11 of 97 asymptomatic United States military personnel.[7] Only 2 of the men had *N. gonorrhoeae* infection, and 1 of them was also infected with *C. trachomatis*. None of the men had symptoms of urethritis or a detectable discharge on reexamination 3 to 6 weeks after culture results were obtained. Pyuria was present in 2 of 11 men with *C. trachomatis*, compared with 8 of 86 without *C. trachomatis* infection. Only a history of prior urethritis was significantly more frequent in men with *C. trachomatis* (6 of 11) than in men without *C. trachomatis* (15 of 86) ($P < 0.02$). In another study, when male contacts to women with chlamydial cervical infection were cultured, approximately 50% of the infected men were asymptomatic.[8] These latter two studies highlight the importance of asymptomatic *C. trachomatis* infection in men. By analogy with other infections, these asymptomatic or minimally symptomatic men are a major reservoir of infection in the community and undoubtedly contribute significantly to the spread of disease.

Unless an individual patient demonstrates seroconversion, a fourfold or greater rise in antibody, or the presence of IgM antibody to *C. trachomatis*, serologic data is difficult to interpret in an individual because a high proportion of sexually active men have antibody without currently detectable infection.[5] Indeed, there is a suggestion that men with antibody may be relatively (but not absolutely) protected against *C. trachomatis* infection. Nevertheless, in studies of men with NGU, men with *C. trachomatis* infection usually have more antibody to *C. trachomatis*, and in carefully selected men, a primary antibody response can be demonstrated much more often in men from whom *C. trachomatis* is isolated, compared with men from whom *C. trachomatis* is not isolated. Similarly, among men with NGU, blood lymphocyte transformation to *C. trachomatis* antigen is more frequent in men with *C. trachomatis* than in men without *C. trachomatis* identified.

Primates inoculated in the urethra with *C. trachomatis* do not develop florid disease, but do develop urethral PMN and *C. trachomatis* replication with positive cultures for up to three months. Urethral follicles have been seen.

Concurrent presence of *C. trachomatis* and *N. gonorrhoeae* provides an opportunity to prospectively assess the ability of *C. trachomatis* to cause disease. Infection with *N. gonorrhoeae* can be diagnosed much more rapidly than *C. trachomatis* infection, so that only gonorrhea would be diagnosed at the initial visit. Until recently most gonorrhea treatment regimens utilized were active against *N. gonorrhoeae*, but not against *C. trachomatis*. Thus when men were treated with single-dose penicillin or aminocyclitols, which do not normally eradicate *C. trachomatis*, men with *C. trachomatis* would usually develop postgon-ococcal urethritis within 1 to 3 weeks after treatment of the gonorrhea. In contrast, among those treated with tetracyclines or trimethoprim-sulfamethoxazole (TMP-SMX), drugs which usually eradicate *C. trachomatis*, postgonococcal urethritis is very infrequent.[9] It can be argued that these data detract from the role of *C. trachomatis* as a primary pathogen, and indicate that *C. trachomatis* may require reactivation by some stimulus, in this case *N. gonorrhoeae*, to produce clinically apparent disease. An alternative explanation is simply that both organisms were acquired simultaneously, but *C. trachomatis* infection becomes symptomatic later because it replicates more slowly.

Treatment studies of men with NGU are also consistent with the role of *C. trachomatis* as a pathogen. The overall efficacy in treatment of NGU with antimicrobials like sulfonamides, rifampin, and multiple-dose penicillin regimens that eradicate *C. trachomatis*, but are not very active against other causes of urethritis, is poor.[24] They are usually effective at curing urethritis in men with *C. trachomatis*, but not against the urethritis in men without *C. trachomatis*. This is consistent with a role for *C. trachomatis*. Of interest, even tetracyclines, which have considerable activity against *U. urealyticum* as well, result in better response in men with *C. trachomatis* than in those without. However, in men without *C. trachomatis* results with tetracyclines are better than with the other antimicrobials.

Ureaplasma urealyticum

Unlike *C. trachomatis* and *N. gonorrhoeae*, which are considered pathogens meriting treatment whenever identified, *U. urealyticum* is frequently present in apparently normal men, and its presence is not by itself an indication for treatment. Indeed, by the time apparently normal men have had vaginal intercourse with 3 to 5 partners, over 40% are colonized with *U. urealyticum*.[10] This high prevalence in sexually active men without disease complicates assessment of its role as a urethral pathogen. Even if *U. urealyticum* was not a pathogen, isolation studies that utilize a control group with fewer sex partners could show an increased rate of isolation in men with NGU. However, if men in the control group have had many partners, the high rate of detection of *U. urealyticum* in the control group will make it hard to identify a subgroup of men who have disease. This is also a problem with the evaluation of other components of the normal flora. Thus, many of the earlier studies that did not match for sexual activity cannot be adequately evaluated. The absence of a good serologic test and the existence of numerous serotypes further complicate assessment.

Nevertheless, isolation studies, antimicrobial treatment results, serotyping data, and animal and human inoculation studies support a role for *U. urealyticum* as a urethral pathogen.[10] When men with urethritis are adequately matched with men without urethritis for number of sex partners, *U. urealyticum* has usually been isolated more often, and in higher concentrations, from men with urethritis. Furthermore, among men with NGU, rates of isolation are usually greater in men without *C. trachomatis* than in men with *C. trachomatis*, in men who have never had urethritis before compared to men with prior urethritis, and in men who have had five or fewer sex partners in their lifetimes compared to men with six or more partners. As with *C. trachomatis*, treatment data in initially *U. urealyticum*-positive men also supports its role in some studies where persistence of *U. urealyticum* correlates with increased likelihood of short-term persistence of urethritis, while eradication or suppression results in improvement. Drugs like sulfonamides, rifampin, and penicillins are not active against *U. urealyticum*, and when *U. urealyticum* persists on them, urethritis also persists. In contrast, aminocyclitols eradicate *U. urealyticum* in approximately two thirds of cases, and disease improves in those in whom it eradicates *U. urealyticum*, and does not improve when *U. urealyticum* is not eradicated. Treatment trials with tetracyclines are also interesting because some isolates are now resistant to tetracyclines. The likelihood of persistent urethritis at the end of treatment is significantly greater when tetracycline therapy fails to eradicate *U. urealyticum*. Follow-up studies 2 to 3 weeks posttreatment also support a role. Among initially *U. urealyticum*-positive men, urethritis 2 to 3 weeks posttreatment is significantly more frequent in those who have *U. urealyticum* recur than in those in whom it does not. Studies evaluating *U. urealyticum* as a cause of postgonococcal urethritis have generally revealed either no or only weak association.

The existence of at least 14 serotypes of *U. urealyticum* further complicates the assessment of its importance. It is quite possible that only one or a few serotypes are pathogenic. In one study that used a system recognizing 8 serotypes, serotype 4 was present in 52% of 122 isolates from men with NGU, compared with 24% of 125 isolates from asymptomatic men.[11] Of interest, in the asymptomatic men, some of the men with serotype 4 had asymptomatic pyuria. These results have not been duplicated by other investigators.

Inoculation of *U. urealyticum* into several nonhuman primates and two men has resulted in colonization of some animals for various periods of time, often with at least transiently increased numbers of polymorphonuclear leukocytes. Both men developed an increased number of polymorphonuclear leukocytes, and one became symptomatic with dysuria and frequency.

The role of *U. urealyticum* requires further evaluation. The author believes that *U. urealyticum* is usually not a pathogen, but that it can be. Because of its high prevalence, even if it only causes urethritis in a small proportion of men who become colonized with it, it could still cause a significant proportion of cases of NGU. Indeed, it is possible that initial contact with *U. urealyticum*, or certain serotypes of *U. urealyticum*, may result in self-limited symptomatic or asymptomatic urethritis in many men. This would be consistent with the increased rate of isolation in NGU patients who have had relatively few sex partners. Despite the inability to demonstrate humoral antibody, lower rates of isolation in men with more partners or prior urethritis may indicate some degree of effective host response.

Other Infective Causes of Urethritis

Despite use of viral cultures, aerobic and anaerobic microbiology, media that would support most fungi, and cultures for *Trichomonas vaginalis*, the etiology of cases not due to *Chlamydia trachomatis* and *U. urealyticum* is not usually elucidated. Occasionally herpes simplex virus and *T. vaginalis* are shown to be important.

T. vaginalis is definitely capable of causing urethritis in men. Despite this capacity to cause urethritis, in North America it is rarely identified in men with urethritis where urine sediment is examined for motile trichomonads or urethral swabs are cultured. Thus, it was identified in only 1 of 113 men with NGU, 0 of 69 men with gonorrhea, and 0 of 68 men without urethritis in one study,[3] from 0 to 69 men with NGU and 0 of 39 men without urethritis in another study,[12] from 0 of 82 asymptomatic men, 2 of 63 men with NGU, and 2 of 99 men with gonorrhea in a third study,[13] and 3 of 179 men in a fourth study.[14] In this last study, however, 9 (11%) of 85 men with NGU demonstrated seroconversion or increased indirect hemagglutination titers to *T. vaginalis* ($\geq$1:80) in paired sera. Thus, at least in

this last study, although the response of urethritis to metronidazole was not determined, the serologic data suggest that *T. vaginalis* may be more a frequent cause of urethritis in North America than appreciated. In marked contrast to North American and European studies, *T. vaginalis* is reported frequently from Africa, South America, India, and the USSR. These studies have not usually employed diagnostic tests for *C. trachomatis* and *U. urealyticum*, but even if they had been used, it would not explain away the presence of trichomonads. Because trichomonads persist on tetracycline or erythromycin treatment, *T. vaginalis* becomes a relatively more important cause of persistent urethritis.

Herpes simplex virus, especially in primary infection, often causes urethritis, although there is usually no problem in making a diagnosis of herpes. Among 63 men with primary herpes, dysuria was present in 44% (lasting for 2 to 20 days), urethral discharge was noted in 27%, and urethral cultures were positive in 28%.[15] Among 218 men with recurrent HSV, they were present in 9%, 4%, and 4% respectively. Because HSV is self-limited, even if external lesions were not visible, the urethritis would usually subside quickly. However, sometimes it persists and is one of the causes of persistent urethritis. Because of its tendency to recur, it can also be a cause of recurrent self-limited urethritis. The diagnosis of HSV is usually obvious.

The etiologic significance of other organisms detected in the genital tract is uncertain. The meatus and anterior urethra have their own aerobic and anaerobic bacterial flora. In general, total aerobes are similar or less in men with NGU compared to controls, and total anaerobes are usually less in men with NGU.[12,16] However, several groups have demonstrated associations between some aerobes and anaerobes and presence of NGU, and especially *C. trachomatis*-negative NGU. These organisms include *Staphylococcus saprophyticus, Co-*

rynebacterium genitalium type I, and *Haemophilus equigenitalis*. For all of these organisms, subsequent studies have not supported a role. There are no data that *G. vaginalis*, Group B streptococci, or yeasts are primary causes of urethritis, and certainly they are usually not causes even if isolated. Occasionally urethritis can be demonstrated in conjunction with balanitis in which these organisms are recovered. In occasional men with urethritis, *N. meningitidis* and various *Haemophilus* species are recovered. Since coliforms can cause cystourethritis in women, it is surprising that they are not identified in men, especially homosexual men who practice active anal intercourse. In a recent study, an anaerobic gram-negative bacillus was isolated from 50% of men with NGU, compared with 14% of men with gonococcal urethritis and 13% of men without urethritis.[17] Further information is required.

Our knowledge of the etiology of NGU progressed considerably in the 1970s, but has not advanced greatly since. It is likely that there are other infective causes of urethritis. Some cases may be due to mixed aerobic and anaerobic infection, and some may be due to a known organism whose significance has not been recognized. However, I believe that there are also presently unknown causes of urethritis and cervicitis, and also cases where the inflammatory response is not due to actual ongoing infection.

Noninfective Causes of Urethral Irritation

Although infection is the most frequent cause of urethritis, other conditions can also produce dysuria and sometimes even discharge. These include congenital abnormalities, mechanical causes, and urethral neoplasms. Congenital abnormalities include urethral valves, urethral diverticuli, and meatal stenosis. Meatal stenosis should be obvious clinically. Mechanical causes include urethral stricture, urethral foreign bodies, and self-instrumentation or introduction of chemicals into the urethra. The urethral neoplasms include benign polyps and fibroma, and malignant transitional cell or squamous cell carcinoma. Infective urethritis that is presumably not related to sexually acquired pathogens can also arise in chronically catheterized men. In this case the pathogens are usually obvious.

There are numerous other factors that have been postulated as causes of urethritis. Though individual patients may note an apparent association, there is no firm support for any of the following factors as being causes of urethritis. The factors include "too frequent" sex, "too infrequent" sex, masturbation, caffeine, alcohol, spicy food, other specific foods, and allergies.

CLINICAL DIAGNOSIS

Diagnosis of NGU requires demonstration of a urethral polymorphonuclear leukocyte response, and exclusion of *N. gonorrhoeae*. Urethritis is suggested by the history of urethral discharge, pain on urination, and itch in the meatal region, or by a history of a genital infection in a male or female partner. When urethritis is present or suspected, there are numerous features that may suggest the diagnosis of NGU rather than gonorrhea, but none will always differentiate between the causes of urethritis. There is no useful feature that differentiates between chlamydial and nonchlamydial urethritis. It is important to note that presence or absence of urethritis does not correlate entirely with the presence or absence of urethral pathogens. Stated differently, urethral infection with *C. trachomatis* and *N. gonorrhoeae* can be present without any apparent polymorphonuclear leukocyte response.

Historical Features

As mentioned earlier, the age groups affected by gonococcal and nongonococcal urethritis as seen in STD clinics are virtually identical. In a study performed in the mid-1970s, the pattern was slightly different for patients seen outside of STD clinics, where men with both gonococcal and nongonococcal urethritis tended to be slightly older, with a greater tendency toward older age in men with NGU.[18] The overlap in age was considerable, however. NGU tends to have a longer incubation period (1–5 weeks) than gonorrhea (<1 week), and symptoms with NGU are less florid and arise more gradually.[19] Consequently, men with NGU tend to delay longer after onset of symptoms before seeking medical attention.

Men with NGU are more likely to have had NGU in the past, while men with gonorrhea are more likely to have had gonorrhea in the past.[19] However, rates of past urethritis with either gonococcal or nongonococcal urethritis are significant with either presentation, and even if the previous diagnosis was correct, many men cannot remember what the previous diagnosis was. Among men with NGU, those with one or more prior episodes of urethritis, or six or more sex partners in their lifetime are less likely to have *U. urealyticum* isolated.[4] Men with two or more prior episodes of urethritis are less likely to have *C. trachomatis* isolated.

Men may be seen because of a history of genital infection in the partner, or because an infant developed a compatible syndrome. Absence of symptoms does not exclude infection in the male. A specific history of gonococcal or chlamydial infection in the partner is of some help, but because of frequent coexistence of both infections, the history is not specific. History of *T. vaginalis* infection in the partner, however, may be the only clue that *T. vaginalis* may be present.

The urethra has only a limited repertoire of symptoms: primarily discharge, dysuria, and itch. These are useful in recognizing urethritis and differ quantitatively between gonococcal and nongonococcal urethritis, but are similar qualitatively. With gonorrhea, discharge may be quite profuse, green or yellow, and noted all day long. Less obvious discharge is also frequent with gonorrhea, and is typical for NGU. In these situations, discharge is usually described as being clear or mucoid, most marked in the morning, and occasionally present only intermittently or simply noted as staining on the underclothing. Dysuria is frequent with both gonorrhea and NGU, but is more likely to be present without discharge in men with NGU. Although occasionally severe, dysuria is typically mild. The third major symptom is a sensation of an itch or an irritation in the distal urethra or meatus. As a single symptom, this is more often noted with NGU. Other symptoms of urethritis are very unusual, and indicate either other diagnoses, development of complications, or need for urologic intervention. Systemic complaints, frequency, urgency, nocturia, hematuria, scrotal swelling, inguinal lymphadenopathy, genital ulcers or rashes, and perineal pain should not be attributed to urethritis.

Examination

The pattern of medical practice often dictates that men will be examined for urethritis under suboptimal conditions. Men with symptoms suggestive of urethritis are often examined in the afternoon, without regard to when they last voided. Under these conditions, it is often difficult to demonstrate more subtle episodes of urethritis. However, it has been repeatedly demonstrated that at least 50% of men who seek medical attention because of recent onset of dysuria or urethral discharge, but who are not initially shown to have urethritis, will have evidence of increased numbers of polymorphonuclear leukocytes when reevaluated in the morning prior to voiding. In one study of 200 men who were reevaluated in this manner, 103 had NGU and 5 had gonorrhea.[20] In another study, almost 80% of such men who had *C. trachomatis* identified were shown to have significant pyuria, or else developed pyuria within weeks when reexamined under optimal conditions.[6] In contrast, pyuria was demonstrated in only one third of men without *C. trachomatis*. Thus, the need for an optimal examination cannot be overstressed. When the diagnosis is in doubt, this will require reassessment in the morning prior to voiding.

When patients are examined for the possibility of urethritis, a thorough genital examination should be performed both to detect clues to the etiology of the urethritis, and to recognize the presence of concurrent infections. The whole genital region should be examined for lesions and rashes, the inguinal lymph nodes should be palpated, the scrotal contents should be palpated, and the perianal region should be examined for lesions and discharge. In homosexual or bisexual men, anoscopy is usually indicated. The penile shaft and glans should be carefully examined to detect warts, trauma, or other lesions. The glans and meatus should be examined to detect evidence of lesions or balanitis. The urethra should be palpated throughout its accessible length to detect localized areas of tenderness suggestive of herpes, foreign bodies, or other indurated regions. Finally, to detect urethral discharge, the urethra should be milked from the base to the meatus at least 3 or 4 times if discharge is not present spontaneously.

In most men with urethritis, the only abnormalities detected will be meatal inflammation, and the presence of a urethral discharge. Presence of urethral discharge does not specifically indicate the presence of urethritis. Similarly, absence of urethral discharge does not exclude the presence of urethritis. However, in general, when there is green, yellow, or white urethral discharge, there are almost always increased numbers of polymorphonuclear leukocytes.[21] Mucoid discharge usually has increased numbers of polymorphonuclear leukocytes, but may not, especially if ejaculation has occurred recently. Clear discharge, especially after treatment, often does not have increased numbers of polymorphonuclear leukocytes.

DIFFERENTIAL DIAGNOSIS

As discussed earlier, numerous features are quantitatively, but not qualitatively, different between groups of men with gonococcal urethritis compared to nongonococcal urethritis. However, the ultimate distinction requires laboratory evaluation. Among men with NGU there are neither quantitative nor qualitative differences between men with and without *C. trachomatis* infection, so that this distinction requires laboratory evaluation as well. However, unusual causes of urethritis and other syndromes may be strongly suspected on clinical grounds.

In the absence of external genital lesions, herpes should be suspected when dysuria is marked, inguinal lymphadenopathy is present, there are systemic symptoms, or there is point tenderness on palpation of the urethra. The possibility of urethritis concurrent with balanitis should be considered if balanitis is present, or if the partner is known to have vaginal candidiasis or *Gardnerella vaginalis* infection and the male has symptoms of irritation or erythema of the glans or distal shaft. Urethritis is often present concurrently with epididymitis, but presence of scrotal swelling especially of recent onset, and scrotal or inguinal pain in association with evidence of epididymal inflammation on examination should prompt management for epididymitis. Urethral discharge can occur with prostatitis. In this circumstance, there is often a history of discharge with hard bowel movements. Other symptoms can include vague inguinal, scrotal, or perineal discomfort, myalgias, altered frequency or force of voiding, and chills and fever. Occasionally men with urethritis will complain of vague discomfort in the genital area, and no other cause is found. Frequency, nocturia, and hematuria with or without fever suggest the possibility of cystitis. Gross hematuria alone can be due to both benign and severe problems, and should prompt rapid urologic evaluation. The possibility of Reiter's syndrome, or reactive arthritis, should be considered when conjunctivitis, arthralgias or arthritis, balanitis, or skin rash especially involving the palms and soles occur with urethritis. A history of recent diarrhea would also be consistent with the diagnosis of Reiter's syndrome or reactive arthritis.

Mechanical or structural abnormalities should be considered when problems arise at a young age, when foreign bodies like catheters have been in place, if there is a history of trauma, if self-instrumentation or installation of chemicals has occurred, with hematuria, or when urethritis persists unresponsive to reasonable treatment regimens.

LABORATORY DIAGNOSIS

Laboratory diagnosis of NGU requires identification of urethritis (an increased number of polymorphonuclear leukocytes in urethral material), and exclusion of *Neisseria gonorrhoeae*. Specific additional studies can also be performed to establish the presence or absence or other organisms that could cause or contribute to the urethritis. Similar diagnostic tests can be utilized to detect organisms when urethritis is absent.

Demonstration of Increased Numbers of Polymorphonuclear Leukocytes

The most convenient specimens are urethral smears obtained from meatal exudate or endourethral swabs, and the first voided urine. For both specimens, the patient should be examined after as long an interval without voiding as possible. If the diagnosis is in doubt, overnight is best, but an interval of four or more hours is a reasonable compromise that most men find acceptable. In most situations only the smear is required.

For Gram stain, a swab of exudate is adequate if present, but an endourethral swab inserted 3–4 cm into the urethra is required if discharge is minimal or absent. The swab is then rolled gently back and forth over the slide to cover an area approximately 1 cm.^{2} The slide is then Gram-stained or stained with methylene blue. It is then scanned at a magnification of $\times 100$ and then areas that have the largest numbers of polymorphonuclear leukocytes are examined under oil ($\times 1000$). The number of polymorphonuclear leukocytes in each of five fields is then recorded. The presence of a mean of more than four polymorphonuclear leukocytes per field appears to provide the best correlation with urethritis.[16,21] While enumerating the number of polymorphonuclear leukocytes, the slide should also be examined for gram-negative diplococci by Gram stain, or diplococci by methylene blue stain.

To detect polymorphonuclear leukocytes in urine sediment, the first 10–15 ml of voided urine should be collected.[21] This is then centrifuged at 400 $\times$ G for 5 to 10 minutes, all but 0.5 ml of the supernatant is discarded, and the sediment is resuspended in the residual urine. Sufficient sediment is placed on the slide to cover approximately 1 cm^2 and then a coverslip is placed over it. The number of polymorphonuclear leukocytes in each of 5 $\times$ 400 power fields is counted. The presence of 15 or more polymorphonuclear leukocytes in one or more of the five fields appears to be the best cutoff between normal and abnormal, and correlates well with the number of polymorphonuclear leukocytes in urethral smears.

Although the number of polymorphonuclear leukocytes in smear or urine correlate well, results are most likely to differ when urethritis is mild or minimal. Under these circumstances, only one test may be abnormal, and on consecutive dates it may not always be the same test. A much greater concern, however, is that men with proven gonococcal or chlamydial urethral infection may not have any polymorphonuclear leukocyte response, and analysis of the number of urethral polymorphonuclear leukocytes will always lack both sensitivity and specificity if used as an indication of infection with a specific organism.

Detection of *Neisseria gonorrhoeae*

Smears of urethral exudate or material obtained with an endourethral swab provide the most rapid and least expensive test to detect *N. gonorrhoeae*. For experienced microscopists evaluating specimens from STD clinic populations, the sensitivity and specificity of detection of typical gram-negative intracellular diplococci as indicating gonorrhea, and the presence of increased numbers of polymorphonuclear leukocytes without any evidence of typical or atypical gram-negative diplococci as indicating NGU, are close to 100%.[19] In populations with a lower prevalence of gonorrhea, the predictive value of positive Gram stains are lower. The predictive value of a negative Gram stain for exclusion of *N. gonorrhoeae* remains high, however.

Until penicillinase-producing strains of *N. gonorrhoeae* became more prevalent, culture conformation of gonococcal infection was not necessary when Gram stains were unequivocal. However, penicillinase-producing *N. gonorrhoeae* are becoming more prevalent, and some isolates as well are relatively resistant to penicillin, so that, when feasible, cultures should be obtained from all men with urethritis. The same specimen as is used for Gram stain is adequate. Cultures should definitely be obtained when the Gram stain is interpreted as being equiv-

ocal, when the person reading the Gram stain is not experienced, for test of cure, for treatment failures, and when penicillinase-producing *N. gonorrhoeae* infection is suspected on epidemiologic grounds.

Numerous media and transport systems are available for culture of *N. gonorrhoeae*. Cultures are often performed on selective media incorporating vancomycin. Since vancomycin-sensitive isolates are frequent in some regions, and overgrowth is not usually a problem with male urethritis specimens, use of nonselective media may be preferable in men. If transport media are utilized, the specimens should be inoculated onto growth media as soon as possible. With delays of 12 to 24 hours or greater, a negative culture does not exclude the presence of gonorrhea. Once inoculated, cultures are incubated at 36°C in increased carbon dioxide tension. Most isolates can be identified in 1 to 3 days. Oxidase-positive colonies are identified as *N. gonorrhoeae* by fluorescent antibody or by sugar fermentation. Isolates should be tested for beta-lactamase production.

Nonculture techniques to detect *N. gonorrhoeae* infection are presently being evaluated. These are especially useful in situations where transport of specimens may be suboptimal or culture facilities are not available. Use of the limulus lysate assay to detect lipopolysaccharide in urethral secretions correlates well with the presence of the organism. Tests to detect other gonococcal products, presence of oxidase, and presence of plasmid DNA require further evaluation.

Detection of *Chlamydia trachomatis*

Until very recently, specific diagnosis of *C. trachomatis* infection usually required isolation and cell culture. Because of a high prevalence of antibody to *C. trachomatis* in the population, and especially in sexually transmitted diseases clinic populations, serology is rarely diagnostic. The major exception is in men with their first episode of urethritis, who have the acute sera obtained within 10 days of onset of symptoms. The appropriate specimen for culture is endourethral material rather than urethral exudate because *C. trachomatis* is an intracellular parasite of columnar epithelial cells rather than polymorphonuclear leukocytes. The yield on culture of exudate is much lower than the yield from endourethral specimens. The endourethral swab should be inserted 3 or 4 cm into the urethra and then placed into specific chlamydial transport media. Special calcium alginate swabs on flexible aluminum shafts are generally used to obtain cultures, because in most studies they provide an adequate sample and are the least toxic to chlamydiae. The specimen should be transported to the laboratory as quickly as possible and then immediately inoculated onto cell culture, or else frozen at −70°C. The shorter the delay prior to freezing or culturing the better. With delays beyond 24 hours, the yield drops markedly. Depending upon the methodology utilized, preliminary results from cultures are often available within 1 to 3 days after inoculation. Availability of commercially prepared cell culture systems is a major advance because they can provide good cells and media to smaller laboratories that do not have or cannot contribute the necessary resources to make their own. High-quality antisera to detect *C. trachomatis* inclusions facilitates the recognition of *C. trachomatis* inclusions in culture, and circumvents much of the problem with false positive interpretations that many new laboratories experience with iodine stains.

The advances facilitating greater access to cultures are very beneficial. However, it is likely that nonculture tests will have a greater ability to improve management of chlamydial infection. They should facilitate diagnosis when specimen transport or culture facilities are lacking or suboptimal, and provide more rapid diagnosis. At least two new tests have been released. They appear promising, but need much more evaluation to assess their benefit both in research laboratories, and in routine laboratories. One test utilizes monoclonal antibody to detect elementary bodies in genital secretions. Preliminary data with this test are very encouraging, and for some investigators provides sensitivity as good as with cell culture. For others sensitivity is less than culture. The major problem will be specificity, especially when there are low numbers of chlamydiae. The second type of test uses immunoenzyme technology and spectrophotometers to detect chlamydial antigens. There are fewer data available on the sensitivity and specificity of this test. Results take hours with this test, rather than under a hour with the direct test using fluorescein-conjugated monoclonal antibody.

Detection of *Ureaplasma urealyticum*

Detection of *U. urealyticum* is within the realm of feasibility for most diagnostic laboratories, although its usefulness in the routine management of men with urethritis is questionable. In patients with obvious urethritis, diagnostic yield from cultures of the first voided urine is similar to that obtained with an endourethral swab, but in men with no or minimal urethritis, an endourethral swab is preferable. *U. urealyticum* is cultured in both broth and agar media. In broth, its presence is identified by a pH shift. On agar, it produces typical colonies, which can be identified directly on differential agar or by addition of a reagent making use of the urease production. Serology is not useful for diagnosis of *U. urealyticum* infection.

Because *U. urealyticum* is so often detected in apparently normal men, interpretation of a positive culture for *U. urealyticum* in an individual patient is difficult. Thus, isolation of *U. urealyticum* from a man with acute urethritis does not necessarily mean that it is causing urethritis. It is most significant when isolated at the end of a course of treatment from a male with persistent urethritis.

Detection of *Trichomonas vaginalis*

Detection of *T. vaginalis* infection in men is suboptimal. Culture, using modified Diamond's media, or other similar media is the best available technique, but its sensitivity in men has yet to be established, primarily because it is never certain how often *T. vaginalis* is missed. These cultures are not difficult to perform. Motile *T. vaginalis* can be detected in the first voided urine sediment, but the sensitivity of this procedure has yet to be established. In women, sensitivity of saline preparations for diagnosing vaginal trichomoniasis is less than the sensitivity of culture.

TREATMENT

Most individuals agree that tetracyclines are the initial antimicrobial of choice, that they should be given for a minimum of 7 days, and that sex partners of heterosexual men should be treated.[22,23] Although failure to eradicate *C. trachomatis* with this approach is very unusual, urethritis persists at the end of treatment in approximately 5% of men, and recurs in another 25–35% by 5 to 6 weeks after cessation of therapy if pyuria at follow-up is used as the determinant of failure.[4] Recommendations for follow-up (or even need for follow-up in asymptomatic men), and management of failures and their contacts are not well defined and are subject to the particular impressions of the person or group making the recommendation.

Recommendations will likely become easier to make once specific infections are treated, rather than a whole syndrome with multiple etiologies. Furthermore, as more

becomes known about the significance of individual organisms to men, women, and offspring, it will become easier to know how diligently to attempt to eradicate specific organisms. For example, it is appropriate to try to eradicate *C. trachomatis* and *T. vaginalis* from a couple, but it is usually not indicated to try to eradicate *U. urealyticum* from a woman.

There are numerous potential methodologic pitfalls with studies attempting to evaluate the optimal management of NGU.[24] Definition of cases is relatively standard, but definition of treatment failures is not. Microbiology should be used at follow-up as well as initially, because many treatment failures do not have significant pyuria, despite having positive cultures. The duration of follow-up in studies continues to be source of contention. A short follow-up period facilitates follow-up, and decreases the likelihood of resumption of sexual intercourse. Since in my experience *C. trachomatis* microbiologic failure on suboptimal regimens was frequently not detected until more than 3 weeks posttreatment, I recommend at least 6 weeks of follow-up.[24] This is more time-consuming, and increases the likelihood that patients will be reexposed, but it is a better indicator of the in vivo efficacy of antimicrobials against certain pathogens that may take weeks to become apparent. All agree that total abstinence is the best for the duration of treatment and follow-up. However, that is not always practical. If sexual intercourse is resumed with a previously exposed partner, the partner should have been treated before resumption of intercourse. Even then, if a condom is not used, or is used improperly, then the male will be reexposed to the contact's flora. A partner treated with a tetracycline or erythromycin regimen is not likely to be infected with *C. trachomatis*, but will often continue to be colonized by *U. urealyticum*. She can then reinfect the male, with the possible outcome being a recurrence of the urethritis. Presumably a similar sequence of events could occur with other unknown causes of urethritis. Finally, all treatment studies are subject to the vagaries of patient compliance with medication use.

Suspectibility of *Chlamydia trachomatis* and *Ureaplasma urealyticum* to Antimicrobials

Tetracyclines are active in vitro and in vivo against all isolates of *C. trachomatis*,[24] and approximately 90% of isolates of *U. urealyticum* are eradicated from the male urethra.[24] In about half of the cases, tetracyclines fail to eradicate *U. urealyticum* from the vagina. Erythromycins are somewhat less active than tetracyclines in vitro against *C. trachomatis*, but usually, though not always, eradicate *C. trachomatis* in vivo. Erythromycin is usually active against *U. urealyticum*, including tetracycline-resistant isolates, in men, but almost never eradicates *U. urealyticum* from the vagina.

No other groups of antimicrobials have equivalent or better activity against both organisms. Good in vivo activity of antimicrobials against *C. trachomatis* is demonstrated by sulfonamides and rifampin, while multiple-dose penicillins and clindamycin will frequently, but not always, eradicate *C. trachomatis*. With the exception of clindamycin which sometimes eradicates *U. urealyticum*, none of the other antimicrobials have any activity against *U. urealyticum*. While lacking in useful activity against *C. trachomatis*, aminocyclitols will often eradicate *U. urealyticum*. Cephalosporins, single-dose penicillins, nalidixic acid, and metronidazole are essentially inactive against both organisms.

Initial Antimicrobial Treatment for Nongonococcal Urethritis

The preferred treatment is 7 days of either tetracycline 500 mg four times daily, or doxycycline or minocycline 100 mg twice daily.[22] Although lower daily doses have shown similar results to these regimens, the number of patients studied have not been large, so that the possibility of a beta error (failure to identify a true difference) is high. Furthermore, the larger doses are better against gonococcal infections.

Data on the optimal duration of treatment are contradictory, with one investigator reporting good results with a single 300-mg dose of doxycycline. This regimen results in considerable vomiting, and the results have not been confirmed. It is not a recommended regimen. Other studies have shown that tetracycline treatment is better than treatment with a placebo, or no treatment, and that 7 days of tetracycline therapy is better than 4 days of tetracycline therapy. The major question is the benefit of prolonging initial treatment beyond 7 days. Data are conflicting, but at least in one relatively large double-blind study comparing 21-day regimens with 7-day regimens, there was no demonstrable benefit in prolonging treatment beyond 7 days.[4] Longer treatment simply delayed the time to recurrence as defined by time after treatment was initiated, but did not delay it from the time treatment ceased. Another study comparing different durations of treatment showed a better outcome with longer treatment, but did not have comparable follow-up after cessation of treatment.[25]

Tetracyclines have become the drug of choice because of their safety, and their activity against *C. trachomatis* and *U. urealyticum*. Tetracycline is sometimes poorly tolerated, with gastrointestinal upset being the major side effect. Furthermore, it should be taken four times daily on an empty stomach. Compared to tetracycline, doxycycline and minocycline are more active against *C. trachomatis* and *U. urealyticum* on a weight basis. They have long half-lives, which means that they can be taken less often, and the consequences of missing one or more doses may be less important. They need only be taken twice daily, and can be taken with food. Their major problems are expense, and predisposition to causing photosensitivity. In some studies use of minocycline has been associated with significant neurologic side effects that are occasionally incapacitating. These side effects have not been evaluated as carefully with doxycycline, but have been described.

However, as noted earlier, tetracyclines are not universally successful in the treatment of NGU. Treatment outcome is very dependent upon the initial etiology. Using tetracyclines, numerous studies have shown that men with positive cultures for *C. trachomatis* initially have had a more favorable outcome (20% persistence or recurrence of urethritis) than men in whom *C. trachomatis* was not initially identified (40% persistence or recurrence of urethritis). These failures are not due to failure to eradicate *C. trachomatis*. In some studies men with *U. urealyticum* isolated initially have done less well than men with *C. trachomatis* alone or *C. trachomatis* plus *U. urealyticum*. In one study men with neither *C. trachomatis* nor *U. urealyticum* did least well (50% persistent or recurrent urethritis).[4] About one half of the men with persistent *U. urealyticum* on tetracycline treatment have tetracycline resistant *U. urealyticum* isolates, but the microbiologic cause for most of the cases of recurrent urethritis is unexplained.

Use of Other Antimicrobials for Treatment of Acute Nongonococcal Urethritis

If for some reason only treatment of *C. trachomatis* is desired, there are several options available beside tetracyclines, but for treatment of NGU, only erythromycins are useful. They have been less well studied than tetracyclines, but erythromycin 500 mg four times daily for 7 days, or 500 mg twice daily for 10 to 14 days likely have similar efficacy as the 7-day tetracycline regimens. Occasionally men with *C. trachomatis* may not have the *C. trachomatis* eradicated, but erythromycin may be more active against *U. urealyticum* and is certainly more active against tetracycline-resistant isolates.

Erythromycin tends to be less well-tolerated than tetracyclines, although that is less of a problem in men than women. Erythromycin estolate should not be used. Erythromycin base, stearate, or ethyl succinate can all be used. Erythromycin is useful for treatment of sex partners. However, in women, erythromycin almost always fails to eradicate *U. urealyticum*.

Management of Sexual Partners

If at all possible, investigation and treatment should be arranged for all recently exposed sex partners of heterosexual men. In most cases, this will only be a steady partner, and the contact from whom the male acquired the problem. Because the physical sequelae in women can be so disastrous, this should be done as quickly as possible. Because many sexually transmitted pathogens can be present concurrently, because management of pelvic inflammatory disease is different from management of NGU contacts, and because investigation of the female may provide clues to the etiology in the male, the woman should be examined rather than just treated. The male should be asked if he is aware of symptoms in the partner. Symptoms in the woman of pain with intercourse, low abdominal pain, unusual vaginal bleeding, or pregnancy should prompt an immediate assessment.

The appropriate management of male partners of men with NGU is less well defined. *C. trachomatis* and *U. urealyticum* are less likely to be recovered from the urethra of the index case. However, at least in sexually transmitted disease clinic populations, *C. trachomatis* is recovered from the rectum in at least 5% of homosexual men, even without symptoms of proctitis. The most aggressive approach would be to examine, investigate, and treat male partners with one week of a tetracycline regimen. Pending further data, this is likely the best approach.

Additional Measures

Men should be advised not to have sexual intercourse until both the male and any previously exposed sex partners with whom he may have sexual intercourse in the future are treated. It is a hard concept for patients and physicians to comprehend that even if symptoms and signs disappear at the end of therapy, the symptoms or signs can recur in up to one third of men. This complicates the recommendations for how long to avoid sexual intercourse posttreatment. If the male is symptomatic at the end of treatment, he should be reinvestigated and sexual intercourse not resumed. If asymptomatic, and partners have taken a regimen that will eradicate *C. trachomatis*, then there is likely little long-term risk in resuming sexual intercourse. However, if urethritis recurs, it is not possible to reliably exclude reinfection from relapse. Since *C. trachomatis* is not likely to be present, this is a nuisance, but not a major risk. If a patient does not want to resume having sexual intercourse until after the period during which recurrence is likely to arise is over, then he should wait about two months.

If sexual intercourse is resumed, using condoms likely decreases the risk of reinfection. However, since organisms like *U. urealyticum* are present in large numbers, and are present at the introitus, the condom should be applied before there is any genital contact.

Patients are often told to drink lots of water, and avoid alcohol. With NGU, there is no proven scientific rationale for either approach. The only obvious danger to treatment of NGU in using alcohol in excess is the concern that medications may be forgotten, or sexual intercourse resumed prematurely. It is more important to tell patients about their infection, and to stress the importance of completing the course of therapy, than to spend the time on discussions about drinking water and avoiding alcohol.

POSTTREATMENT EVALUATIONS

In keeping with standard sexually transmitted disease management, posttreatment evaluation would normally be recommended. However, it is difficult to define the best time for evaluation and to define why follow-up of all cases is indicated. As discussed above, these uncertainties arise because the clinical improvement after treatment does not guarantee that urethritis will not recur, and recurrence of urethritis does not mean that significant known pathogens are present. In contrast, absence of symptoms or signs of urethritis does not preclude persistence of urethral pathogens.

A definite indication for follow-up is the persistence or recurrence of symptoms. Even in asymptomatic men, other reasons for follow-up 3 to 5 weeks posttreatment are an initial positive urethral culture for *C. trachomatis*, a question about the patient's compliance, or atypical features of the urethritis initially. A need for follow-up of asymptomatic men who take medications reliably and whose sex partners are appropriately treated is debatable. Although about half of the men with pyuria at follow-up are asymptomatic, the benefit of detecting and treating asymptomatic pyuria is likely marginal.

The rates of detection of potential pathogens in persistent and recurrent urethritis are summarized in Table 5-1.

Examination for Persistent or Recurrent Urethritis

For men seen at follow-up, procedures similar to those used at the initial visit should be utilized. In addition, the patient should be questioned about compliance in taking medication, and about resumption of sexual intercourse or genital contact with new or previous partners. Although the risk of transmission of pathogens is not well-defined, it is likely that intercourse with a previous, untreated partner is probably a greater risk than sexual intercourse with a new partner. If he has had intercourse with a previous partner, it should be clarified if the partner was treated, what medication was utilized, and the timing of the treatment and resumption of intercourse. He should then be carefully examined as before, again paying special attention to clues that might suggest an unusual etiology for the urethritis. Presence of symptoms does not by itself indicate that urethritis is present. An increased number of polymorphonuclear leukocytes should be documented. In men with pyuria or an initial positive diagnostic test for *C. trachomatis*, diagnostic tests should be repeated for *C. trachomatis*. Examination and culture of exudate, urethral swabs, and/or first voided urine should be performed for *T. vaginalis*. Cultures for herpes simplex virus should be performed if indicated. In unusual situations, urethral specimens should be cultured for yeasts, *Gardnerella vaginalis*, and aerobes. If the etiology is still not apparent, every attempt should be made to evaluate the sex partners.

Antimicrobial Treatment

In the absence of pyuria, retreatment is not indicated unless a culture is positive for *C. trachomatis*, *N. gonorrhoeae*, or *T. vaginalis*. Very occasionally it may be prudent to retreat a male without pyuria if he has

been repeatedly exposed to an untreated partner.

In the absence of positive tests for definite urethral pathogens (*C. trachomatis*, *N. gonorrhoeae*, and *T. vaginalis*), the benefit of treating men with asymptomatic pyuria is very uncertain. It is probably indicated to give them a second course of antimicrobial, but further treatment is not likely indicated unless a cause is found.

When men have symptomatic pyuria, if a treatable cause is found, then specific treatment should be initiated. Most often no cause is definitely proven. Management at this stage is very empirical. Because tetracycline-resistant *U. urealyticum* is a cause of persistent urethritis, and *U. urealyticum* is a probable cause of recurrent urethritis, then treatment with erythromycin 500 mg four times daily for 7 to 14 days is as reasonable as any other treatment. Unless the partner has some other indication for treatment, the author does not retreat partners at this stage. Most men improve on erythromycin, but some will have a further recurrence of urethritis. If only asymptomatic pyuria is present, in the great majority of men no further investigation or treatment is indicated. If symptomatic pyuria persists, the management becomes more difficult. Sometimes a thorough discussion of the problem, as discussed below, allays fear, but in other situations further studies are required to exclude urethral abnormalities. These are rarely abnormal, but include studies to detect prostatic infection, possibly voiding cystourethrograms to detect strictures or other abnormalities, and finally urethroscopy to detect endourethral lesions. If antimicrobial therapy is required, then some men will benefit from an empirical course of minocycline or doxycycline 100 mg once or twice daily, or tetracycline 250 mg or 500 mg four times daily for 4 to 6 weeks. If symptoms persist after this approach, and all other investigations have been negative, then it is probably better to follow the patient without further treatment than to initiate more antimicrobial therapy blindly.

COMPLICATIONS

The most frequent complications are consequences in partners, and patient or physician frustration. Physical complications to the male are fortunately unusual.

Physical Complications

Even when urethritis persists, if a patient with NGU has received a course of therapy that will eradicate *C. trachomatis*, physical problems are exceedingly unusual. Although urethral stricture was frequently described in the preantimicrobial era, it is an exceedingly infrequent complication in the 1980s. Less than 1% of men with NGU develop epididymitis in association with urethritis. *C. trachomatis* is a major cause of epididymitis in sexually active men, but epididymitis should not arise very often after treatment. Urethritis is one of the stimuli that precipitates Reiter's syndrome in immunologically susceptible men. It is not yet clear whether early treatment of nongonococcal urethritis diminishes the risk of subsequent development of Reiter's syndrome.

Consequences in Partners

Perhaps one of the major reasons for identifying urethritis in males is that it offers an opportunity to detect potential disease in female partners. Approximately 10% of women with lower genital tract infection with *C. trachomatis* will develop spread to the endometrium, fallopian tubes, or peritoneum. Such infections are frequently followed by involuntary infertility, an increased risk of ectopic pregnancy, and persistent pelvic pain. Since only one third of women who are seen with involuntary infertility and evidence of tubal obstruction give any history at all suggestive of previous pelvic inflammatory disease, it may be that the only way disease could have been prevented in these women would have been recognition of disease in the male. Women with *C. trachomatis* infection are also very likely to transmit it to infants after vaginal delivery.

A very high proportion of female contacts to men with nongonococcal urethritis have positive vaginal cultures for *U. urealyticum*. The *U. urealyticum* frequently persists after treatment as a NGU contact. This is not usually of concern to the women. However, because *U. urealyticum* is occasionally associated with recurrent spontaneous abortions in early pregnancy, and possibly involuntary infertility, it is prudent to ascertain if these have been problems for the female contact. Under these circumstances, it may be necessary to attempt to eradicate the *U. urealyticum* from the woman.

Psychological Complications

Confusion and psychological distress are frequent with NGU. This is especially the case when NGU arises when a couple have apparently had a monogamous relationship for many months or even years, and when urethritis persists despite antimicrobial therapy. It is further compounded when patients receive misinformation. Fortunately, the psychological distress can usually be reduced or even prevented by a thorough discussion of the typical concerns. The usual concerns are mistrust of the partner, fear of becoming infertile, fear of spreading sexually transmitted diseases when urethritis persists, fear of impotence, and fear of physical sequelae.

With respect to mistrust of the partner, when there has been a monogamous relationship, it is important for both the male and female to recognize that genital pathogens can persist asymptomatic for a relatively prolonged period of time before they become symptomatic. Thus, when one or both partners have had previous partners, it is always possible that one of them may have been an asymptomatic carrier. The other situation where mistrust of the partner is sometime a problem is when there are repeated recurrences. Although recurrences can be related to reexposure, most recurrences are not, and it is important that the male recognize that in most cases his partner should not be identified as the cause of the recurrences. With time it usually becomes apparent that the recurrences can occur without reexposure.

Some men are concerned that persistent urethritis will result in infertility. This is a relatively infrequent event, even if epididymitis arises. It is possible that *U. urealyticum* infection may cause involuntary infertility if the ureaplasma persists, but this needs to be studied in much more detail. Presumably, if there is an association then this type of infertility can be eradicated by appropriate antimicrobial therapy.

One of the most difficult issues to deal with is the concern that the male poses a risk to sex partners. Once a male has received a course of tetracycline followed by a course of erythromycin, it is exceedingly unusual to detect significant sexually transmitted pathogens. Even in the very unusual situation where the male's problem is due to *Trichomonas vaginalis*, or possibly *Gardnerella vaginalis* or yeasts, and the male transmits the pathogen to a female, the disease produced in the partner is a nuisance rather than a severe threat. Thus, it is very unlikely that such a male with persistent urethritis can transmit a serious infection to the partner. However, there is no way that one can tell a patient with persistent urethritis that he poses absolutely no risk to female partners.

Impotence on the basis of a physical cause is not a complication of NGU. Other long-term complications such as prostatic cancer do not appear to be a complication, although that has been less well studied. It is not clear what the relationship is between urethritis and prostatitis, but it seems most likely that prostatitis is not a complication of ongoing urethritis. The distinction may, however, be very difficult to establish.

REFERENCES

1. Wiesner PJ: Selected aspects of the epidemiology of nongonococcal urethritis. p 9. In Hobson D, Holmes KK (eds): Nongonococcal Urethritis and Related Infections. The American Society for Microbiology, Washington DC, 1977
2. Cates W Jr: Sexually transmitted diseases: The national view. Cutis 33:69, 1984
3. Holmes KK, Handsfield HH, Wang SP, et al: Etiology of nongonococcal urethritis. N Engl J Med 292:1199, 1975
4. Bowie WR, Alexander ER, Stimson JB, et al: Therapy for nongonococcal urethritis: double-blind randomized comparison of two doses and two durations of minocycline. Ann Intern Med 95:306, 1981
5. Schachter J: Chlamydial infections. N Engl J Med 298:428, 490, 540, 1978
6. Bowie WR: Unpublished data
7. Podgore JK, Holmes KK, Alexander ER: Asymptomatic urethral infections due to Chlamydia trachomatis in male U.S. military personnel. J Infect Dis 146:828, 1982
8. Thelin I, Wennstrom A-M, Mardh P-A: Contact-tracing in patients with genital chlamydial infection. Br J Vener Dis 56:259, 1980
9. Stamm WE, Guinan ME, Johnson C et al: Effect of treatment regimens for Neisseria gonorrhoeae on simultaneous infection with Chlamydia trachomatis N Engl J Med 310:545, 1984
10. Taylor-Robinson D, McCormack WM: The genital mycoplasmas. N Engl J Med 302:1003, 1063, 1980
11. Shepard MC, Lunceford CD: Serological typing of Ureaplasma urealyticum isolates from urethritis patients by an agar growth inhibition method. J Clin Microbiol 8:566, 1978

12. Bowie WR, Pollock HM, Forsyth PS, et al: Bacteriology of the urethra in normal men and men with nongonococcal urethritis. J Clin Microbiol 6:482, 1977

13. Wong JL, Hines PA, Brasher MD, et al: The etiology of nongonococcal urethritis in men attending a venereal disease clinic. Sex Transm Dis 4:4, 1977

14. Kuberski T: Trichomonas vaginalis associated with nongonococcal urethritis and prostatitis. Sex Transm Dis 7:135, 1980

15. Corey L, Adams HG, Brown ZA, Holmes KK: Genital herpes simplex virus infections: Clinical manifestations, course, and complications. Ann Intern Med 98:958, 1983

16. Swartz SL, Kraus SJ, Herrmann KL, et al: Diagnosis and etiology of nongonococcal urethritis. J Infect Dis 138:445, 1978

17. Fontaine EA, Taylor-Robinson D, Hanna NF, Coufalik ED: Anaerobes in men with urethritis. Br J Vener Dis 58:321, 1982

18. Gale JL, Hinds MW: Male urethritis in King Country, Washington, 1974–75:I. Incidence. Am J Public Health 68:20, 1978

19. Jacobs NF, Kraus SJ: Gonococcal and nongonococcal urethritis in men. Clinical and laboratory differentiation. Ann Intern Med 82:7, 1975

20. Simmons PD: Evaluation of the early morning smear investigation. Br J Vener Dis 54:128, 1978

21. Bowie WR: Comparison of Gram stain and first voided urine sediment in the diagnosis of urethritis. Sex Transm Dis 5:39, 1978

22. Centers for Disease Control: 1985 STD treatment guidelines. MMWR (4S) 34:75S, 1985

23. Jaffe HW: Nongonococcal urethritis: Treatment of men and their sexual partners. Rev Infect Dis 4:S772, 1982

24. Bowie WR: Treatment of chlamydial infections. p 231. In Mardh P-A, et al (eds): Chlamydial Infections. Elsevier Biomedical Press, Amsterdam, 1982

25. Thambar IV, Simmons PD, Thin RN, Darougar S, Yearsley P: Double-blind comparison of two regimens in the treatment of nongonococcal urethritis. Seven-day versus 21-day courses of triple tetracycline (Deteclo). Br J Vener Dis 55:284, 1979

6

Pelvic Inflammatory Disease

Yehudi M. Felman
James A. Nikitas

The rising incidence of sexually transmitted diseases, coinciding with the widespread use of the intrauterine contraceptive device, has heightened the incidence of pelvic inflammatory disease. The term pelvic inflammatory disease (PID) refers to a clinical syndrome that originates as an infection in the lower genital tract, usually the endocervix, and causes an inflammatory response in adjacent tissues, including the endometrium, endosalpinx, ovaries, perimetrial tissues, and peritoneal cavity. The morbidity produced by PID in young women is greater than that produced by all other serious infections. In the United States, PID occurs in about 850,000 women every year, requiring more than 212,000 hospital admissions and 115,000 surgical procedures.[1] The economic loss resulting from this infection is estimated to be approximately 2.7 billion dollars annually.[1] This cost includes management of patients and outpatients, including long-term sequelae such as chronic pelvic pain, ectopic pregnancy, and infertility.

Chronic pelvic pain is thought to be caused by the formation of pelvic adhesions secondary to the associated pelvic adhesions. The increased incidence of ectopic pregnancy cases, another complication of PID, reflects the increased number of cases of PID.

A major complication of PID is infertility, which has been demonstrated to increase in frequency with each subsequent bout.[2] An alteration of the tubal tissue caused by infection is thought to induce fertility. Early diagnosis and prompt treatment appear to be crucial in preventing infertility and the other long-term sequelae.

ETIOLOGY

The microbial etiology of PID in any individual patient cannot be predicted from the clinical picture alone. The syndrome is the same regardless of the organism(s) causing the disease. Usually the cause of the infection is assumed to be a potential pathogen isolated from the endocervical canal. Two sexually transmitted microorganisms that have been implicated are *Neisseria gonorrhoeae* and *Chlamydia trachomatis*. However, endocervical cultures do not reliably reveal the organism(s) that cause the pelvic infection. Inaccessibility of the infected sites is a major problem in establishing a microbiologic etiology, unless culdocentesis or laparoscopy is performed. When culdocentesis or laparoscopy is performed, the organisms isolated from the fallopian tubes do not always correspond to those cultured from the cervix or vagina.

In a group of 30 patients with PID, Thompson and coworkers[3] found the gonococcus in 80% of the patients in cultures from the cervix, and only in 33% from the peritoneal cavity. In most United States populations, cervical *N. gonorrhoeae* has been isolated in only 40 to 50% of women with acute PID.[4] In Scandinavian countries where gonococcal infection has been less common, *N. gonorrhoeae* has been isolated in 10 to 20% of women with PID.

N. gonorrhoeae is rarely found as the only pathogen when cultures are taken from the infected pelvis. Other aerobic and anaerobic organisms are also present. It has been estimated that one fourth to one third of abdominal cultures will grow nongonococcal organisms either alone or associated with the gonococcus.[4,6] The significance of the nongonococcal organisms is difficult to assess unless they appear in pure culture. However, a number of nongonococcal organisms have in recent years been implicated as primary incitants of PID.

Of the sexually transmitted pathogens, *Chlamydia trachomatis*, an acknowledged cause of nongonococcal urethritis, has been documented as a primary pathogen that causes PID.[7–10] In the United States about 20% of women with PID harbor *C. trachomatis*.[4] In Scandinavian countries, at least 40% of acute PID is caused by this intracellular organism.[8] Specimens from the infected pelvis of women with nongonococcal PID have also grown pure cultures of *Mycoplasma* species,[11] *Ureaplasma urealyticum*,[11] and cytomegalovirus.[4] The role of these organisms in acute PID must await further study.

A variety of aerobic and anaerobic bacteria have been recovered from the peritoneal cavity and have been implicated as causative agents of PID. These include Enterobacteriaceae, *Pseudomonas*, enterococcus, *Bacteroides*, *Peptostreptococcus*, and *Peptococcus* species. A polymicrobial infection is the usual result when these organisms are involved.[11]

With the exception of *C. trachomatis*, nongonococcal PID is often associated with trauma, pregnancy, and gynecologic surgical procedures; PID due to *N. gonorrhoeae* and *C. trachomatis* is usually the result of sexually transmitted infection.

With this variety of etiologic agents involved in PID, some of them only equivocally important, PID is best divided into gonococcal and nongonococcal forms, depending on the presence or absence of *N. gonorrhoeae* in the endocervical and abdominal cultures.

EPIDEMIOLOGY

Several risk factors have been cited as being important in the development of PID. Age is one factor. Active PID is estimated to develop in 1% of sexually active women annually. However, 1.5 to 2% of the patients are sexually active teenagers between 15 and 19 years of age.[5] This is also the age group that has the highest prevalence of organisms that cause PID.

Patients at increased risk of acquiring gonorrhea is another factor; 10 to 17% of women who contract gonorrhea and are not promptly and/or properly treated will develop PID. About one half of women with PID have endocervical gonorrhea, and the gonococcus is the most common organism isolated from the abdomen of women with PID.[4] Thus, women with untreated gonorrhea are at great risk to develop PID, and the greater the number of sexual partners, the greater the risk of contracting gonorrhea.[12] It follows that women who have multiple sexual partners are at increased risk for developing PID.

A woman's marital status is another factor. Single women are more likely to develop PID than their married counterparts.[13] This factor may reflect the likelihood of multiple sexual partners in single women versus one or very few in married women.

Patients who use intrauterine contraceptive devices (IUD) are at increased risk of developing PID, especially of the nongonococcal type.[3] IUD users have a relative risk of acquiring PID 150 to 400% higher than non-IUD users.[14] On the other hand, the use of oral contraceptive decreases the risk of developing PID, as compared with women using IUDs or no contraceptive method.[14,15] The suggestion has been made that the use of oral contraceptives changes the properties of the cervical mucus, thus making it impermeable to bacteria.[16] A recent study has also found that women using oral contraceptives had significantly milder degree of inflammation of the fallopian tubes as compared with nonusers.[17]

Use of barrier forms of contraception also decreases the risk of acquiring sexually transmitted diseases.[18,15] These forms of contraception (condom, diaphragm, spermicidal foam or jelly) may prevent pathogens from ascending to the upper genital tract.

Patients who appear to be at increased risk of developing PID are nulligravid women using IUDs as compared with women who have been pregnant.[20]

Asymptomatic gonococcal infection in either sexual partner is another factor for increased risk of developing PID. Male sexual partners of women with PID have an increased likelihood of being asymptomatic.[21] It has also been shown that up to 17% of asymptomatic women harboring the gonococcus and who are not brought to treatment will eventually develop PID.[22]

One episode of PID increases the risk for developing subsequent episodes. This may be attributed to tubal damage resulting from the initial episode consequently interfering with normal host defense mechanisms.

SYMPTOMS AND SIGNS

Pelvic inflammatory disease presents the same signs and symptoms regardless of the etiologic agent. The classical presenting symptoms are moderate fever (generally above 99°F), bilateral lower abdominal pain that is maximal in the region of the fallopian tubes and generally lasts no longer than 14 days, increased vaginal discharge, and irregular bleeding. However, only about 20% of PID patients show all of these symptoms, each of which may also occur in other pathologic conditions. Objective findings that may occur in patients with PID are rebound tenderness, adnexal masses, displacement of the cervix, and abnormal vaginal discharge. A third of PID patients may complain of recent abnormal uterine bleeding and dyspareunia.[3] Once PID has occurred, the woman is vulnerable to recurrences of the disease and each occurrence increases the risk of associated complications such as infertility, ectopic pregnancy, pelvic abscesses, chronic pelvic pain, and menstrual irregularities. Two or more of these complications will develop in many women after a single episode of PID.

Certain clinical differences may be observed between gonococcal and nongonococcal PID. The acute onset of pain that occurs at the time of menstruation is seen more often in gonococcal PID than in the nongonococcal form. In the latter, pain is milder, more insidious, and generally not associated with the menses. Purulent discharge is more commonly seen in gonococcal PID, which responds more quickly to therapy than does the nongonococcal form. A foul-smelling vaginal discharge, abdominal bleeding, and cramplike abdominal pain may precede the onset of the disease in nongonococcal PID, especially when an intrauterine device (IUD) is involved.

DIAGNOSIS

The diagnosis of PID is not a simple matter. Clinical diagnosis is frequently inaccurate and laboratory tests, with the exception of culdocentesis and laparoscopy, are nonspecific. The classical symptoms upon which clinical diagnosis depends occurs only in 20% of the patients.[6] Bilateral pain and adnexal tenderness may not be demonstrated on bimanual examination, and fever and vaginal discharge may be absent. When abdominal pain and adnexal tenderness are present, these symptoms may not be diagnostic, as they occur in many other disease states (e.g., endometriosis, ovarian cyst).

Jacobson and Westrum[23] found that only in two thirds of patients with PID was the diagnosis confirmed by laparoscopy, 23% had abdominal pain without any laparoscopic abnormality and 12% had other diseases.

Nevertheless, with a good history, awareness of the disease, and a well-performed bimanual pelvic examination supported by laboratory findings, a correct diagnosis can be made in the majority of cases. Bilateral lower abdominal pain, adnexal tenderness, and often cervical motion tenderness will usually be demonstrated by bimanual examination. Examination for adnexal masses to rule out pelvic abscess is necessary, though a mass may represent an ovarian cyst, ectopic pregnancy, or endometriosis. A yellowish endocervical discharge may be seen on speculum examination. Some patients may have a temperature above 99°F.

Some laboratory tests, though not specific, may help to establish the diagnosis. There may be a leukocytosis (>10,800), but this finding is present only in 30% of patients.[6] The erythrocyte sedimentation rate is elevated to over 15 mm/nm in 75% of the PID patients. Culture of the endocervix and anal canal for *N. gonorrhoeae* should be performed in all cases, and when positive, the patient is considered to have gonococcal PID. A cervical Gram stain, taken so as to exclude vaginal bacteria, is a quick diagnostic assist when it is positive for gram-negative diplococci. A negative smear, however, does not exclude gonococcal PID. A gonococcal culture for definitive identification of the organism on MTM or NYC media is always in order. Endocervical cultures for other organisms are not indicated, since the opportunistic pathogens involved in PID are often found in the vaginas and cervices of normal women. However, when culdocentesis or laparoscopy are performed, the aspirate obtained should be cultured for the gonococcus, chlamydia, mycoplasmas, aerobic, and anaerobic bacteria. Culdocentesis and laparoscopy are the more accurate of the diagnostic methods and are indicated for difficult diagnostic cases. In all cases of gonococcal PID, the male partner should be examined, cultured, and treated with full therapeutic doses of the recommended medications as listed on the CDC or NYC treatment schedule.

DIFFERENTIAL DIAGNOSIS

PID may be confused with other abdominal pathologic conditions. PID must be differentiated from appendicitis, ectopic pregnancy, septic abortion, rupture of an ovarian cyst, pyelonephritis, and other conditions.

Appendicitis usually presents with severe vomiting and nausea. The pain in the right lower quadrant is unilateral in appendicitis and usually bilateral in PID. The white blood count in appendicitis is only moderately elevated, unless the infected appendix is ruptured.

Ectopic pregnancy is associated with menstrual irregularities, unilateral pain without fever unless rupture has occurred.

The exudate, obtained by culdocentesis in ruptured ectopic pregnancy contains non-clotting blood; in PID it is purulent. An enlarged uterus suggests ectopic pregnancy.

Patients with septic abortion present a history of intrauterine manipulation. Examination of the patient shows evidence of the products of conception and/or a dilated cervical.

Patients with ruptured ovarian cysts are afebrile and the abdominal pain is usually unilateral.

Costovertebral angle tenderness is the hallmark of acute pyelonephritis. A positive urine culture obtained, of course, under sterile conditions, will confirm the diagnosis.

Abdominal pain in PID is of short duration; pain that lasts longer than 3 weeks is not likely to be PID. Though a temperature >99°F is often present in 40% of patients, a normal temperature does not preclude the possibility of PID; neither does a negative smear for *N. gonorrhoeae* excludes gonococcal PID.

SEQUELAE

PID has been reported to be the most common cause of involuntary infertility in women.[5] As each recurrence of the disease occurs, the probability of this complication increases.[2] Approximately 10% of patients may become infertile after one episode of PID. With more than one episode of PID, as many as 35% of patients may become infertile.[6] With three or more episodes, the likelihood of remaining infertile approximates 75%. Infertility occurs more in nongonococcal PID than in gonococcal PID.

In about 2 to 4% of patients with PID, the pelvic infection may disseminate to the liver resulting in a perihepatitis. The patient presents with severe pleuritic upper quadrant abdominal pain, and a "friction rub" can be heard over the liver. "Violin strings" may form between the abdominal wall and liver

capsule. This complication, known as the Fitz-Hugh–Curtis syndrome, may occur in both gonococcal and nongonoccal types of PID. Wang and associates[24] have confirmed an etiologic relationship of acute *C. trachomatis* infection with the Fitz-Hugh Curtis syndrome.

Unilateral or bilateral ovarian abscesses are a common complication of PID due to the spilling of exudate from the infected bubo to the ovary and peritoneum. A major cause of death due to PID is the rupture of such an abscess. Abscess formation occurs more often in nongonococcal PID. Tubal occlusion, scarring, and adhesions are long-term complications of PID. Death due to PID following the use of IUD has also been reported.[25]

TREATMENT

Treatment of PID is dependent upon the etiologic organisms causing the infection. This can be established definitely by direct examination of the intraabdominal site by culdoscopic or laparoscopic procedures. However, this is often inappropriate or infeasible. Definitive diagnosis is thus unascertainable. The choice of treatment depends instead on the clinical assessment as to which microorganisms are most likely to be involved at each clinical stage of the disease. Under these conditions, strict and rigid follow-up examination of the patient is required within 48 to 72 hours after start of treatment to assess the result of the chosen therapy. Such early examination may prevent further extension of the infection and the development of sequelae because of inadequate or improper treatment.

Most women with acute PID can be treated on an ambulatory basis. Hospitalization is required (1) in questionable diagnosis, (2) for patients that can not be treated with oral medication, (3) in the presence of an adnexal mass, (4) when there is evidence of peritonitis or pregnancy, (5) for patients who did not respond to treatment as outpatients, (6) for patients who will not follow instructions, (7) and patients for whom follow-up examination cannot be arranged 48 to 72 hours after initiation of treatment.[26]

The recommended treatment of acute salpingitis for outpatients is 0.5 g of tetracycline four times daily for 10 days. Tetracycline is preferable to 4.8 million units of intramuscular aqueous procaine penicillin G, or 3.5 g of oral ampicillin or 3.0 g of oral amoxicillin. Each of these antibiotics is administered with 1.0 g of oral probenecid and followed by 0.5 g of ampicillin or 0.5 g of amoxicillin given orally four times a day for 10 days. Since early PID is more likely to be caused by *N. gonorrhoeae* and *C. trachomatis*, and since both organisms (except penicillinase-producing *N. gonorrhoeae*) are susceptible to the tetracyclines,* the treatment of choice under these conditions would be a tetracycline regimen.

Outpatients should be reexamined at 3 and 7 days after the start of treatment and also after completion of therapy. They should be cultured for *N. gonorrhoeae* and *C. trachomatis*, if culture is available, after treatment.

Single-drug therapy is not adequate for the treatment of polymicrobial PID. Additionally, PID due to a single organism resistant to the penicillins or the tetracyclines require alternate forms of therapy. Combinations of drugs are thus necessary to eradicate the infection. However, as of the present, no field studies have confirmed any experimental work with combinations of oral antibiotics. Theoretically, at least, the combination of trimethoprim-sulfamethoxazole and tetracycline appears to be more efficacious than tetracycline alone.[26]

For hospitalized patients, the recommended regimens[26] for the treatment of acute salpingitis are aqueous procaine penicillin G, 20 million units administered daily until improvement occurs, followed by 500

mg of oral ampicillin or amoxicillin four times daily to complete 10 days of therapy; or 250 mg intravenous tetracycline four times a day until improvement occurs, followed by 500 mg of oral tetracycline four times a day for a total of 10 days of therapy. Either of these two drug regimens is recommended for patients with PID due to *N. gonorrhoeae*. For PID due to *C. trachomatis*, the tetracycline regimen is strongly recommended.

PID due to polymicrobial etiology requires multiple drug therapy. For the polymicrobial infections, a number of newer broad-spectrum antibiotics have been proposed and tried in a few patients. Among these agents, cefamandole nafate, a cephalosporin derivative, showed in vitro activity against important anerobes. Like cefoxitin, cefamandole is resistant to β-lactamase and thus may be active against PPNG; both, however, are not very effective against enterococci. Another recent derivative of cephalosporin, moxalactam, is similar in its antibacterial spectrum to that of cefamandole and cefoxitin. It is also active against *Bacteroides fragilis* and other *Bacteroides* species. Unfortunately, none of these newer drugs is effective against *C. trachomatis*.

A triple-drug combination that is effective against the multiple pathogens likely to be associated with PID consists of a penicillin or cephalosporin, an aminoglycoside, and either clindamycin or chloramphenicol. The last two antibiotics, however, have caused rare, though severe, untoward reactions and must be used with vigilance and care.

The combination doxycycline and cefoxitin form an effective combination against most organisms responsible for PID, including many of the important anaerobes. This combination is without the toxicity shown by chloramphenicol and should be the combination of choice. Patients allergic to penicillin may be given doxycycline or tetracycline alone or possibly together with clindamycin.[26]

---

* Not to be used for pregnant women.

As gonorrhea due to PPNG increases in the United States, it is likely that more cases of PPNG PID will occur. No information is available regarding the treatment of PPNG-associated PID. However, since spectinomycin and cefoxitin are effective in the treatment of uncomplicated PPNG infections, these drugs should also be effective in PPNG-associated PID.

Although some investigators[3,6] consider the removal of the IUD, when used, as part of the therapy, others[26] claim that the benefits of such removal are not clearly defined and that the problem remains a controversial issue.

Pregnant women with PID should be hospitalized and treated with penicillin (if not allergic to it) in the dosages recommended for acute salpingitis. For penicillin allergic patients, the recommended regimen is a single intramuscular dose of spectinomycin along with intravenous erythromycin, followed by oral erythromycin therapy until resolution of symptoms.[26] Tetracyclines in pregnancy are contraindicated; spectinomycin, though not associated with teratogenicity in a single 2.0-g dose, has not been examined in larger repetitive doses. The erythromycin estolate preparations should not be used during pregnancy.

Patients who do not improve or who have increasing abdominal pain need to be reevaluated with repeat pelvic examination. Laparoscopy should be considered for patients who show no response to treatment or worsen.

CONCLUSION

Any woman who is a contact to gonorrhea, or has a positive gonorrhea culture, or has recent onset of lower abdominal pain can be a candidate for PID. It is essential that we start to see most pelvic infections as foci of gonorrhea prevention. Pelvic inflammatory disease is a complex and poorly understood syndrome, which often is a sequel to gonococcal or chlamydial infection. It causes serious morbidity in young women, and it is often difficult to diagnose. Since mild cases, which often present themselves at sexually transmitted clinics, are easily missed, awareness of the disease must remain very high. There is no substitute for an adequate history and a bimanual pelvic examination for all women attending these clinics as well as hospital emergency rooms.

Treatment, to a large extent, depends upon the physician's judgment regarding the clinical stage of the disease and his assessment of which microorganisms are most likely to be involved. Single-drug therapy is generally adequate in early uncomplicated PID. Tetracycline would appear to be the drug of choice, since it is effective in both gonococcal and chlamydial PID. Later and recurrent stages of the disease are generally due to polymicrobial etiology. Penicillin (or cephalosporin) combined with an aminoglycoside—generally used in this situation—is ineffective against *C. trachomatis* and many of the anaerobes. Tetracyclines combined with cefoxitin, though not yet clinically tested, appear to be effective against the organisms mainly involved in PID (gonococcus, chlamydia, anaerobes) and should (until proven otherwise) be the drugs of choice.

Additionally, the identification and treatment of asymptomatic males with gonococcal urethritis is of tremendous importance in the control of PID. The asymptomatic male can infect any number of females who subsequently develop gonorrhea and PID. Condoms and spermicidal jellies reduce the risk of transmission of both *N. gonorrhoeae* and *C. trachomatis* in the first place. Oral contraceptives reduce the risk of the complications of pelvic inflammatory disease.[5] As with all sexually transmitted diseases, serologic tests for syphilis should be performed on all PID patients.

Considering the multiplicity of possible etiologic agents involved in the causation of

PID, therapy cannot be dependent upon microbiologic data. The clinical parameters are the essential monitors for the effectiveness of therapy.[6]

REFERENCES

1. Curran JW: Economic consequences of pelvic inflammatory disease in the United States. Am J Obstet Gynecol 138(part 2):848, 1980
2. Westrom L: Effect of acute pelvic inflammatory disease on fertility. Am J Obstet Gynecol 138:88, 1980
3. Thompson SE III, Hager WD, Kwai-Hay W, et al.: The microbiology and therapy of acute pelvic inflammatory disease in hospitalized patients. Am J Obstet Gynecol 136:179, 1980
4. Eschenbach DA, Buchanan TM, Pollack HM, et al.: Polymicrobial etiology of acute pelvic inflammatory disease. N Engl J Med 293:166, 1975
5. Forslin L, Falk V, Danielson DP: Changes in the incidence of acute gonococcal and nongonococcal salpingitis. Br J Vener Dis 54:247, 1978
6. Smith MS, Eschenbach DA: Pelvic inflammatory disease. Clin Pediatr 19:791, 1980
7. Taylor ES, McMillan JH, Greer BE, et al.: The intrauterine device and tubo-ovarian abscess. Am J Obstet Gynecol 123:338, 1975
8. Mardh PA, Ripa T, Swensson L, et al.: Role of Chlamydia trachomatis infection in acute salpingitis. N Engl J Med 296:1377, 1977
9. Paavonen J: Chlamydia trachomatis in acute salpingitis. Am J Obstet Gynecol 138(part 2):848, 1980
10. Holmes KK, Eschenbach DA, Knapp JS: Salpingitis: Overview of etiology and epidemiology. Am J Obstet Gynecol 138(part 2):839, 1980
11. Mardh PA, Westrom L: Tubal and cervical cultures in acute salpingitis with special reference to Mycoplasma hominis and T-strain mycoplasms. Br J Vener Dis 46:179, 1970
12. Darrow WW: Changes in sexual behavior and venereal diseases. Clin Obstet Gynecol 18:255, 1975
13. Westrom L: Incidence, prevalence and trends of acute pelvic inflammatory disease and its consequences in industrialized countries. Am J Obstet Gynecol 138:880, 1980
14. Senanayake P, Kramer DG: Contraception and the etiology of pelvic inflammatory disease: New perspective. Am J Obstet Gynecol 38(part 2):852, 1980
15. Senanayake P, Kramer DG: Contraception and pelvic inflammatory disease. Sex Transm Dis 8:89, 1981
16. Eschenback DA: Acute pelvic inflammatory disease: Etiology, risk factors and pathogenesis. Clin Obstet Gynecol 19:247, 1976
17. Svensson L, Westrom L, Mardh P-A: Contraceptives and acute salpingitis. JAMA 251:2553, 1984
18. Keith L, Berger GS, Moss W: Cervical gonorrhea in women using different methods of contraception. J Am Vener Dis Assoc 3:17, 1976
19. Kelaghan J, Rubin GL, Ory HW, et al.: Barrier-method contraceptives and pelvic inflammatory disease. JAMA 248:184, 1982
20. Westrom L, Bengtsson LP, Mardh P-A: The risk of pelvic inflammatory disease in women using intrauterine contraceptive devises as compared to non-users. Lancet 2:221, 1976
21. Handsfield HH, Lipman TO, Harnish JP, et al.: Asymptomatic gonorrhea in men. Diagnosis, natural course, prevalence, and significance. N Engl J Med 290:117, 1974
22. Eschenbach DA, Holmes KK: Acute pelvic inflammatory disease: Current concepts of pathogenesis, etiology, and management. Clin Obstet Gynecol 18:35, 1975
23. Jacobson L, Westrum L: Objectivised diagnosis of acute pelvic inflammatory disease. Am J Obstet Gynecol 105:1088, 1969
24. Wang SP, Eschenbach DA, Holmes KK: Chlamydia trachomatis infection in Fritz-Hugh-Curtis syndrome. Am J Obstet Gynecol 138(2):1034, 1980
25. Scott R: Critical illness and death associated with intrauterine devices. Obstet Gynecol 31:322, 1968
26. Goodrich JT: Pelvic inflammatory disease: Considerations related to therapy. Rev Infect Dis 4:5778, 1982

7

Lymphogranuloma Venereum

Margaret R. Hammerschlag

Lymphogranuloma venereum (LGV) is a systemic infection caused by certain specific serotypes of *Chlamydia trachomatis.* As with other chlamydial infections, LGV is almost exclusively transmitted by sexual contact. However, unlike other oculogenital chlamydial infections, LGV is characterized by a significant systemic component and a trophism for lymphoid tissue.

HISTORICAL BACKGROUND

Although LGV was probably described by John Hunter in 1786, it was first clearly recognized as a separate venereal disease by Durand, Nicolas, and Favre in 1913.[1] At that time the authors proposed the term *lymphogranulomatose inguinale* for a new syndrome characterized by the development of inguinal adenitis following a transient penile ulcer. The adenitis eventually suppurates, then drains externally, leading to fistulae. The histology of the lesions were unique, with multinucleated epitheloid cells. The structure was definitely different than that typical of the syphilitic gumma. In later reports, the authors described the clinical characteristics of the disease; they found it to be limited almost exclusively to men, identifying only one case in a woman and none in children. At that time Durand and his colleagues were unable to identify the causative agent of the disease. Subsequently, Frei[2] introduced a specific skin test in 1925. The antigen was originally made from the pus of the adenitis of a patient (who concurrently had syphilis). Frei injected 0.1 cc of this material intracutaneously into the original patient from whom he had aspirated the pus, and into other patients with the disease; three healthy subjects (including Dr. Frei himself) served as controls. Within 36–48 hours, a 2- to 3-cm area of erythema developed at the site of infection in all three patients, but not in the controls. Frei also tested antigens prepared from lymph nodes of patients with syphilis, tuberculosis, leukemia, and Hodgkin's disease, all of which gave negative results.

In 1929 Hellerstrom and Wassen[3] transmitted the infection to monkeys by the intracerebral route. In addition, they inoculated the prepuces of two rhesus monkeys who developed inguinal adenopathy within two weeks. In 1931 Levaditi, Marie, and Lepine[4] produced an experimental infection in a human subject after urethral inoculation of material obtained from passage through monkey brains. Earlier work by Levaditi and Hellerstrom and Wassen suggested that the causative agent of LGV was a virus, and in 1933 Findlay noted similarities between the developmental cycle and that previously described for the agent of psittacosis. The complement-fixation test was introduced in the 1930s. Several studies by Rake, Eaton, Shaffer, and Tygeseson in 1941 and 1942[5] demonstrated antigenic similarities between the agents of LGV, psittacosis, and trachoma inclusion conjunctivitis.

BIOLOGICAL CHARACTERISTICS OF THE ORGANISM

The etiologic agent of LGV is now classified as a biovar or serovar of *Chlamydia trachomatis*. Serologically, the LGV biovar falls with the B complex and is considered to be a junior antigen with extensive cross-reactions.[6] Three serotypes have been identified by the microimmunofluorescence test by Wang and Grayston.[6] LGV and other strains of *C. trachomatis* share a cross-reacting antigen group with a molecular weight of 1.55×1.0^5. They also share 100% DNA homology. LGV differs from other strains of *C. trachomatis* in its behavior both in cell culture and in vivo.[7] LGV appears to be much more virulent. In cell culture LGV strains are capable of unrestricted multiplications without mechanical assistance such as centrifugation, which is required for the propagation of the other strains of *C. trachomatis*. Infection with LGV is not enhanced by pretreatment of host cells with DEAE-dextran, or inhibited by neuraminidase. In vivo, LGV is lethal when injected intracerebrally into mice, whereas the other strains of *C. trachomatis* are not. LGV strains frequently infect macrophages and appear to have a predilection toward lymph node involvement. The oculogenital strains of *C. trachomatis* are primarily limited to infection of squamocolumnar cells. These characteristics suggest that LGV strains have a less restricted host range, which may be a function of less specialized host cell receptor requirements.

EPIDEMIOLOGY

LGV probably has a worldwide distribution, although reliable data on prevalence and incidence using specific serologic and cultural methods are not available. The disease appears to be more prevalent in certain parts of South America, the West Indies, southeast Asia, India, and west and east Africa.[8] However, LGV is probably underreported owing to difficulties in diagnosis secondary to lack of facilities. LGV accounted for 6% of all cases of sexually transmitted diseases reported in Madras, India between 1968 and 1977.[8] Osoba[9] reported from Nigeria a 2% prevalence of LGV in patients seen at special clinic at the University Hospital in Ibadan over a 6-month period. In an earlier study,[10] using the LGV complement-fixation test, Osoba found the prevalence of seropositivity in Ibadan to range from 53% to 11.5%, while in Benin it ranged from 7.3% to 18.3%. Similar prevalences have also been reported from Lusaka, Zambia.[9] In a study from southern Africa, Piot and coworkers[11] identified LGV in 3 to 10% of male patients with genital ulcerations. LGV is thought to be an uncommon diagnosis in industrialized countries, but this is probably due again to underreporting. In the United States, from 1941 to 1947 approximately 1300 to 2600 cases of LGV were reported each with a rate per 100,000 population of 1.0 to 2.2.[12] After 1947 the incidence dropped dramatically; from 1966 to 1979 the number of reported cases ranged from 250 to 756 (rate 0.2 to 0.4). During the Vietnam conflict, it was reported that American military personnel acquired LGV at a rate of 14 cases per 1,000. Schachter and Osoba[8] recently reported that 29 cases of LGV were diagnosed at his laboratory and reported to physicians, while during the same period only 20 cases were reported throughout California. This observation confirms that many cases are not being reported to the public health authorities.

Cases of LGV in the United States may not always be limited to servicemen or to individuals of lower socioeconomic class. A small outbreak of LGV involving four students was reported from a midwestern college town.[13] Scattered cases of LGV have been reported from New Zealand, Australia, and Northern Europe.[14–16]

Another feature that probably contributes to underreporting is the differences in the presentation of LGV between men and women. The classical acute bubonic form is usually seen in young men, who are more likely to attend the venereal disease clinics. Of 148 patients diagnosed as having LGV at the venereal disease clinic at the University Hospital in Kingston, Jamaica, only 5 were women.[17] The women were more likely to come in later to the University clinic. Since the later sequelae in women usually involves the anorectal syndrome, women are more likely to seek attention at general medical or gastroenterology clinics.

LGV is also becoming recognized as a significant infection among homosexuals, where it frequently causes proctocolitis. Since the other serovars of *C. trachomatis* may also be isolated from the gastrointestinal tract, the differentiation of LGV in the laboratory becomes more important. The two major diagnostic tests available, the Frei test and the complement-fixation test (CF), are not specific for the LGV biovar. Schachter and Dawson[18] have reported that 15% of men with chlamydial urethritis and 40% of women with chlamydial cervical infection will have complement-fixation titers $\geq 1:16$. Surveys that have only used the complement-fixation test for determining the prevalence of LGV may have actually been detecting antibody from previous, but unrelated, chlamydial infections.

CLINICAL MANIFESTATIONS

The clinical course of LGV is usually divided into three stages. The primary stage involves the incubation period and the initial lesion; the secondary stage includes the lymph node involvement; and the tertiary state includes the late sequelae of the disease.

The Primary Lesion

The incubation period after exposure to LGV appears to range from 3 to 30 days. Following this period a primary lesion may develop. This lesion is usually transient and nonpainful. It is frequently not noticed by the patient. In men, most often the primary lesion is on the penis, usually the glans. In women, it may be on the vaginal wall, on the labia, or occasionally on the cervix. The primary lesion may take several forms; the most common being a herpetiform lesion, but ulcers, vesicles, papules, or pustules have also been described. The lesions are usually 5 to 6 mm in diameter. After a few days, there is healing without scar formation. In several series, less than 40% of confirmed cases of LGV had a primary lesion on examination or gave a history of a lesion.[8,19] Primary lesions may also occur on extragenital sites such as the fingers and the tongue.[8] This is probably a reflection of the type and mode of exposure.

Histopathologically, the primary lesions demonstrate an acute inflammatory reaction with loss of superficial epithelium and a base of acute inflammatory reaction containing polymorphonuclear leukocytes (PMNs) and fibrin. In the deeper tissues there can be a sprinkling of plasma cells, histiocytes, lymphocytes, polymorphonuclear leukocytes, and capillaries.[20] These findings are nonspecific and can be seen with other pathogens.

Considering the infrequent history of a

primary lesion obtained from patients presenting with lymphadenopathy and the infrequent observation of such lesions by physicians, some investigators have suggested that LGV may not be associated with a primary lesion. The lesions observed could be secondary to other causes such as abrasions, common ulceration, or misdiagnosed herpetic infection. Perline and associates[21] reported from Ethiopia in 1980 that genital lesions were observed only in 3 of 17 (18%) patients with laboratory-confirmed LGV (either isolation of LGV from bubo aspirate or serology). In each case these lesions were either a small papule or abrasion, which was inconspicuous and painless. In contrast, genital lesions were present in 68% of the non-LGV patients with inguinal buboes. These lesions tended to be painful and usually preceded the onset of the lymphadenopathy.

In a recent study from southern Africa, Piot and colleagues[11] describe an ulcerative genital lesion from which they were able to isolate *C. trachomatis*. Inguinal lymphadenopathy, usually unilateral, was present in 50% of these cases. Only one patient had fluctuant buboes. The lesions had an appearance that was different from ulcers that were chlamydial-negative. The ulcers were described as deep, 4 to 6 mm in diameter with elevated edges. The base was purulent or indurated in one half of the lesions and over half were tender. Whether these lesions represented the primary lesion of LGV or were a different disease process was not clear.

The Secondary Lesion: Lymphadenitis or Lymphadenopathy

Most patients with LGV come to medical attention because of the complaint of painful inguinal lymphadenopathy. Many patients will also have systemic symptoms such as fever, headache, malaise, and anorexia, in addition to the presence of enlarging buboes. As previously mentioned, this presentation is seen mainly in men. The male:female ratio in most series is approximately 10:1[5,8,17] The lymphadenopathy usually occurs from one to several weeks after infection. Since a primary lesion is frequently not mentioned by the patient, the incubation period really cannot be determined with any degree of precision. The buboes are usually unilateral, but lymphangiography frequently demonstrates involvement of the contralateral side.[22]

The inguinal nodes are most frequently involved. When the femoral nodes are also involved, one may see the so-called "groove sign," which results when the two groups of nodes are separated by Pupart's ligament. Although this sign is considered pathognomonic for LGV, it has been found in only 15 to 20% of patients.[8] In women, the primary infection is thought to occur on the labia or intravaginally. The drainage of this area is usually to the retroperitoneal lymph nodes, thus women infrequently present with inguinal buboes. Lymphographic studies of males with acute LGV also demonstrated involvement of the iliac nodes in all cases.[22] Lymphadenopathy at other sites, such as superclavicular, axillary, submaxillary, and cervical nodes have also been reported in LGV, presumably after infection at an extragenital site.[23–26] One case of cervical lymphadenopathy reported by Thorsteinsson and coworkers[25] occurred in a 31-year-old male homosexual who practiced fellatio frequently.

Initially, the inflammation is usually restricted to a single lymph node which eventually extends to the entire chain of nodes which become matted. Histological examination of these nodes reveal the presence of stellate microabscesses surrounded by histiocytic cells and epitheloid cells. These abscesses may expand and coalesce leading to suppuration and perinodular fibrosis.[20] The lymphadenopathy may regress spontaneously or may rupture, leading to draining fistulae. Chronic lymphadenopathy can develop, which may persist for many years.

The Tertiary Stage: The Genitoanorectal Syndrome

The tertiary stage is actually a misleading term, since many patients may not have had preceding lymphadenopathy. The tertiary stage covers a variety of the late sequelae of LGV, including rectal stricture, rectovaginal fistulae, esthiomene, and elephantiasis. In contrast to the bubonic form of LGV where the majority of patients are male, the genitoanorectal syndrome occurs most frequently in women.[8] This sexual distribution is probably secondary to the observation that women tend not to present with clinically detected lymphadenopathy, thus the disease is unrecognized and untreated and progresses. Another reason is related to the fact that in women the rectoperitoneal lymphatics are involved.

Rectal strictures are among the commonest manifestations of LGV. Strictures may be secondary to either chronic inflammatory reaction and granulation or late scarring. The strictures are anular, the majority occurring within 3 to 10 cm of the anus.[8,20] Histopathology demonstrates a complete loss of the mucosal epithelium with replacement by granulation of the surrounding tissue. Penile fistulas may occur in the male and rectal or rectovaginal fistulas in the female to give the so called "watering-can" perineum.

The genital syndrome of hypertrophic ulceration of the pudenda includes the condition esthiomene, which is from the Greek for "eating away." This condition was first described by Frei and Koppel in 1928 as enlarged edematous and violaceous labia. The swelling has been attributed to both lymphatic stasis and to a chronic inflammatory process. Although it is seen more frequently in women, hypertrophic lesions involving the penis, scrotum, and anus may

be seen in males. Dan and associates[27] described one patient, an elderly man with a 20-year history of multiple perianal, ulcerative granulomatous polypoid lesions with perianal fistulas. *C. trachomatis*, assumed to be an LGV strain, was isolated from lesions. Elephantiasis of varying degree may also be present in both women and men, frequently involving the scrotum in the latter.[8] As with the development of the hypertrophic ulceration, elephantiaisis may be secondary to lymphatic stasis or direct activity of the LGV. Women may also experience destruction of the urethra as a late manifestation of LGV.

Proctitis—Proctocolitis

The association of LGV with acute proctocolitis has recently received a great deal of attention, due in part to renewed interest in infectious disease associated with homosexuality, especially the "gay bowel" syndrome. However, this association was recognized over 40 years ago by Grace,[28] who found LGV to be a relatively common venereal disease among male homosexuals. Many of these men presented with proctitis. Both the LGV and trachoma biovars may infect the rectal mucosa, but the disease associated with LGV strains appears to be significantly more severe. Quinn and colleagues,[29] in Seattle, cultured 171 homosexual men, 96 of whom had symptoms of proctitis and 75 who were asymptomatic. *C. trachomatis* was isolated from the rectal cultures of 14 (8%) of these men, and 3 of the isolates had LGV immunotypes. Of the 11 men with the non-LGV isolates, 8 (73%) were symptomatic. Their findings included fecal leukocytes and mild abnormalities of the mucosa present at sigmoidoscopy. Mild nongranulomatous inflammatory changes were seen on rectal biopsy. In contrast, the three men with LGV isolates had signs and symptoms of severe proctitis, including anorectal pain, tenesmus, fever, abdominal pain, diarrhea, and purulent or bloody discharge. Leukocytosis and an elevated erythrocyte sedimentation rate were also present. Sigmoidoscopy revealed focal or diffuse friability and ulcerations. Rectal biopsies demonstrated granulomatous inflammation, including crypt abscesses with granulomas and giant cells. In two of the men, the rectal biopsy was initially thought to be suggestive of Crohn's disease. The pathologic process in LGV colitis is always restricted to the lower 10 cm of the intestinal tract. The similarity between the pathologic findings in LGV colitis, Crohn's disease, and ulcerative colitis were noted by Bras and colleagues in 1962.[20] Unlike Crohn's disease, most patients will respond to therapy with tetracycline. Depending on the population, the prevalence of LGV from rectal cultures may be more frequent. Schachter[8] recently reported from San Francisco that 20 of 27 (74%) chlamydial isolates recovered from rectal biopsies of 127 men with proctitis were LGV immunotypes. If untreated, anorectal LGV may progress and cause rectovesicular and other rectal fistulas, perirectal abscess, or rectal strictures that may be misdiagnosed as carcinoma.[8]

Systemic Complications and Extragenital Infection

Infection with LGV outside the gastrointestinal or genitourinary tract are uncommon. Sabin and Aring[33] reported several cases of meningitis probably due to LGV in 1942. Cardiac involvement (pericarditis) has been observed clinically and at autopsy.[34] Arthritis with synovial effusion has also been reported.[5]

Schachter and Dawson[5] observed several cases of pneumonia resulting from laboratory infection and one case in a 77-year-old woman without an obvious source. She had fever and pneumonia. Acute and convalescent chlamydial complement-fixation titers were 1:16 and 1:256, and an LGV L_2 biovar was isolated from her blood. This woman denied any recent sexual activity. Hilar and mediastinal lymphadenopathy have been described following accidental exposure in the laboratory.

Hepatic involvement, including hepatitis, has also been reported. In 1941 Barth and Alexenco[35] were the first to describe a case of LGV associated with acute hepatitis. Inclusion bodies were found in a liver biopsy specimen. Individual cases of hepatitis complicating LGV has also been described by Schachter and coworkers[36] in 1969 and Bjerke and Hovding[37] in 1977.

The similarities between the pathology seen in LGV proctocolitis and Crohn's disease has suggested to some that LGV may be involved in the etiology of the latter. An initial report[8] found that 69% of 55 patients with Crohn's disease had serum antibodies specific for LGV serovars detected by the microimmunofluorescence test. However, several subsequent studies have failed to detect any excess antibody among individuals with Crohn's disease. Studies based on serology alone can frequently be misleading, since LGV infection typically results in a high titer of antibodies broadly reactive to many *C. trachomatis* serotypes, not the specific of low-grade titers that have been reported in these studies.

LGV may also cause immunologic reactions, probably secondary to diffuse elevations of serum immunoglobulins seen in the disease. *C. trachomatis* appears to be a polyclonal B-cell activator.[6] Erythema nodosum and erythema multiforme have been described as well as the presence of cryoglobulins.

Another controversial association is the possible relationship of LGV with neoplastic degeneration.[8] A high incidence of vulval carcinoma is frequently reported from populations where the incidence of LGV and other sexually transmitted diseases are also very high. Sengupta[38] has stated that vulval carcinoma is associated with lack of hygiene, promiscuity, and low socieconomic status; thus the presence of LGV may be a confounding variable.

DIFFERENTIAL DIAGNOSIS

Since sexually active individuals may be exposed to many sexually transmitted pathogens, multiple infections are not uncommon. This observation also applies to patients with LGV. Individuals with LGV should be tested routinely for gonorrhea and syphilis; as many as one third of patients with LGV in one study concurrently had syphilis.[8]

Another reason for this approach in the differential diagnosis of LGV is the possibility that the patient may have another sexually transmitted disease with clinically similar symptomatology. Syphilis is a prime example, since inguinal lymphadenopathy is common and a healed chancre may look like the primary lesion of LGV. However, the lymphadenopathy associated with syphilis is usually discrete and hard in contrast to the matted nodes seen in LGV. Serology may be misleading; biologic false positive VDRL's have been reported in patients with LGV.[5] This may also be related to the observation that *C. trachomatis* is a polyclonal B-cell activator.

Genital herpes may be confused with the primary lesion of LGV; however, herpetic lesions are frequently painful. Regional inguinal lymphadenopathy in genital herpes is not uncommon and is often accompanied by low-grade fever and malaise. The clinical course of genital herpes is usually self-limited and shorter (10 days to 2 weeks).

Other sexually transmitted diseases often considered in the diagnosis of LGV are granuloma inguinale (GI) and chancroid. Clinically there is little resemblance between these infections and LGV. Granu-

loma inguinale, also called donovanosis, is caused by *Calymmatobacterium granulomatis*, a gram-negative pleomorphic organism.[39] Clinically, granuloma inguinale is characterized by a velvety and beefy red granulomatous ulcer with wavy margin, usually involving the skin and mucous membranes of the genitalia. Although it is a local disease, it can become systemic. Actually only 25% or less of granuloma inguinale cases demonstrate inguinal involvement. Unlike LGV, there is no true bubo formation. The diagnosis of granuloma inguinale is confirmed by the demonstration of Donovan bodies in tissue, usually with stained smears from lesions.

Chancroid is caused by *Hemophilus ducreyi*, a small, nonmotile gram-negative, non-spore-forming rod. Clinically, chancroid usually presents initially with a small inflammatory papule on the preputial orifice or frenulum in men and on the labia, fourchette, or perianal region in women. The lesion becomes pustular and ulcerative within 2 to 3 days. In contrast with syphilitic chancre, the chancroidal ulcer usually is extremely painful and tender and not indurated. Over 50% of cases of chancroid will also have acute, painful, tender inflammatory inguinal adenopathy. It is unilateral in approximately two thirds of patients and may suppurate. Unlike LGV, the characteristic ulcer of chancroid is concurrent with lymphadenopathy. A specific diagnosis of chancroid may be made by deep scraping the ulcer and demonstrating the presence of *H. ducreyi* by specific fluorescent antibody staining[40] or by culture. In the study of Piot and associates[11] of genital ulceration in southern Africa, chancroid was the most common diagnosis (42 to 48%) for the three populations studied.

Other conditions that must be considered in the diagnosis of LGV include cat-scratch disease, bacterial lymphadenitis, and, rarely, lymphoma. Najafi and coworkers[41] reported on a patient with LGV whose signs and symptoms simulated an incarcerated hernia and was operated upon.

DIAGNOSIS

The Frei Test

Frei introduced his skin test in 1925. He originally aspirated the pus from the bubo of a patient with LGV. When he injected this material intradermally into another patient with LGV, it elicited a delayed hypersensitivity skin reaction. The Frei test has been the classical diagnostic test for LGV. Once the organism was successfully isolated, antigen grown in mouse brain or yolk sac was substituted for pus. Standardized procedures for preparing the antigen were introduced in the 1940s.[5]

The Frei test is a genus-specific test, which may be positive in a number of individuals infected with any chlamydia, including those of the trachoma biovar. Schachter and associates[36] have also isolated LGV from the buboes of patients who have had negative skin tests. Only 36% of their patients with LGV had a positive Frei test. Because of its low sensitivity and specificity, the Frei antigen is no longer commercially available in the United States.

The Complement-Fixation Test

The complement-fixation (CF) test for chlamydia was introduced in the 1930s. Like the Frei test, the CF test is genus-specific and will detect antibodies to either *C. trachomatis* or *C. psittaci*. In fact the CF antigen may be prepared from either organism. The CF antigen is a heat-stable, acidic polysaccharide common to all members of the *Chlamydia* genus, prepared from yolk-sac cultures. In LGV, the CF test usually becomes positive within the first two weeks of infection. Titers may be positive for life. Treatment may result in a dramatic fall of

the CF titer in some patients and early intensive treatment may prevent the development of any CF response. Most patients with LGV will have CF titers $\geq 1:16$. Schachter and associates[36] found that 10 of 12 (83%) of patients with LGV in one study had a titer of $1:16$ or greater. More recently, Perine and coworkers,[21] in their study from Ethiopia, reported that 13 of 15 (87%) of patients with LGV had CF titers of this magnitude. The demonstration of seroconversion or a 4-fold or greater rise in titer is unusual because of the long clinical course of LGV. Usually the CF titers seen in LGV are significantly higher than those in individuals with other *C. trachomatis* infections, such as nongonococcal urethritis, cervicitis, or conjunctivitis. CF titers in these illnesses are usually less than $1:16$, whereas most individuals with LGV have titers $> 1:64$ or even $>1:256$. In many STD clinics, there usually is a high background rate of CF titers $>1:16$, which probably reflects the non-LGV *C. trachomatis* infections so prevalent in these populations.[8]

The Microimmunofluorescence Test

The microimmunofluorescence (MIF) test was developed by Wang and Grayston[6] to serotype strains of *C. trachomatis*, but was soon adapted to detect antichlamydial antibodies. The antigens are purified elementary bodies, usually grown in yolk sacs. At present there are 15 identified serotypes of *C. trachomatis*, including the three LGV serotypes, L1, L2, and L3. The MIF test detects type-specific antibodies produced against the individual chlamydial serotypes and can therefore differentiate between antibodies produced by *C. trachomatis* and *C. psittaci*. The type-specific antigens are trypsin-labile proteins, which are part of the major outer membrane protein of the chlamydial elementary body.[7] The type-specific antigens are destroyed during the procedures used to prepare the complement-fixation antigen.

Patients with LGV usually will have a very broadly reacting antibody response. The LGV serotypes extensively cross-react with the trachoma biovar, especially the B complex.[6] The MIF test is significantly more sensitive than the complement-fixation test in the diagnosis of all *C. trachomatis* infections. Most individuals with LGV will have very high MIF titers, usually >1:1000 (IgG antibody) and IgM titers >1:32. Perine and associates[21] reported that 82% of their patients with LGV had MIF titers of this magnitude. Males with nongonoccal urethritis usually will not have such high MIF titers. However, Schachter[42] found MIF IgG titers >1:1000 in several men with proctitis due to non-LGV strains of *C. trachomatis*. He suggested that the elevated antibody responses seen in these men were a function of the site of infection.

Isolation of *Chlamydia trachomatis*

The most definitive diagnostic test for LGV is the isolation of the organism from the patients. The best site appears to be the pus from a fluctuant lymph node. However, there are few reported data of the relative sensitivity of culturing buboes in LGV. Schachter and coworkers[36] isolated *C. trachomatis* from aspirates of lymph nodes in 6 of 11 (55%) individuals with LGV. Perine and coworkers[21] isolated LGV from the buboes of 4 of 18 patients with LGV, but the actual number of patients who had negative aspirates was not given. Culture of swabs or biopsies from other involved sites, such as the rectal mucosa, may also be helpful in the diagnosis.

To obtain bubo pus for culture, the recommended technique is to aspirate the node through healthy adjacent tissue. After the pus is obtained, the viscous material should be ground and at least a 1:5 to 1:10 dilution

of the material be made in tissue culture media or saline.[5] Dilution is necessary to avoid possible cytotoxic effects. The material may then be inoculated onto tissue culture. The method used most widely today is cycloheximide treated McCoy cells.[8] The growth cycle of the LGV biovar is shorter than for other chlamydial strains, therefore cultures should be examined at 24 to 48 hours instead of 48 to 72 hours.

LGV has also been isolated from the urethras of men with urethritis and from the cervix of asymptomatic women.[8] Hubrechts and coworkers[16] have reported a case of possible LGV in a young woman, where they isolated a strain of *C. trachomatis* identified as serotype K. Biologically serotype K appears to be closely related to the LGV serotypes.[6]

Noncultural Methods of Antigen Detection

Recently several methods have been introduced that detect chlamydial antigen directly in clinical or histopathologic specimens. One method being evaluated extensively in genital specimens from adults is the use of fluorescein-conjugated monoclonal antichlamydial antibodies. This method appears to have a greater than 90% correlation with tissue culture. Recently Klatz and coworkers[43] reported the diagnosis of hemorrhagic proctitis due to LGV L_2 by identification of the intracellular organisms and inclusions in a rectal biopsy using fluorescein-tagged monoclonal antibodies directed toward the chlamydial group antigen and the L_2 serotype antigen. This patient, a 23-year-old man, also had inguinal adenopathy. Cultures of his lymph node aspirates were negative. The patient also had an MIF IgG titer of 1:2048 and a complement-fixation titer of 1:128.

In a similar case, Schuch and coworkers[44] identified *C. trachomatis* in a rectal biopsy of a 36-year-old woman with proctitis and a painful vaginal mass. The chlamydia were identified using a peroxidase-conjugated monoclonal antichlamydia antibody. Serology was not performed, but it was assumed, based on her clinical presentation, that she probably had infection with an LGV serotype.

TREATMENT

The major modality of therapy available for LGV is antimicrobial. However, the response to chemotherapy is extremely variable and is complicated by the natural history of the disease. Surgical therapy of the late lesions is also disappointing, largely due to their extent, fibrosis, and impairment of the local blood supply.[8]

LGV was shown to be susceptible to sulfonamides in the late 1930s, which became the first chemotherapeutic agents to be tried, and they are still recommended. Many reports of different regimens are difficult to interpret because the stage of the disease will influence the response to therapy. Treatment in the early stages of the disease has a better response than therapy begun at the later, chronic stages. After appropriate therapy, constitutional symptoms such as fever, malaise, chills, and headache disappear rapidly. The buboes usually take several weeks to resolve.

The only controlled trial of chemotherapy available in the literature was reported in 1963 by Greaves and coworkers.[45] They studied a group of 43 men with LGV, diagnosed by the presence of inguinal buboes and high CF titers. They did not demonstrate any significant difference between treatment with chloramphenicol, chlortetracycline, oxytetracycline, or sulfadiazine given for 14–18 days. A more recent study conducted in Ethiopia[21] demonstrated a very good response to a 7- to 14-day course of either tetracycline or trimethoprim-sulfamethoxazole. Their patients had a rapid response of systemic symptoms and prompt relief of bubo pain. Sowmini and associates[46] in a study from India, treated 80 patients with LGV with minocycline, 200 mg twice a day for 10 days. They reported that the healing time in uncomplicated cases was less than 10 days. However, 37.5% of their patients complained of either nausea, vomiting, or dizziness.

Most recent recommendations for treatment of LGV suggest that patients be treated for 2 to 3 weeks. The drugs of choice are tetracycline, 1 or 2 g/day or sulfisoxazole with a loading dose of 4 g followed by 500 mg four times a day for 21 days.

PREVENTION AND CONTROL

The observation that LGV strains may be isolated from the urethras of men with urethritis and from the cervices of asymptomatic women suggests that this may represent a reservoir for the spread of the infection. The only forseeable way in which control of LGV can be achieved is if screening tests are easily available in the populations at risk. Awareness of LGV, as a result of comprehensive laboratory investigation, should help to prevent the spread of infection in the community and the development of the late sequelae.

REFERENCES

1. Durand M, Nicolas J, Favre M: Lymphogranulomatose inguinale subaigue d'origine genital probable, peut-être venérienée. Bull Mem Soc Med Hosp 35:274, 1913
2. Frei W: Eine neue Hautreaktion bei Lymphogranuloma inginale. Klin Wochenschr 4:2148, 1925
3. Hellerstrom S, Wassen E: Meningo-encephalitische Veranderungin bei aflen nach intracerebraler Impfung mit Lymphogranuloma inguinale. Haut kr 37:732, 1930
4. Levaditi C, Marie A, Lepine P: Conservation de la virulence du virus lymphogranu-

lomateux. CR Soc Biol (Paris) 108:1496, 1931

5. Schachter J, Dawson CR: Human Chlamydial Infections. PSG Publishing, Littleton, MA, 1978

6. Wang S-P, Grayston JT: Micro-immunofluorescence antibody response, in Chlamydia trachomatis infection. A review. p 301. In Mardh P-A, Holmes KK, Oriel JD, et al (eds): Chlamydial Infections. Elsevier Biomedical Press, Amsterdam, 1982

7. Ward ME: Chlamydial classification, development and structure. Br Med Bull 39:109, 1983

8. Schachter J, Osoba AO: Lymphogranuloma venereum. Br Med Bull 39:151, 1983

9. Osoba AO: Lymphogranuloma venereum. p 193. In Holmes KK, Mardh P-A (eds): International Perspectives on Neglected Sexually Transmitted Diseases. McGraw-Hill, New York, 1983

10. Osoba AO: Sero-epidemiological study of lymphogranuloma venereum in Western Nigeria. Afr J Med Sci 6:125, 1977

11. Piot P, Ballard RC, Fehler HG, et al: Isolation of Chlamydia trachomatis from genital ulceration in southern Africa. p 115. In Mardh P-A, Holmes KK, Oriel SD (eds): Chlamydial Infections. Elsevier Biomedical Press, Amsterdam, 1982

12. Centers for Disease Control: STD Fact Sheet. 35th Ed. U.S. Department of Health and Human Services, Atlanta, 1981

13. McLelland BA, Anderson PC: Lymphogranuloma venereum. Outbreak in a university community. JAMA 235:56, 1976

14. Vogel MJ: Lymphogranuloma venereum. Med J Aust 2:175, 1973

15. Graham DM, Praszkier J, Rollo DJ: Lymphogranuloma venereum in Australia. I. Clinical aspects of the disease and isolation and identification of the causal agent from a patient in Melbourne. Med J Aust 2:239, 1974

16. Hubrechts J-M, Blondeel A, Demaubege J, et al: Isolation of Chlamydia trachomatis in lymphogranuloma venereum. Acta Clin Belg 35:75, 1980

17. Sigel MM, Burgoon CF, Sutherland ES, Grant LS: LGV as seen in the VD clinic. p 43. In Sigel MM (ed): Lymphogranuloma venereum. University of Miami Press, Coral Gables, FL, 1962

18. Schachter J, Dawson CR: Lymphogranuloma venereum. JAMA 236:915, 1976

19. Abrams AJ: Lymphogranuloma venereum. JAMA 205:199, 1968

20. Bras G, Brook SEH, Hill KR: The pathology of lymphogranuloma venereum in Jamaica. p 13. In Sigel MM (ed): Lymphogranuloma venereum. University of Miami Press, Coral Gabales, FL, 1962

21. Perine PL, Anderson AJ, Krause DW, et al: Diagnosis and treatment of lymphogranuloma venereum in Ethiopia. p 1280. In Nelson JD, Grassi C (eds): Current Chemotherapy and Infectious Disease. American Society of Microbiology, Washington, DC, 1980

22. Osoba AO, Beetlestone CA: Lymphographic studies in acute lymphogranuloma venereum infection. Br J Vener Dis 52:399, 1976

23. Curth H: Extragenital infection with the virus of lymphogranuloma inguinale. Arch Dermatol 28:377, 1933

24. Andrada MT, Kanti-Dhar J, Wilde H: Oral lymphogranuloma venereum and cervical lymphadenopathy. Case report. Milit Med 139:99, 1974

25. Thorsteinsson SB, Musher DM, Min K-W, Gyorkey F: Lymphogranuloma venereum. A cause of cervical adenopathy. JAMA 235:1882, 1976

26. Walzer PD, Armstrong D: Lymphogranuloma venereum presenting as superclavicular and inguinal adenopathy. Sex Transm Dis 4:12, 1977

27. Dan M, Rotmensch HH, Eylan E, et al: A case of lymphogranuloma venereum of 20 years' duration. Br J Vener Dis 56:455, 1980

28. Grace AW: Anorectal lymphogranuloma venereum. JAMA 122:74, 1943

29. Quinn TC, Goodell SE, Mkrtichian E, et al: Chlamydia trachomatis proctitis. N Engl J Med 305:195, 1981

30. Geller SA, Zimmerman MJ, Cohen A: Rectal Biopsy in early lymphogranuloma venereum proctitis. Am J Gastroenterol 74:433, 1980

31. Levine JS, Smith PD, Burgge WR: Chronic proctitis in male homosexuals due to lymphogranuloma venereum. Gastroenterology 79:563, 1980

32. Bolan RK, Sands M, Schachter J, et al:

Lymphogranloma venereum and acute ulcerative proctitis. Am J Med 72:703, 1982

33. Sabin AB, Aring CD: Meningoencephalitis in man caused by the virus of lymphogranuloma venereum. JAMA 120:1376, 1942

34. Sheldon WH, Wall MJ, Slade JD, Heyman A: Lymphogranuloma venereum in a patient with mediastinal lymphoadenopathy and pericarditis. Arch Intern Med 82:410, 1948

35. Barth C, Alexenco W: Beitrag zur Frage der Lymphogranulomatosis inguinalis. Klin Wochenschr 20:102, 1941

36. Schachter J, Smith DE, Dawson CR, et al: Lymphogranuloma venereum. Comparison of the Frei test, complement fixation test, and isolation of the agent. J Infect Dis 120:372, 1969

37. Bjerke JR, Hovding G: Lymphogranuloma venereum with hepatic involvement. Acta Derm Venerol (Stockh) 57:90, 1977

38. Sengupta BS: Vulval cancer following or coexisting with chronic granulomatous disease of the vulva. Trop Doct 11:110, 1981

39. Sowmini CN: Donovanosis. p 205. In Holmes KK, Mardh P-A (eds): International Perspectives on Neglected Sexually Transmitted Diseases. McGraw-Hill, New York, 1983

40. Ronald AR, Wilt JC, Albritton WL: Haemophilus ducreyi. p 93. In Holmes KK, Mardh P-A (eds): International Perspectives on Neglected Sexually Transmitted Diseases. McGraw-Hill, New York, 1983

41. Najafi JA, Guzman LG, Fields J: Surgical aspects of inguinal lymphogranuloma venereum. Milit Med 144:697, 1979

42. Schachter J: Confirmatory serodiagnosis of lymphogranuloma venereum proctitis may yield false-positive results due to other chlamydial infections of the rectum. Sex Transm Dis 8:26, 1981

43. Klatz SA, Drutz DJ, Tam MR, Reed KH: Hemorrhagic proctitis due to lymphogranuloma venereum sero-group L2. Diagnosis by fluorescent monoclonal antibody. N Engl J Med 308:1563, 1983

44. Schuch RJ, Musich JR, Nelson RL: Chlamydial proctitis: Unusual presentation as a symptomatic vaginal mass. Obstet Gynecol 63:132, 1984

45. Greaves AB, Hilleman MR, Taggart SR, et al: Chemotherapy in bubonic lymphogranuloma venereum. A clinical and serological evaluation. Bull WHO 16:277, 1963

46. Sowmini CN, Gopalan KN, Rao GC: Minocycline in the treatment of lymphogranuloma venereum. J Am Vener Dis Assoc 2:19, 1976

8

Chancroid

Axel W. Hoke

Chancroid is an acute autoinoculable infectious disease usually affecting the genital region. It is characterized clinically by multiple painful ulcerations often accompanied by suppurative regional lymphadenopathy. Chancroid has been recognized as a clinical entity for centuries, and was, and often still is, confused with other sexually transmitted diseases.

In 1852 Bassereau[1] first clearly differentiated chancroid from syphillis, and seven years later Ducrey[2] identified the causative organism that still bears his name. In 1900 Bezancon and his colleagues[3] were the first to culture *Haemophilus ducreyi* in vitro.

ETIOLOGY

The causative organism of chancroid is *Haemophilus ducreyi*, a small gram-negative bacillus with rounded ends, 0.5 μm in width by 1.5 to 2.0 μm in length. It is often considered a streptobacillus because of its tendency to develop chain formations, especially in culture. *H. ducreyi* is non-spore-bearing and non-acid-fast. The organism requires hemin (X factor) for growth, but, unlike some species of *Haemophilus, H. ducreyi* does not require nicotinamide adenine dinucleotide (V factor). The hemin concentration required (200 to 500 μg/m) is much higher than for other *Haemophilus* species. Maximal growth is at 33 to 35°C, in contrast to other bacteria, which grow best at 35 to 37°C. High humidity and 5% CO_2 enhance growth of *H. ducreyi*.

On culture, the colonies appear nonmucoid yellow-gray and are cohesive, which enables them to be pushed across the agar surface.[4] Microscopic examination from cultures show the gram-negative organisms in parallel and tangled chains. Longer chains form on liquid media such as clot preparations because of reduced interfacial tension.

H. ducreyi is nonhemolytic. Biochemical tests for indole, H_2s, catalase, arginine dihydrolase, lysine decarboxylase, ornithine decarboxylase, and urease are all negative. Tests for alkaline phosphatase and nitrate reduction are positive.[5]

EPIDEMIOLOGY AND INCIDENCE

Chancroid is found throughout the world, but is most common in tropical and subtropical countries. Historically, seamen have acquired it in seaports, usually from prostitutes. During times of war the incidence has risen. During the Korean conflict Asin[6] reported the incidence 14 times that of syphilis and nearly twice that of gonorrha. He personally observed 1,402 cases. Among American soliders in Vietnam it was second only to gonorrhea in frequency.[7] In 1982 the incidence of chancroid among American troops stationed in Korea was still nearly as great as gonorrhea.[8] Recent introduction of more reliable culture techniques[9,10] has led to more reports of outbreaks of chancroid throughout the world.[11–16]

The Centers for Disease Control reported 1,392 cases in 1982 and 847 in 1983. However, since chancroid is not considered a reportable infectious disease in the United States, these statistics are not accurate. Many cases of chancroid are still diagnosed primarily on clinical grounds without adequate laboratory confirmation. Even well-trained venereologists may be in error almost half of the time.[17]

In most reports of chancroid males outnumber females more than 10:1,[18] but during a recent epidemic in Greenland, the ratio was 1.6:1.[12] This was attributed to a low prostitute population, prostitution being considered a major factor in the usual preponderance of chancroid in males. Chancroid is much more common in uncircumcised men, maceration beneath the prepuce perhaps reducing the normal integumental barrier to infection.

CLINICAL CHARACTERISTICS

The incubation period of chancroid varies from 1 to 14 days, with most cases occurring 2 to 6 days following sexual contact. Incubation in females tends to be somewhat longer than in males for reasons that are not clear.[12]

The lesion first appears at the site of inoculation as a tender papule or small vesicopustule. This rapidly breaks down to form an ulcer, which varies in size from several millimeters to several centimeters. The typical ulcer is sharply punched out with an erythematous halo. The edges are often ragged, undermined, and characteristically soft (as opposed to the hard chancre of syphilis). The base is usually covered with a mucopurulent exudate giving the ulcer a "dirty" appearance (Plate 8-1) (as opposed to the cleaner ulcer of classic primary syphilis). Pain is the most frequent presenting complaint, although older lesions tend to become less painful, and some cases are entirely painless. In a series of 500 cases of chancroid observed by Tan and coworkers[19] pain was reported in only 19% of the patients! Also, as the lesion ages, fibrosis may alter the initially soft margins to produce a cartilaginous feel not unlike that of a syphilitic chancre. The majority of the patients we have seen have presented with two or more ulcers, often at readily traumatized sites such as the frenulum. Autoinoculation produces the so-called "kissing ulcers" (Plate 8-2). However, Asin[6] reported multiple ulcers in only 30% of his 1,402 cases. In size the ulcers vary from 1 mm to several centimeters.

In males the most common locations for ulcers are, in order of frequency, the frenulum (Plate 8-3) and coronal sulcus, internal surface of the prepuce, preputal margins, glans penis, shaft of the penis, and corona. Less frequently, lesions are seen on the scrotum, pubis (Plate 8-4), anus, or thighs.[6] Urethral discharge may mask a rare intraurethral chancroid lesion.[20] In women lesions occur on the labia, clitoris, fourchette (Fig. 8-1) vestibule, and anus. As can be seen, the most common sites in both men and women are the areas most often traumatized during sexual contact. A frequent presenting complaint of a typical male patient is that he got a "hair cut" from his partner's pubic hair. Extragenital ulcers are rare, but have been reported on the tongue, lips, eyelids, breasts,[17] and finger.[21]

A number of clinical variants of chancroid have been described. "Dwarf chancroid" with multiple small, shallow, painful

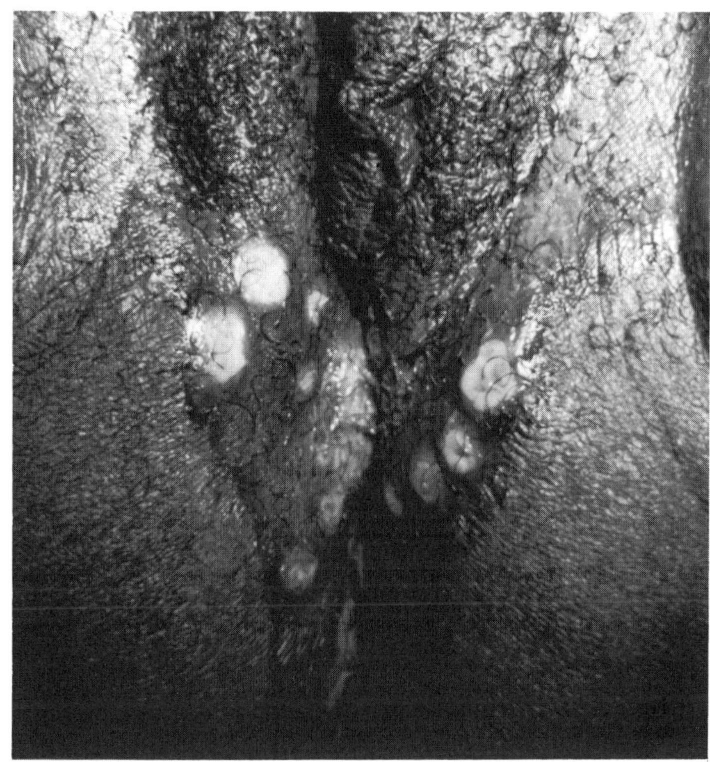

Fig. 8-1 Multiple painful chancroid ulcerations of the anogenital area in a woman. (Courtesy of Antoinette F. Hood, M.D.)

ulcerations, usually on the prepuce, is easily confused with herpes genitalis. Giant or serpiginous chancroid (Fig. 8-2), with lesions spreading by autoinoculation, may extend to the groin or thigh. Less common forms include transient chancroid (chancre mou volant). This rare type consists of a small ulcer that resolves spontaneously in 4 to 6 days and is followed 10 to 20 days later by an acute regional lymphadenitis

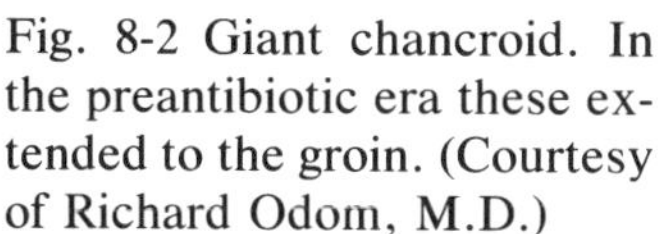

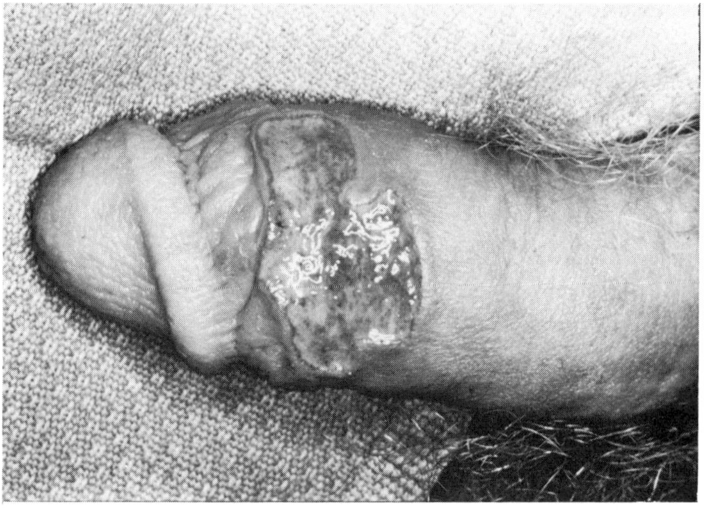

Fig. 8-2 Giant chancroid. In the preantibiotic era these extended to the groin. (Courtesy of Richard Odom, M.D.)

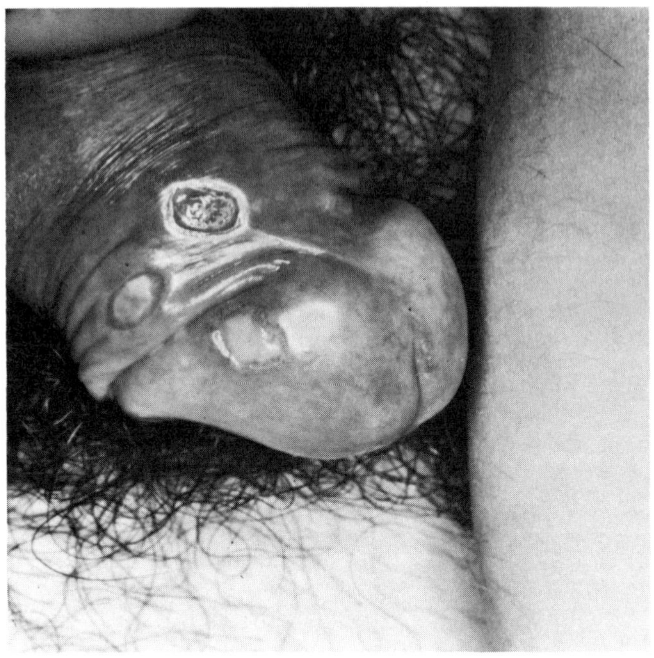

Fig. 8-3 Mixed infection of chancroid and syphilis. Note positive skin test on the arm (Ito-Reenstierna); this test is no longer used because of poor specificity.

mimicking lymphogranuloma venereum. Phagadenic chancroid (Plate 8-5), a rapidly destructive type believed to occur secondarily to a superimposed fusospirochetal infection, is now fortunately rare.

Inguinal adenitis is seen in about half the patients. It appears 1–2 weeks after the onset of the primary lesion, is usually unilateral and painful, and may become fluctuant and rupture (Plate 8-6). Other complications of chancroid include balanitis, paraphimosis (Plate 8-7), and phimosis (Plate 8-8). Urethral fistulas have been reported. Mixed infections with other venereal diseases, especially herpes genitalis and syphilis (Fig. 8-3), must be kept in mind, since they alter the clinical picture and response to therapy. Low-grade fever and mild malaise are present only on rare occasions.

DIAGNOSIS

The diagnosis of chancroid is usually made when the clinical presentation is suggestive (i.e., multiple, painful genital ul-

cerations appearing several days after sexual contact) and other venereal diseases such as genital herpes and primary syphilis have been ruled out. Unfortunately, diagnoses based solely on the above are often erroneous.[18] A presumptive diagnosis of chancroid is supported by the following laboratory procedures.

SMEARS.[22] Prior to obtaining the specimen, the lesion must be carefully cleansed with isotonic saline to reduce contaminating organisms. The material should be collected from an undermined edge of the ulcer with a cotton-tipped applicator, which is then rolled across the slide in one direction so as to preserve the morphologic integrity of the organisms. On Gram-stain the organisms of *H. ducreyi* are found in small clusters or in short parallel chains along strands of mucus. At times larger groups may assume a "school-of-fish" configuration (Plate 8-9). Interpretation of these smears has to be done with care, since other genital flora including *Gardnerella vaginalis* (usually not found in chains) and *Bacteroides* species

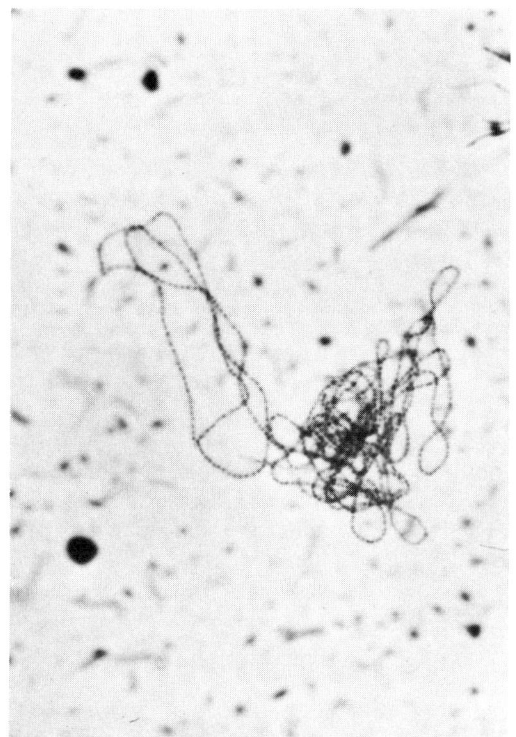

Fig. 8-4 Long twisting chains of *Haemophilus ducreyi* from clot culture. *Note:* liquid media allow longer chains to develop than solid media.

(usually shorter and not in chains) could be mistaken for *H. ducreyi*. Stains other than gram such as Barritt's modification of Pappenheim's pyronin methyl green stain may be helpful. This stains pus cells bluish green and bacteria a brilliant red.[23]

Cultures. *H. ducreyi* is a fastidious organism but may be cultured on selective media recently introduced. Hammond and coworkers[13] used an enriched chocolate agar to which vancomycin was added to prevent overgrowth by contaminants. Sottnek and associates[10] had good results with a heart infusion agar to which fetal bovine serum and vancomycin had been added. Human blood either from the patient or a volunteer is a readily available liquid culture medium. The technique[22] consists of inoculating serum from a well cleaned ulcer in 10 ml of blood that has been previously heated to 56°C for 30 minutes. (*Note:* Heat inactivation may not be necessary.) The serum is incubated at 35°C for 48 hours and gram stained smears from the pellicle examined for *H. ducreyi* (Fig. 8-4, Plate 8-10). Overgrowth with contaminating organisms may be reduced by the addition of vancomycin 3 mg/L. A newly developed rapid-identification system, the Rap I D N H system (Innovative Diagnostic Systems, Inc., Decatur, Ga) with a database for *Haemophilus, Neisseria*, and other fastidious gram-negative bacilli may become a useful confirmatatory diagnostic tool.[24] Indirect fluorescent antibody techniques for the cultural identification of *H. ducreyi* may show promise.[25]

Most recently, Hansen and Loftus have described the use of monoclonal antibodies to detect *H. ducreyi* in skin lesions of animals. They suggest that monoclonal antibodies, either through direct or indirect immunofluorescent techniques, have the potential for use as a rapid immunodiagnostic test for chancroid (Fig. 8-5).

BIOPSY. Biopsy may be a diagnostic aid but is not indicated in most cases. Three vertically arranged zones proceeding from the floor of the ulcer include the following:

1. Superficial necrotic zone composed of necrotic debris, fibrin, red blood cells, polymorphonuclear leukocytes and in appropriately stained sections, rod-shaped organisms;

2. A midzone of proliferating blood vessels with endothelial swelling which may result in occlusion with subsequent tissue necrosis;

3. A deep zone of diffuse infiltrate of plasma cells and lymphocytes.

MISCELLANEOUS TESTS OF HISTORICAL INTEREST. The intradermal skin test (Ito-Reenstierna) proved to be nonspecific and

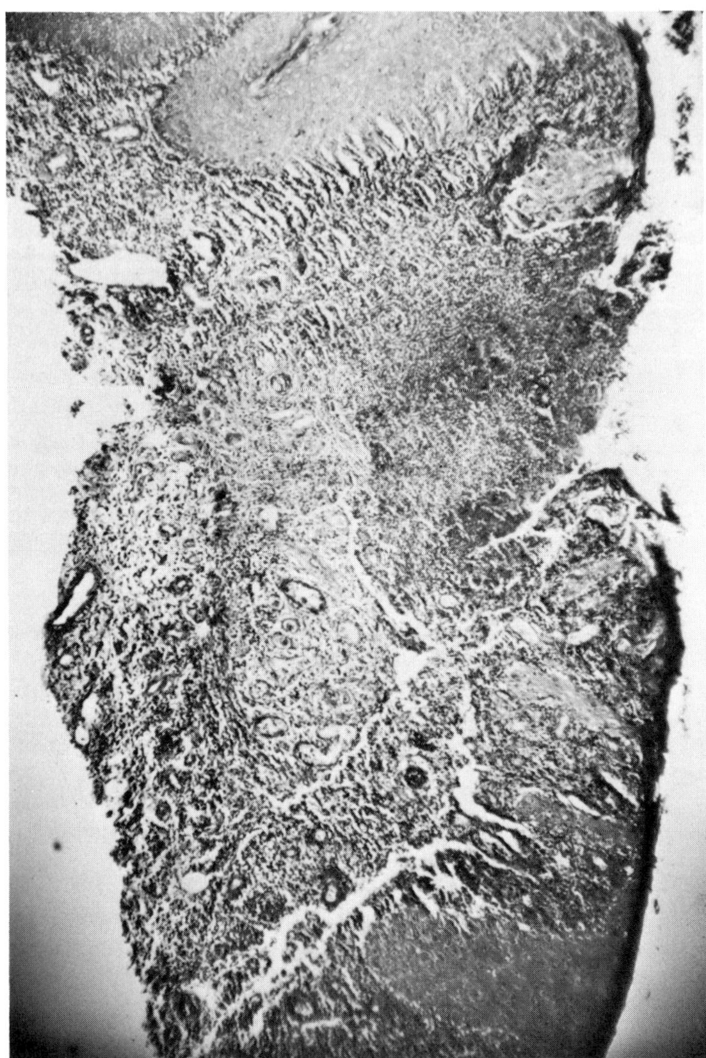

Fig. 8-5 Biopsy of chancroid. *Note*: The superficial necrotic zone, and a midzone with proliferating blood vessels, some showing occlusion.

is no longer available. Autoinoculation may produce serious infection at the site of inoculation and is no longer used.

DIFFERENTIAL DIAGNOSIS

Causes of painful genital lesions other than chancroid include trauma (the all too common zipper cut) human bites (Fig. 8-6), herpes genitalis, atypical primary syphilis, lymphogranuloma venereum and granuloma inguinale.[28] Less common considerations are primary cutaneous gonococcal infection, infected scabies, microaerophilic streptococci[29] and Behçet's syndrome.

TREATMENT

The Centers for Disease Control recommends erythromycin 500 mg given orally four times a day for 10 days as the treatment of choice for chancroid.[16] An alternate re-

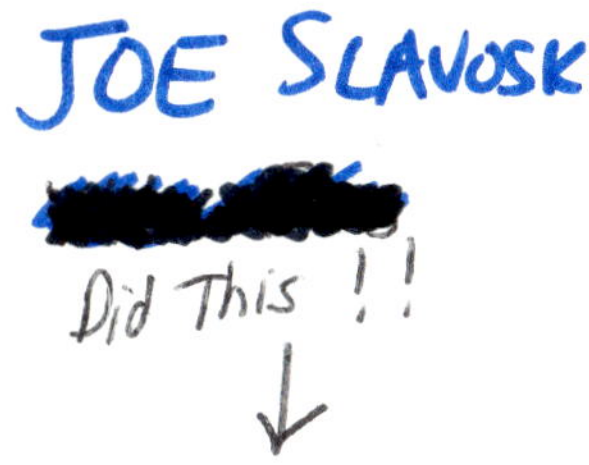

Fig. 8-6 Human bite of penis. Painful multiple infected ulcers mimicking chancroid.

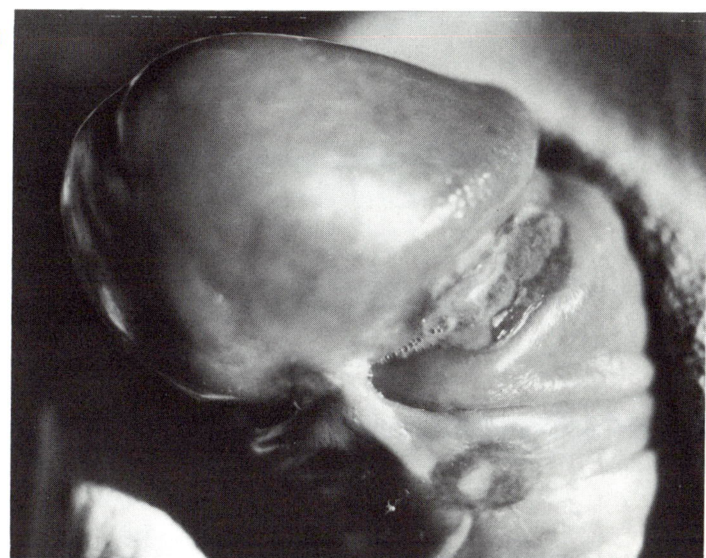

gime is trimethoprim (160 mg)/sulfamethoxazole (800 mg) twice a day for 10 days. Duration of therapy may have to be longer in the presence of large ulcerations or lymphadenitis and should be continued till lesions have healed. Most strains of *H. ducreyi* are now resistant to tetracycline. Many strains of *H. ducreyi* are also susceptible to aminoglycosides, cephalosporins, and cephamycins.[30]

Fluctuant lymph nodes should be carefully aspirated through an 18-gauge needle. Moist cool compresses help debride the ulcers and reduce pain. Dorsal slit for relief of phimosis should be avoided since extension of infection may ensue. Sexual contacts should be examined and even if no evidence of chancroid is found, they should be treated with a 10-day course of erythromycin or sulfamethoxazole-trimethoprim.

REFERENCES

1. Bassereau P: Traité des Affections de la Peau Symptomatiques de la Syphilis. Ballière, Paris, 1852
2. Ducrey A: Experimentelle Untersuchungen über den Ansteckungsstoff des Weichen Schankers und über die Bubonen. Monatsshr Prakt Dermatol 9:387, 1892
3. Bezancon F, Griffon V, Le Sourd L: Culture du Bacille du Chancre Mou. CR Soc Biol (Paris) 52:1048, 1900
4. Hammond GW, Chang JL, Wilt JC, et al: Antimicrobial susceptibility of Hemophilus ducreyi. Antimicrob Agents Chemother 13:608, 1978
5. Kilian M: Taxonomic study of the genus Hemophilus, with the proposal of a new species. J Gen Microbiol 39:9, 1976
6. Asin J: Chancroid: A report of 1,402 cases. Am J Syph 26:483, 1952
7. Kerber RE, Rowe CE, Gilbert KR: Treatment of chancroid: A comparison of tetracycline and sulfasoxazole. Arch Dermatol 100:604, 1969
8. Fitzpatrick JE, Aeling JL: Chancroid: A review with emphasis on recent changes in incidence and treatment. J Assoc Mil Derm 8:31, (Spring) 1982
9. Hammond GW, Lian CT, Wilt JC, et al: Comparison of specimen collection and laboratory techniques for isolation of Hemophilus ducreyi. J Clin Microbiol 7:39, 1978
10. Sottnek FO, Biddle JW, Kraus SJ, et al: Isolation and identification of Hemophilus ducreyi in a clinical study. J Clin Microbiol 12:170, 1980
11. Nayyar KC, Stolz E, Michel MF: Rising in-

cidence of chancroid in Rotterdam. Epidemiological, clinical, diagnostic, and therapeutic aspects. Br J Vener Dis 55:439, 1979

12. Lykke-Olsen L, Larsen L, Pedersen TG, et al: Epidemic of chancroid in Greenland 1977–1978. Lancet 1:654, 1979

13. Hammond GW, Slutchuk M, Scatlift J, et al: Epidemiologic, clinical, laboratory, and therapeutic features of an urban outbreak of chancroid in North America. Rev Infect Dis 2:867, 1980

14. Hansfield HH, Totten PA, Fennel CL, et al: Molecular epidemiology of Hemophilus ducreyi infections. Ann Intern Med 95:315, 1981

15. Hafitz A, Kinghorn GR, McEntegart M: Chancroid in Sheffield: A report of twenty-two cases diagnosed by isolating Hemophilus ducreyi in a modified medium. Br J Vener Dis 57:382, 1981

16. Centers for Disease Control: Chancroid—California. MMWR 31:173, 1982

17. Chapel TA, Brown WJ, Jeffries G, Stewart JA: How reliable is the morphologic diagnosis of penile ulcerations? Sex Transm Dis 4:150, 1977

18. Hart G: Chancroid, donovanosis, lymphogronulome venereum. DHEW Publication No (CDC) 17:8302, 1975

19. Tan T, Rajan VS, Koe SL, et al: Chancroid 1977: A study of 500 cases. Asian J Infect Dis 1:27, 1977

20. Coombes FC: Chancroid disease and its treatment. NY State J Med 46:1700, 1946

21. Brandt R, Sanderson ES, Hicks DV: Extragenital chancroid: A case report. Vener Dis Inform 22:89, 1941

22. Borchardt KA, Hoke AW: Simplified laboratory technique for diagnosis of chancroid. Arch Dermatol 102:188, 1970

23. Barritt MM: An improved Pappenheim stain for detection of gonococci in smears of pus. Br Med J 1:254, 1943

24. Hannah P, Greenwood JR: Isolation and Rapid Identification of Hemophilus ducreyi. J Clin Microbiol 16:861, 1982

25. Denys GA, Chapel TA, Jeffries CD: An indirect fluorescent antibody technique for Hemophilus ducreyi. Health Lab Sci 15:128, 1978

26. Hansen EJ, Loftus TA: Monoclonal antibodies reactive with all strains of Haemophilus ducreyi. Infect Immun 44:196,1984

27. Margolis RJ, Hood AF: Chancroid: Diagnosis and treatment. J Am Acad Dermatol 6:493, 1982

28. Werman BS, Herskowitz LJ, Olansky S, et al: A clinical variant of chancroid resembling granuloma inguinale. Arch Dermatol 119:890, 1983

29. Leibovitz A: An outbreak of pyogenic penile ulcers associated with microaerophilic streptococcus resembling Haemophilus ducreyi. Am J Syphil Gonorr Vener Dis 38:203, 1954

30. Kraus SJ, Kaufman HW, Albritton WL, et al: Chancroid therapy: A review of cases confirmed by culture. Rev Infect Dis 4(Suppl):S848, 1982

9

Granuloma Inguinale

Ted Rosen
Jaime A. Tschen

DEFINITION

Granuloma inguinale, also known as granuloma venereum, donovanosis, ulcerating granuloma of the pudenda, granuloma donovani, and granuloma pudenda tropicum, is a sexually transmitted disease characterized by chronic, indolent, ulcerogranulomatous lesions of the skin and mucous membranes.

ETIOLOGY

Although Koch's postulates have not been completely fulfilled, granuloma inguinale is widely accepted to be caused by *Calymmatobacterium granulomatis*, previously known as *Donovania granulomatis* or *Klebsiella granulomatis*. This organism is a small (1.0 to 1.5 μm × 0.5 to 0.7 μm) gram-negative pleomorphic bacillus with serologic cross-reactivity with both *Klebsiella rhinoscleromatis* and some Enterobacteriaceae.[1]

The disease has reputedly been reproduced in human subjects by direct innoculation of lesion exudate or tissue fragments.[2–5] The incubation period under experimental condition varies from several weeks to nearly 2 months—closely correlating with clinical observations on probable incubation duration. It is noteworthy, however, that transfer of material from culture media to either animals or humans rarely, if ever, results in development of experimental infection.[6] Thus, all features of Koch's postulates remain unsatisfied.

The possibility of a contributory defect in cellular immunity among affected individuals has been proposed by some authorities.[7] This seems feasible in view of disease despite detectable circulating antibodies and the presence of intracellular organisms. This consideration remains to be fully investigated.

EPIDEMIOLOGY

The usual age range for patients with granuloma inguinale is the second and third decades of life, which corresponds with the peak age of incidence for most other sexually transmitted diseases.[7–10] A predilection for dark-skinned individuals has been suggested,[11] but this likely relates more to the usual areas of endemic disease rather than to actual racial susceptibility. The disease is also commonly seen among individuals of low socioeconomic status; again, this probably relates to poor hygiene and/or social habits rather than any genetic predisposition. There is clearly a male sex bias with a ratio of about 2:1. Nonetheless, the disorder is certainly seen in female patients in all parts of the world.[12–14]

Granuloma inguinale was first recognized as a distinct disease in India by McLeod.[15] Earliest morphologic/histologic studies were reported from India in 1905 by Donovan.[16] The disease is encountered primarily, though not exclusively, in tropical and semitropical regions of the world. Granuloma inguinale remains endemic in portions of Africa and southeast Asia, in southern India, and in New Guinea.[17] In contrast, the disease is virtually unknown in Europe and Japan. Grindon[18] first reported the presence of granuloma inguinale in the United States in 1913. Most cases have been reported from southern or southeastern states in a sporadic fashion. The overall American incidence of this disease has been steadily declining, with only an estimated 50 cases annually.[19,20] A localized epidemic was recently reported from Houston, Texas during 1982–1983.[21]

Sexual contact remains the most likely most of transmission of granuloma inguinale. Nonetheless, the exact mechanisms of infection/transmission remains controversial. Several studies highlight aspects that suggest a nonvenereal etiology: low incidence among prostitutes, occurrence in both elderly and very young sexually inactive individuals, and the occasional presence of only extragenital lesions.[9,22] Moreover, some authorities maintain that granuloma inguinale is rare among sexual partners of patients with active and presumably contagious lesions. Packer and Goldberg[1] reported that the sexual partner was infected in only two of approximately 500 cases. Proponents of this viewpoint contend that organisms—which have been reportedly recovered from the gut[23]—become pathogenic when fecal contamination comes into contact with breaks in the genital, perineal, or perianal skin.

While the foregoing lines of evidence suggest that transmission may not be entirely venereal in the usual sense, more recent epidemiologic data support the proposition that granuloma inguinale is generally a sexually transmitted disease. For example, Lal and Nicholas[10] note the frequent occurrence of concomitant STD's, involvement in sexual partners in 52% of cases, and genital lesions in 90% of cases. During the recent outbreak in Texas, a female prostitute, her husband, and four "customers" all developed the disorder. Such a cluster of cases is difficult to explain unless granuloma inguinale is indeed as STD on the classic sense.

A final epidemiologic facet of this disease that remains unresolved concerns the relationship between granuloma inguinale and genital carcinoma. Cutaneous squamous cell carcinomas have been reported to arise in lesions of granuloma inguinale.[24,25] Complement-fixing antibody to *Calymmatobacterium granulomatis* was detected in about 15% of male patients with penile carcinoma, while antibody was not found among control sera.[26] On the other hand, many patients with genital carcinoma have neither clinical evidence, history, or serologic findings consistent with granuloma inguinale. In addition, some cases of alleged genital carcinoma coincident with or due to granuloma inguinale may actually represent the infection simulating a malignancy.[14]

DIAGNOSIS

The diagnosis of granuloma inguinale depends upon a characteristic clinical appearance coupled with typical histologic findings. Four clinical variants are recognized: ulcerovegetative, nodular, hypertrophic, and cicatricial. Ulcerovegetative lesions, which are the most common, begin as papules or small nodules, which rapidly erode

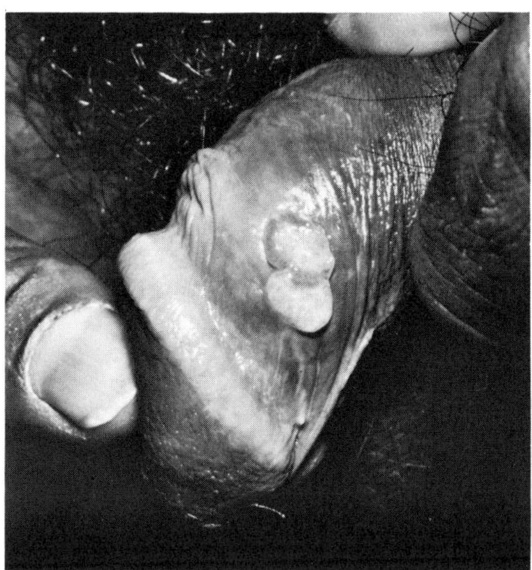

Fig. 9-1 A variant of granuloma inguinale consists of fleshy nodules resembling condyloma accuminatum.

to form a spreading ulcer. Such lesions typically demonstrate a rolled border and a beefy, friable, exuberant granulation tissue at the base (Plates 9-1A,B). Nodular lesions appear as soft, erythematous papules with a granulation tissuelike surface (Fig. 9-1). The rare hypertrophic and cicatricial forms demonstrate large vegetating masses and expanding cicatricial plaques, respectively. Lesions of granuloma inguinale—even extensive ulcerative ones—are generally painless. True lymphadenopathy is not seen; however, involvement of inguinal subcutaneous tissue may produce indurated areas that resemble lymphadenitis ("pseudobuboes"). Constitutional symptoms are absent. In men, lesions are most commonly found on the prepuce or in the coronal sulcus; in women, lesions favor the labia or fourchette, but may also bc found in the vagina or on the cervix. In male homosexuals, perianal lesions are commonly encountered.[27]

Left untreated, genital granuloma inguinale can be mutilating.[6] In men, this disorder may destroy the entire penis. In women, long-standing disease results in elephan-

tiasis-like enlargement of the external genitalia with extensive perineal ulceration. Pregnancy may accelerate the disease process; there is no evidence of congenital transmission.[28]

Extragenital cutaneous[29] and oral[30] lesions have been reported, but fewer than 10% of patients are so affected. Presumably hematogenous dissemination has, rarely, led to osseous involvement[31–33] as well as to involvement of the visceral organs.

In addition to clinically compatible lesions, the diagnosis of granuloma inguinale requires the identification of causative organisms (Donovan bodies) in affected tissue. This is a difficult, time-consuming task, and the yield from touch or crush preparations or biopsy specimens varies from case to case. Lesional tissue should be stained with Wright's, Giemsa, or argentaffin (e.g., Worthin-Starry) stains. Organisms are found intracellularly within mononuclear histiocytes; a safety-pin shape may be apparent due to bipolar staining (Fig. 9-2). The number of intracytoplasmic organisms varies, but there are usually ten or more per cell. Individual organisms or groups of organisms are observed with cytoplasmic compartments presumed to be phagosomes.

Freshly prepared tissue crush specimens are said to demonstrate organisms more readily than formalin-fixed paraffin-embedded biopsy specimens.[34] The use of a plastic-embedded thin section stained with polychrome is an alternative and highly efficient method of identifying Donovan bodies in biopsy specimens.[35] Regardless of the technique employed, repeated sampling may be necessary in order to verify this diagnosis.[36] If the patient has applied over-the-counter topical antibacterial preparations or ingested antibiotics for even a few days, it becomes increasingly difficult to find the causative organisms.

Ultrastructural features are nonspecific and consistent with those common to gram-negative bacilli: a large distinct capsule and absence of a flagellum.[37,38]

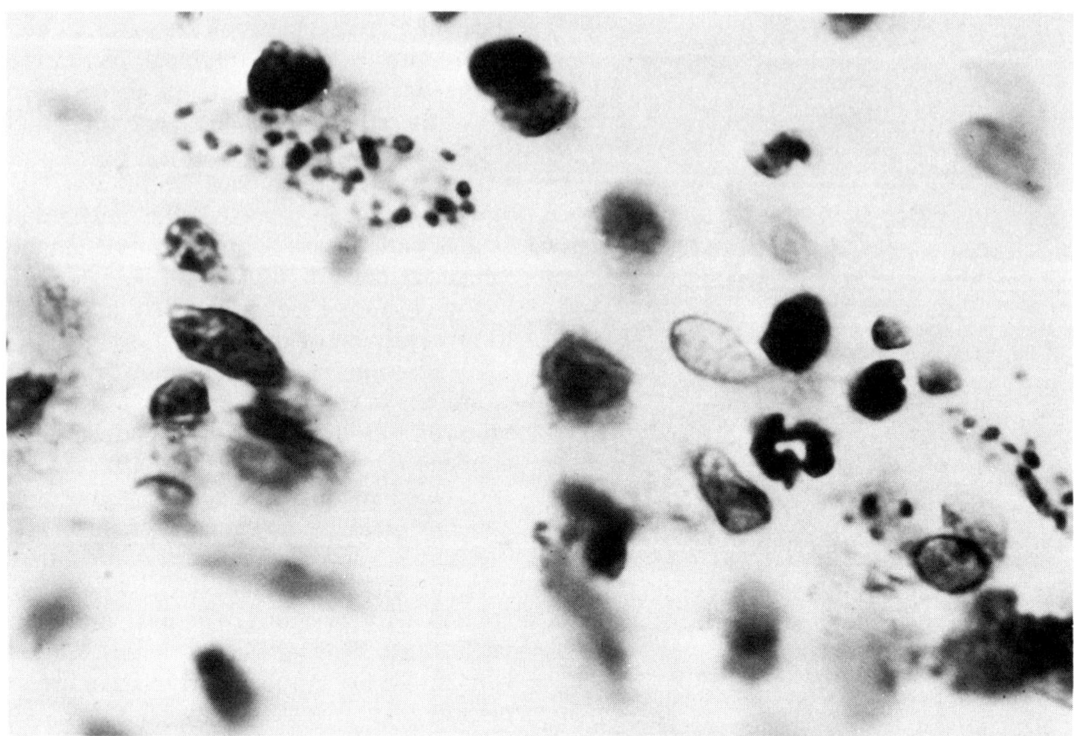

Fig. 9-2 Organisms of granuloma inguinale within macrophages are demonstrated in silver stain.

Culture for *Calymmatobacterium granulomatis* is not practical and therefore is not readily available. Peptidelike materials and an anaerobic or microaerophillic environment facilitate growth of these organisms. The most consistently successful culture technique has been inoculation of infected matter into the yolk sac of a 5-day-old chick embryo at 37°C.[39,40] Organisms can be recovered after 72 hours of incubation in this system. Coagulated egg yolk slants have also been used with some success.[5]

DIFFERENTIAL DIAGNOSIS

Because the laboratory manipulation involved are so tedious, the diagnosis of granuloma inguinale, especially in endemic areas, is based solely on morphologic grounds. Despite the fact that this disorder does indeed present with a characteristic clinical picture, such reliance on observation alone is fraught with many potential errors.[41]

Granuloma inguinale should be considered in the diagnosis of any ulcerative or granulomatous lesion of the perineal region. A complete differential diagnosis should also include tumor, chancroid, syphilis, chronic herpes simplex, and anogenital cutaneous amebiasis. Less likely to be confused with granuloma inguinale would be a host of diseases that result in superficial genital erosions (typical herpes progenitalis, erythema multiforme, fixed drug eruption, pemphigus vulgaris, and so on).

Lesions suspected of being granuloma inguinale should be biopsied if they fail to respond to adequate antimicrobial therapy. Genital carcinoma and granuloma inguinale may closely resemble one another and may even be coexistent.

In contrast to lesions of granuloma inguinale, those of chancroid are generally more acute, considerably more painful, more suppurative than granulomatous at the base, less progressive, and less indurated. Lymphadenopathy is typical of chancroid, but is unusual in granuloma inguinale. While classic lesions of these two diseases are easily differentiated on the above basis, a variant of chancroid exists that almost exactly mimics granuloma inguinale on purely morphologic grounds.[42] Chancroid cultures, though difficult, may be necessary to identify the causative bacteria when clinical confusion exists.

Typical chancres of primary syphilis are cleaner, more indurated, and less progressive than lesions of granuloma inguinale. Lymphadenopathy is the rule in lues as well. Hypertrophic, moist papules or nodules of secondary syphilis—condyloma-lata—may be mistaken clinically for the nodular variety of granuloma inguinale. A darkfield examination readily demonstrates treponemes in condylomata and serologic tests for syphilis are nearly always positive.

Chronic herpes simplex infections—encountered in immunocompromised hosts—present with persistent, progressive, suppurative to granulomatous, erosions in the anogenital area. Viral cultures disclose the true nature of such lesions.

While anogenital amebiasis is rare in the United States, it is likely to be encountered among individuals from tropical regions typically endemic for granuloma inguinale. Chronic cutaneous lesions, known as amebomas, may be clinically indistinguishable from those of granuloma inguinale. In patients from appropriate parts of the world, a history should be obtained for gastrointestinal symptoms which might suggest prior amebic dysentery. Biopsy of suspected lesions will demonstrate causative parasites and thereby distinguish this disease from granuloma inguinale.

TREATMENT

Systemic in-vitro antibiotic sensitivity testing of the presumed causative bacterium has not been performed. Therefore, all treatment protocols herein advanced are based upon empiric results of various antimicrobial agent treats. Therapy usually requires 2 to 4 weeks, the exact duration of treatment being dependent upon clinical response.

Tetracycline remains the consensus drug of choice, administered orally in a total daily dose of 2 g (500 mg four times daily). While prompt involution is the rule, resistance to this agent is well documented both in the United States and elsewhere.[43,44] Nonetheless, the ease of administration, relative safety, and low cost dictate a trial of tetracycline in all proven cases of granuloma inguinale. Minocycline, a close biochemical relative of tetracycline, has been used to treat a small number of patients successfully.[45] This agent is considerably more costly and probably offers no inherent advantage over tetracycline.

Streptomycin, in a total intramuscular dose of 20–30 g given over 5 to 10 days, is generally regarded as equally efficacious in this disorder.[46–49] However, this therapeutic modality is inconvenient and uncomfortable, requiring multiple injections. Moreover, streptomycin is potentially ototoxic and has been associated with up to a 9% failure rate.[49]

Oral chloramphenicol, in a total daily dose of 2 g, is quite effective with a low, 2%, failure rate.[50,51] However, the real potential for fatal blood dyscrasias (aplastic anemia, granulocytopenia, and others) precludes the use of this drug when safer medications are equally efficacious.

The use of 1–2 g daily of oral ampicillin is justifiable in tetracycline-resistant cases.[43,52] Ampicillin therapy has resulted in clinical cure of cases from both the United States and Asia. However, others feel that the response to ampicillin is inconsistent.[34] Thus, this agent should not be utilized as first-line treatment.

Lincomycin,[43] erythromycin,[53] and sodium methacillin[54] have all been used to successfully treat limited numbers of patients with granuloma inguinale. Neither short-term nor long-term efficacy of these agents has been adequately confirmed. Thus, these antibiotics should be reserved as backup alternatives when conventional therapy fails.

Recent work indicates that a viable, highly effective, convenient and relatively safe therapy may be trimethoprim/sulfamethoxazole (cotrimoxazole). In a preliminary study from India, 10 patients treated with twice daily trimethoprim 160 mg/sulfamethoxazole 800 mg cleared within two weeks.[55] An expanded series of Indian patients was later reported, confirming short-term therapeutic efficacy and verifying long-term cure rates for this drug.[56] Rosen and coworkers[21] also found trimethoprim/sulfamethoxazole to be curative in their series from the United States. Side effects in these studies were minimal, but this agent has the well-known potential to produce cutaneous drug eruptions, including toxic epidermal necolysis.

In pregnant patients, tetracycline, streptomycin, and chloramphenicol would be clearly contraindicated and sulfa derivatives relatively prohibited. In this unusual situation, erythromycin or other macrolide antibiotics (e.g., lincomycin) would be indicated. The combination of lincomycin and erythromycin has been reported to be satisfactory in pregnant patients with granuloma inguinale.[57]

It should be noted that appropriate treatment may also vary due to the geographic origin of the infection. For example, despite an overall high cure rate, streptomycin is ineffective in treating granuloma inguinale acquired in New Guinea.[17] Such regional variations in therapy should be considered before initiating antibiotic treatment.

CONTROL

It is doubtful that granuloma inguinale can be brought under "control" in the immediate future. The vast majority of cases occur in endemic regions of the world where both medical technology and public health resources are, at best, minimally adequate. The relative infrequency of the disorder dictates that available public health manpower and funds would be better directed toward more pressing problems. Moreover, as the organism is so poorly characterized and difficult to culture, it is unlikely that a vaccine will be developed to permit mass inoculation. Sporadic cases in highly developed countries can be adequately managed by prompt antibiotic administration and thus do little to stimulate major investigative work in the field.

It is imperative that those who deliver medical care, particularly in venereal disease clinic situations, be aware of this disease to prevent major epidemics in unusual areas.

REFERENCES

1. Packer H, Goldberg J: Studies of the antigenic relationship of D. granulomatis to members of the tribe Eschericheae. Am J Syph 34:342, 1950
2. Greenblatt RB, Dienst RB, Pund ER, Torpin R: Experimental and clinical granuloma inguinale. JAMA 113:1109, 1939
3. Dienst RB, Reinstein CR, Kupperman HS, Greenblatt RB: Studies on the causal agent of granuloma inguinale. Am J Syph 31:614, 1947
4. Dienst RB, Greenblatt RB, Chen CH: Experimental transfer of chemo-resistant granuloma inguinale. Am J Syph 34:189, 1950
5. Morse SA: Manual of Clinical Microbiology. 3rd Ed. American Society for Microbiology, Washington DC, 1980
6. Fritz GS, Hubler WR Jr, Dodson RF, Rudolph A: Mutilating granuloma inguinale. Arch Dermatol 111:1464, 1975
7. Maddocks I, Anders EM, Dennis E: Donovanosis in Papula, New Guinea. Br J Vener Dis 52:190, 1976
8. Rajam RV, Rangiah PN: Donovanosis. WHO Monograph 24. World Health Organization, Geneva, 1954

9. Goldberg J: Studies on granuloma inguinale. VII. Some epidemiological considerations of the disease. Br J Vener Dis 40:140, 1964

10. Lal S, Nicholas C: Epidemiological and clinical features in 165 cases of granuloma inguinale. Br J Vener Dis 46:461, 1970

11. D'Aunoy R, Von Hamm E: Granuloma inguinale. Am J Trop Med 17:747, 1937

12. Packer H, Turner HB, Dulaney AD: Granuloma inguinale of the vagina and cervix uteri with bone metastases. JAMA 136:327, 1948

13. Stewart DB: The gynecological lesions of lymphogranuloma venereum and granuloma inguinale. Med Clin North Am 48:773, 1964

14. Jofre ME, Webling DD'A, James ST: Granuloma inguinale simulating advanced pelvic cancer. Med J Aust 2:869, 1976

15. McLeod K: Precis of operations performed on the wards of the first surgeon Medical College Hospital during the year 1881. Indian Med Gaz 17:121, 1882

16. Donovan C: Medical cases from Madras General Hospital. Indian Med Gaz 40:411, 1905

17. World Health Organization: Non-gonococcal urethritis and other selected sexually transmitted diseases of public health importance. WHO Tech Rep 660:1, 1981

18. Grindon J: Granuloma inguinale tropicum: Report of three cases. J Cutan Dis 31:236, 1913

19. Hart G: Chancroid, Donovanosis and Lymphogranuloma Venereum. Department of Health, Education and Welfare Publication 75-8302, Atlanta, 1975

20. Lynch PJ: Therapy of sexually transmitted diseases. Med Clin North Am 66:915, 1982

21. Rosen T, Tschen JA, Ramsdell W, et al: Granuloma inguinale. J Am Acad Dermatol 11:433, 1984

22. Peck S: Granuloma inguinale. Arch Dermatol 98:555, 1968

23. Goldberg J: Studies on granuloma inguinale. V. Isolation of bacterium resembling Donovania granulomatis from the faeces of a patient with granuloma inguinale. Br J Vener Dis 38:99, 1959

24. Beerman H, Sonck CE: The epithelial changes in granuloma inguinale. A J Syph 36:501, 1952

25. Alexander LJ, Shields TL: Squamous cell carcinoma of the vulva secondary to granuloma inguinale. Arch Dermatol 67:395, 1953

26. Goldberg J, Annamunthodo H: Studies on granuloma inguinale. VIII. Serological reactivity in sera from patients with carcinoma of the penis when tested with Donovania antigens. Br J Vener Dis 42:205, 1966

27. Goldberg J, Bernstein R: Studies on granuloma inguinale VI. Two cases of perianal granuloma inguinale in male homosexuals. Br J Vener Dis 40:137, 1964

28. Kuberski T: Granuloma inguinale (donovanosis). Sex Transm Dis 7:29, 1980

29. Sehgal VN, Sharma NL, Bhargava NC, et al: Primary extragenital disseminated cutaneous donovanosis. Br J Dermatol 101:353, 1979

30. Rao MS, Komeswari VR, Ramula C, et al: Oral lesions of granuloma inguinale. J Oral Surg 34:1112, 1976

31. Kalstone BM, Howell JA, Cline FX: Granuloma inguinale with hematogenous dissemination to the spine. JAMA 176:530, 1961

32. Sieber PE: Granuloma inguinale with bone involvement. Am J Roentgenol 95:515, 1965

33. Kirkpatrick DJ: Donovanosis: A rare case of osteolytic bone lesions. Clin Radiol 21:101, 1970

34. Davis CM: Granuloma inguinale. A clinical, histological, and ultrastructural study. JAMA 211:632, 1970

35. Dodson RF, Fritz GS, Hubler WR, et al: Donovaniosis: A morphologic study. J Invest Dermatol 62:611, 1974

36. Marmell M, Santora E: Donovanosis—granuloma inguinale. Incidence, nomenclature, and diagnosis. Am J Syph 34:83, 1950

37. Davis CM, Collins C: Granuloma inguinale: An ultrastructural study of Calymmatobacterium granulomatis. J Invest Dermatol 53:315, 1969

38. Kuberski T, Papadimitriou JM, Phillips P: Ultrastructure of Calymmatobacterium granulomatis in lesions of granuloma inguinale. J Infect Dis 142:744, 1980

39. Anderson K: The cultivation from granuloma inguinale of a microorganism having the characteristics of Donovan bodies in the yolk sac of chick embryos. Science 97:560, 1943

40. Anderson K, Goodpasture EW, De-

Monbreun WA: An etiologic consideration of Donovania granulomatis cultured from granuloma inguinale in embryonic yolk. Exp Med 81:25, 1945

41. Chapel TA, Brown WJ, Jeffries C, Stewart J: How reliable is the morphological diagnosis of penile ulcerations? Sex Transm Dis 4:150, 1977

42. Ulerman BS, Herskowitz LJ, Olansky S, et al: A clinical variant of chancroid resembling granuloma inguinale. Arch Dermatol 119:890, 1983

43. Breschi LC, Goldman G, Shapiro SR: Granuloma inguinale in Vietnam: Successful therapy with ampicillin and lincomycin. J Am Vener Dis Assoc 1:118, 1975

44. Pariser RJ: Tetracycline-resistant granuloma inguinale. Arch Dermatol 113:988, 1977

45. Velasco JE, Miller AE, Zaias N: Minocycline in the treatment of venereal disease. JAMA 220:1323, 1972

46. Barton RL, Craig RM, Schwemlein GX, et al: Granuloma inguinale treated with streptomycin. Report of three cases. Arch Dermatol Syphilol 56:1, 1947

47. Kupperman HS, Greenblatt RB, Dienst RB: Streptomycin in the therapy of granuloma inguinale. JAMA 136:84, 1948

48. Robinson HM: The treatment of granuloma inguinale, lymphogranuloma venereum, chancroid, and gonorrhea. Arch Dermatol Syphilol 64:284, 1951

49. Lal S: Continued efficacy of streptomycin in the treatment of granuloma inguinale. Br J Vener Dis 47:454, 1971

50. Greenblatt RB, Barfield WE, Dienst RB, et al: A five-year study of antibiotics in the treatment of granuloma inguinale. Am J Syph 36:186, 1952

51. Greenblatt RB, Wammock VS, Dienst RB, et al: Chloromycetin in therapy of granuloma inguinale. Am J Obstet Gynecol 59:1129, 1950

52. Thew MA, Swift JT, Heaton CL: Ampicillin in the treatment of granauloma inguinale. JAMA 210:866, 1969

53. Robinson H, Cohen MM: Treatment of granuloma inguinale with erythromycin. J Invest Dermatol 20:407, 1950

54. Marmell M, Prigott A: Granuloma inguinale (donovanosis) treated with methacycline. NY J Med 64:804, 1964

55. Garg BR, Lal S, Sivamani S: Efficacy of co-trimoxazole in donovanosis. A preliminary report. Br J Vener Dis 54:348, 1978

56. Lal S, Garg BR: Further evidence of the efficacy of co-trimoxazole in granuloma venereum. Br J Vener Dis 56:412, 1980

57. Ashdown LR, Kilvert GT: Granuloma inguinale in Northern Queensland. Med J Aust 1:146, 1979

10

Yeast Vaginitis

Pierre Dejace
Stephen H. Zinner

Although not always strictly "sexually transmitted," genital infections due to yeast are extremely common, particularly in women. *Candida albicans* is the yeast isolated most frequently and represents at least 80% of infecting species. Other organisms such as *C. tropicalis* and *Torulopsis glabrata* may be associated with vaginitis. Still other *Candida* species may be cultured from the vagina, but their role in vaginal symptoms is unclear.

Hippocrates[1] described oral thrush in debilitated patients, and Galen[2] reported its presence in sickly children. Its origin in the mother's genital tract was not known until the postulate of Veron[3] in 1835, and the demonstrations by Haussmann[4] in 1875. Although the fungus causing thrush had been described in 1839 by Langenbeck and was further characterized under many different names, the first description of vaginal candidiasis was by Wilkinson[5] in 1849. Nystatin was isolated in 1950 as the first antifungal antibiotic. Earlier, various dyes, such as gentian violet, were used for treatment. More recently, amphotericin B and the imidazoles have been developed.

PREVALENCE AND EPIDEMIOLOGY

As documented by culture, the presence of yeasts in the vagina of normal nonpregnant women not using oral contraceptives varies from 4.3% in India to 8.1% in the United States and 13.3% in Denmark. In other settings, the prevalence can be higher. A study of 533 women visiting a London STD clinical reported yeasts on vaginal culture in 26% of patients.[6] In pregnancy the prevalence of vaginal yeasts varies from 30 to 55% and is greatest near term.[7–9] Many disease states (diabetes, hypoparathyroidism, and other endocrine diseases) and drugs (antibiotics, oral contraceptives, corticosteroids, and other immunosuppressing drugs) have been shown to increase colonization and/or infection with yeasts. The details of the relation of colonization to symptomatic infection are unclear.

Many studies utilizing vaginal cultures have reported frequent yeast colonization in otherwise asymptomatic women. In a British study in a STD clinic population 20% of the patients from whom *Candida albicans* was recovered had neither symptoms nor any clinical evidence of vaginitis.[6] In the same study, 55% of women whose vaginal cultures yielded *Torulopsis glabrata* had no symptoms. In another study vaginal yeast colonization was associated with itch and irritative symptoms in 67% of 42 women, but these symptoms were present in only 22% of 102 women whose vaginal cultures did not contain yeasts.[10]

The presence of yeasts in normal individuals at other body sites (e.g., mouth, gastrointestinal tract, skin), has been documented in numerous studies.[11] Anal colonization may be an important source of vaginal yeast.

Candidal vaginitis is also transmitted sexually. Although genital disease due to yeast is much less frequent in men, carriage of yeasts on the penis or in semen has been reported in up to 18% of normal males.[12] Candidal balanitis has been described in sexual partners of women with vaginal candidiasis. A case control study of 50 couples estimated the sexual transmission of genital yeast infection at 42%.[13]

Certainly not all vaginal candidiasis is due to sexual transmission. The source of vaginal candida is often endogenous, and women are more often colonized than men presumably because of the closer proximity of the vagina to the gastrointestinal reservoir.[14,15] Sexual transmission can perpetuate the infection if the asymptomatic colonized male partner is not treated. (Treatment of the male may be problematic if urethral rather than penile colonization is present.)

The incidence of vaginal candidiasis is rising in Great Britain, where statistics on all STDs are available. *Candida* infections are now the most common conditions diagnosed in women attending STD clinics.[16] The heavy use of oral contraceptives, particularly those high in progestational activity, may be partially responsible for this high prevalence.[17] Changing sexual mores and large numbers of sexual partners may also contribute to the increasing occurrence of this infection.

Candida vaginitis often presents clinically in the week prior to the onset of menses. Some authors also have noted an increase of candidal vaginitis in late summer and early fall. This correlates with a similar seasonal increase in STD clinic visits in England,[18] and may relate to seasonal variation in sexual activity.[19]

MYCOLOGY—PATHOGENESIS— IMMUNOLOGY

Candida albicans is the most common cause of yeast vaginitis and is isolated in 80 to 90% of studied cases. However, other yeasts pathogenic for the vagina have been isolated. *Torulopsis glabrata* represented up to 16% of the isolates in one study and *C. tropicalis* also may cause infection. Other species obtained from vaginal cultures, but rarely implicated causally in symptomatic infection, include *C. parapsilosis, C. kruzei, C. stellatoidea,* and *C. guillermondi.*

Most authors report no clinical differences in the diseases produced by different yeasts. The capacity to cause infection may relate to cellular properties that promote fungal adherence to vaginal epithelial cells.

The use of broad-spectrum antibiotics is one of the most important predisposing factors for *Candida* vaginitis. Antibiotics disturb the balance between *Candida* and other vaginal colonizers with resulting yeast overgrowth. The relative invasiveness of mycelial, compared to blastospore, forms of *C. albicans* has been suggested to be a pathogenetic factor, but this remains controversial.[11,20]

There are relatively few studies of host defense mechanisms involved in vaginal candidiasis. Both polymorphonuclear neutrophils[21] and monocytes[22] have been shown to damage *Candida* in vitro, but their importance in vaginal candidiasis is unclear. Vaginal discharges rarely contain abundant white cells in yeast infection.[23]

Some authors have shown elevated serum antibody titers, particularly secretory IgA, in patients with chronic or recurrent vaginal candidiasis and have emphasized the importance of local immunity.[20] Other studies have suggested a decreased cellular immune response to candidal antigens in women with chronic candidal vaginitis.[24] Most women with vaginal candidiasis are immunologically normal.

CLINICAL MANIFESTATIONS

Although yeast can be present in the vagina in the absence of symptoms and clinical signs of infection, most infected patients present with rather nonspecific symptoms and signs. The most frequent symptoms include pruritis, which is often severe and may or may not be associated with a vaginal discharge.[6] Although classical vaginal candidiasis is associated with a white curdlike or cheesy discharge this is not always present. Vaginal pruritis alone is not specific for mycotic vaginitis, but pruritis may be severe and may lead to vulval excoriations. Vaginal discharge alone may be seen in about one third of cases, but discharge also may be associated with other etiologies in the absence of *Candida* on culture.

On physical examination, a nonspecific picture of vulval or vaginal erythema with or without vulval swelling, edema, or excoriation may be present. Vaginal plaques of raised white or yellow curdlike patches adherent to the inflamed vaginal wall is suggestive of yeast infection, but this may occur in some patients with trichomonas vaginitis.[6] Satellite lesions extending beyond the major area of erythema are strongly suggestive of candidiasis. Vaginal pH is usually elevated to 4.5 or greater in other forms of vaginitis. A vaginal pH of less than 4.5 in the presence of signs and symptoms of vaginitis or vulvovaginitis is suggestive of candidiasis.[25]

DIAGNOSIS AND DIFFERENTIAL DIAGNOSIS

The clinical picture of candidal vaginitis is somewhat variable, but the diagnosis is usually established easily. Candidal vaginitis is the most common cause of vaginal discharge in sexually active and/or pregnant women. It frequently presents in the week preceding menstruation and during pregnancy, and it is associated with the use of antibiotics, steroids, immunosuppressants, and oral contraceptives, and with diabetes.

The diagnosis can be confirmed by direct smear of a drop of vaginal fluid mixed with a drop of 10% potassium hydroxide, often with a drop of methylene blue. Typical mycelial and yeast forms may be seen (Plate 10-1). The Gram stain is not very sensitive, but it is helpful because in the presence of symptoms a positive result permits immediate diagnosis and treatment. Yeast pseudohyphae and mycelia are gram-positive. A negative result on Gram stain or KOH preparation does not rule out candidiasis,[17] and a culture must be performed.

Cultures on Sabauraud's or Nickerson's media (antibiotic-containing media) are sensitive, but do not provide an immediate result. Some yeasts require 48 hours or more to grow, but most strains will be cultured in 24 hours.

In practice, a reasonably accurate presumptive diagnosis can be based on several considerations. In a patient who reports a regular sexual partner (who is asymptomatic) and presents with a vaginal discharge with vaginal pH less than 4.5, and a wet mount negative for *Trichomonas* and clue cells, yeast vaginitis is the most likely diagnosis. This should be confirmed by culture, but it is reasonable to proceed with topical therapy. Cultures should be performed to exclude *Neisseria gonorrhoeae* and *Trichomonas vaginalis*, and nonspecific vaginosis can be ruled out by a negative KOH test for a "fishy odor" or by gas chromatography. More than one sexually transmitted condition may be present simultaneously in any single patient. It is also important to exclude coinfection with *Chlamydia trachomatis* and syphilis.

TREATMENT

An incredible array of substances has been used in the treatment of vaginal mycotic infections. These include the relatively obsolete antiseptics (boric acid, gentian violet, povidone—iodine) as well as the more specific topical antifungal agents. The latter are polyene antibiotics and substituted imidazoles. Systemic therapy, primarily with ketoconazole, is also available.

Odds[11,26] has reviewed the therapy of vaginal thrush. His analysis of a large number of clinical trials suggested that imidazole derivatives gave higher cure rates than do polyenes. Odds also showed that the nature of the vehicle in topical therapy did not affect the results, but that in general, longer therapy gave better results than shorter courses of usual doses of these agents.

The major therapeutic modalities in use today include

1. Nystatin and other polyenes (pimaricin, candicidin)
2. Topical imidazole derivatives: clotrimazole, miconazole, and econazole (not marketed in the United States)
3. Systemic ketoconazole

Various formulations of nystatin, 100,000 units, applied intravaginally at bedtime for 14 days have long been used to treat vaginal candidiasis. Odds's[26] analysis showed that a two-week course cures approximately 80% of patients. Most studies of other agents in the treatment of this disease have compared results to those obtained with this regimen. Other polyenes have been used (pimaricin, candicidin) with results comparable to nystatin.[26]

Alternatives to nystatin include the imidazoles, clotrimazole or miconazole. They are now considered the drugs of choice in the treatment of vaginal candidiasis by many authors, including the *Medical Letter* consultants.[27] Both of these imidazoles are used intravaginally as a single daily dose for 7 days.

Clotrimazole (Mycelex G, Gyne-lotrimin) is applied as one 100-mg vaginal suppository nightly or as a 1% vaginal cream for 7 to 14 days. Clotrimazole is negligibly absorbed from the vagina. Miconazole (Monistat) is available as a 2% vaginal cream or a 100-mg vaginal suppository to be applied nightly for 7 days. Some studies showed a lower rate of relapse after treatment with miconazole.[28] Miconazole suppositories should not be used concurrently with a latex diaphragm as the vehicle reacts with rubber. Miconazole may be absorbed in small amounts from the vagina, and its use is therefore limited early in pregnancy and in nursing mothers. Both clotrimazole and miconazole have been associated uncommonly with vulval or vaginal irritation, burning, itching, and pelvic or abdominal cramps. Miconazole-impregnated tampons are available in some countries.[29]

Even with these treatments, compliance remains a problem. Some investigators have tried shortened regimens with higher dosages. For example, doubling the dose of clotrimazole and halving the length of therapy (2% cream or 200 mg for 3 days instead of 1% for 6 days) gave identical results in first episodes of candidal vaginitis.[30–32]

Recently, single-dose treatment with vaginal tablets containing 500 mg of clotrimazole has been used successfully with an 88% response rate.[33,34] This formulation is quite acid (pH 3.5 to 3.8), a feature that permits increased release of clotrimazole. Another study of single-dose regimens showed a cure rate of 85.7% four weeks after completion of treatment, which was very similar to the cure rate of 91.9% in patients treated with the 3-day regimen.[35] Results with econazole and miconazole are comparable.[36,37]

Oral ketoconazole also has been used successfully in the therapy of vaginal candidiasis. Double-blind studies comparing ketoconazole to topical miconazole revealed similar results, but more frequent mycologic relapse occurred in ketoconazole-treated patients.[38] A ketoconazole regimen of 200 mg orally twice daily for 5 days is effective.[38] In the uncomplicated case of candidal vaginitis, it does not appear to offer an advantage over topical therapy, and hepatic toxicity has been described. The place of ketoconazole in the treatment of recurrent candidal vaginitis has not been evaluated thoroughly.

Currently, the treatment of choice of vaginal candidiasis remains topical clotrimazole or miconazole, one dose intravaginally for 7 days.[27] Single-dose higher concentration clotrimazole may become the preferred therapy. An alternative is nystatin, 100,000 units intravaginally at bedtime for 14 days.[27]

SPECIAL PROBLEMS: CANDIDA VAGINITIS IN PREGNANCY AND RECURRENT VAGINITIS

Candidal vaginitis is especially common in pregnancy, perhaps because of hormonal influences, and it is particularly difficult to eradicate. The incidence of neonatal thrush is 2- to 35-fold higher in babies born to infected women than to noninfected women.[39] Topical treatment is preferred over systemic therapy in pregnancy to avoid endangering the fetus.[40]

The problem of recurrent vaginitis can be very serious indeed and can lead to much physical and psychological discomfort. No real satisfactory solution has been devised. Intermittent prophylactic treatment has been recommended to approach the problem of recurrent vaginal candidiasis.

In a recent double-blind study intermittent treatment with antifungal suppository and cream used during menstrual flow and from the fifth to the eleventh day of the menstrual cycle reduced vaginal symptoms, although yeast carriage was not reduced.[41] In some cases of recurrent vaginitis, treatment of the male partner might be helpful.[42]

BALANOPOSTHITIS

Although uncommon, yeast infection of the penis is not rare, particularly in patients with diabetes mellitus or following antibiotic therapy.[43] Symptoms are variable. Although burning and itching of the penis may be described within hours of sexual intercourse and generalized erythema of the glans and prepuce may be noted,[44] most cases are milder. Balanoposthitis usually presents as erythema or "glazed skin" with some lichenification and desquamation or as papular lesions with edema of the prepuce.[11,23,43] It has been described in up to 10% of male sexual partners of infected women.[6,39] If balanoposthitis is present clinically, *Candida* can be isolated from 40% of these patients, but it may also be cultured from 18% of nonsymptomatic sexual contacts of women with vaginal candidiasis. This disease responds readily to local antifungal treatment and, provided the sexual partner also is treated, does not usually recur as often as vaginitis. Clotrimazole 1% cream applied twice daily for 7 days should result in cure of 95% of patients.[45]

SUMMARY AND CONCLUSION

Yeast vaginitis is one of the commonest infectious diseases of women. Many aspects of its epidemiology and pathogenesis are still poorly understood. In the presence of an irritating discharge the diagnosis is usually made by direct vaginal smear, although vaginal culture is preferred.

The optimal treatment includes topical clotrimazole or miconazole for 7 days, although equivalent results may be obtained with single high-dose treatment. Recurrent candidal vaginitis remains a difficult problem. Avoiding predisposing factors and treatment of infected sexual partners offers only limited relief. Prophylactic therapy may be necessary, although it is often unsuccessful and is quite expensive.

REFERENCES

1. Hippocrates: Epidemics Book 3. Translated by F Adams, Williams & Wilkins, Baltimore, 1939
2. Galen: De remediis paralilibus. From Galeni Opera Omnia; edited by DCG Kuehn. G. Olms, Hildeshein, 1965
3. Veron: Mémoire sur le muguet. Arch Gen Med 8:466, 1825
4. Haussmann D: Parasites des organes sexuals femelles de l'homme et de quelques animo ux. Baillière, Paris, 1875
5. Wilkinson JS: Some remarks upon the development of epiphytes with the description of new vegetable formations found in connection with the human uterus. Lancet 2:448, 1849
6. Oriel JD, Partridge BM, Denny MJ, Coleman JC: Genital yeast infection. Br Med J 4:761, 1972
7. Carroll CJ, Hurley R, Stanley VC: Criteria for diagnosis of candida vulvovaginitis in pregnant women. Br J Obstet Gynaecol 80:258, 1973
8. Hopsu-Havu VK, Gronroos M, Punnonen R: Vaginal yeasts in parturients and infestation of the newborn. Acta Obstet Gynecol Scand 59:73, 1980
9. Hurley R, Leask BGS, Fakton JA: deFonseka CI: Incidence and distribution of yeast species and of Trichomonas vaginalis in the vagina of pregnant women. Br J Obstet Gynaecol 80:252, 1973
10. McCormack WM, Starko KM, Zinner SH: Personal communication
11. Odds FC: Candida and Candidiasis. University Park Press, Baltimore, 1979
12. Rodin P, Kolator B: Carriage of yeasts on the penis. Br Med J 1:1123, 1976
13. Thin RN, Rendell P, Wadsworth J: How often are gonorrhea and genital yeast infections sexually transmitted? Br J Vener Dis 55:278, 1979
14. Hilton AJ, Warnock, DW: Vaginal candidiasis and the role of the digestive tract as a source of infection. Br J Obstet Gynecol 82:922, 1975
15. Miles MR, Olsen L, Rogers A: Recurrent vaginal candidiasis: Importance of an intestinal reservoir. JAMA 238:1836, 1977
16. Anonymous editorial: Vaginal candidiasis. Br Med J 1:357, 1976
17. Schnell JD: Investigation into the pathoetiology and diagnosis of vaginal mycoses. Chemotherapy 28(Suppl):1:14, 1982
18. Wilmott FF: Genital yeasts in female patients attending a VD clinic. Br J Vener Dis 51:119, 1975
19. Wright RA, Judson FN: Relative and seasonal incidences of the sexually transmitted diseases. Br J Vener Dis 54:433, 1978
20. Mathur S, Virella G, Koistinent, et al: Candidiasis. Infect Immun 15:287, 1977
21. Diamond RD, Krzesicki R, Wellington J: Damage to pseudohyphal forms of Candida albicans by neutrophils in the absence of serum in vitro. J Clin Invest 61:349, 1978
22. Schuit KE: Phagocytosis and intracellular killing of pathogenic yeasts by human monocytes and neutrophils. Infect Immun 24:932, 1979
23. Rein M, Holmes KK: Nonspecific vaginitis, vulvovaginal candidiasis and trichomoniasis: Clinical features, diagnosis, and management. Curr Clin Top Infect Dis 4:281, 1983
24. Syverson RE, Buckley H, Gibian J, Ryan JGM: Cellular and humoral immune status in women with chronic candida vaginitis. Am J Obstet Gynecol 134:624, 1979
25. Peeters F, Snauwaert R, Segers J, et al: Observations on candidal vaginitis: Vaginal pH, microbiology and cytology. Am J Obstet Gynecol 112:80, 1972
26. Odds FC: Cure and relapse with antifungal therapy. Proc R Soc Med 70(Suppl 4):24, 1977
27. Anonymous: Treatment of sexually transmitted diseases. Med Lett 26:5, 1984
28. Eliot BW, Howat RCL, Mack AE: A comparison between the effects of nystatin, clotrimazole and miconazole on vaginal candidiasis. Br J Obstet Gynecol 86:572, 1979

29. Bergstein NAM: Treatment of vulvovaginal candidal infections with miconazole-coated tampons. Br J Vener Dis 56:408, 1980
30. Granitzka S: Efficiency of various therapeutic concepts in genital mycoses. Chemotherapy 28(Suppl 1):92, 1982
31. Robertson WH: A concentrated regimen for vulvovaginal candidiasis. JAMA 244:2549, 1980
32. Stettendorf S, Benijts G, Vignali M, Kreysing W: Three-day therapy of vaginal candidiasis with clotrimazole vaginal tablets and econazole ovules: A multicenter comparative study. Chemotherapy 28(Suppl): 87, 1982
33. Goormans E, Bergstein NAM, Loendersloot EW, Branolte JH: One-dose therapy of Candida vaginalis. I. Results of an open multicenter trial. Chemotherapy 28(Suppl): 106, 1982
34. Krause U: Results of single-dose treatment of vaginal mycoses with 500 mg Conesten vaginal tablets. Chemotherapy 28(Suppl 1):99, 1982
35. Milsom I, Forssman L: Treatment of vaginal candidiasis with a single 500-mg clotrimazole pessary. Br J Vener Dis 58:124, 1982
36. Bingham JS, Steele CE: Treatment of vaginal candidiasis with econazole nitrate and nystatin: Comparative study. Br J Vener Dis 57:204, 1981
37. Cohen L: Single dose treatment of vaginal candidiasis. Comparison of clotrimazole and isoconazole. Br J Vener Dis 60:42, 1984
38. Levine HB (ed): Ketoconazole in the Management of Fungal Disease. ADIS Press, New York, 1982
39. Hurley R, deLouvois J: Candida vaginitis. Postgrad Med J 55:645, 1979
40. McNellis D, McLeod M, Lawson J, Pasquale SA: Treatment of vulvovaginal candidiasis in pregnancy: A comparative study. Obstet Gynecol 50:674, 1977
41. Davidson F, Mould RF: Recurrent genital candidiasis in women and the effect of intermittent prophylactic treatment. Br J Vener Dis 54:176, 1978
42. Fleury FJ: Recurrent candida vulvovaginitis. Chemotherapy 28(Suppl):48, 1982
43. Waugh MA: Clinical presentation of candidal balantis: Its differential diagnosis and treatment. Chemotherapy 28(Suppl 1):56, 1982
44. Thin RN, Leighton M, Dixon MJ: How often is genital yeast infection sexually transmitted? Br Med J 2:93, 1977
45. Waugh MA, Evans EGV, Naygar KC, Fong R: Clotrimazole in the treatment of candidal balantis in men: With incidental observation of diabetic candidal balanoposthitis. Br J Vener Dis 54:184, 1978

11

Genital Herpes

Benjamin Raab

Genital herpes is one of the most prevalent, publicized, feared, and misunderstood of the sexually transmitted diseases. Climbing from relative obscurity in recent decades to its present prominent position, genital herpes has been surrounded by numerous myths, fallacies, and misconceptions. It has transcended the medical realm to become at times a major psychosocial, moral, religious, or political issue. The concern of many patients transcends the usually mild irritation of the periodic clinical lesions, to the fear of spreading an "incurable disease" with its associated sexual and psychologic problems, passing on a fatal or permanently damaging infection to the newborn, and the development of cervical cancer.

A constructive organized approach to the management of the acute infection and prevention of potential complications (transmission, neonatal infection, cervical cancer morbidity) is necessary. With this broader understanding of the problem by the patient, his or her loved ones, and the public, much of the exaggerated fear of genital herpes can be allayed. It can and should be put into perspective as an annoying condition that, with proper education and responsible management, should not impede a person from leading a healthy, happy, "normal" life.

EPIDEMIOLOGY

There is no question that the incidence of genital herpes is on the rise and at an alarming rate. Why this recent increase has occurred is not known, but possible causes include the more liberal sexual attitudes of the past few decades, with increasing exposure to multiple sexual partners, the extensive use of oral contraceptives (allowing direct mucous membrane contact during intercourse), the decreased use of barrier contraception (condoms, spermicidal foams), a possible increase in the practice of oral sex, and, of course, a constantly increasing pool of carriers.

Since genital herpes is not a reportable venereal disease, exact figures are not available, and one must rely instead on calculated estimates, individual clinical surveys, and anecdotal observation.

An analysis performed by the Centers for Disease Control (CDC) on data collected by the National Disease and Therapeutic Index (NDTI) supports the contention that an epidemic of genital herpes infection occurred in the United States from 1966 to 1979. The estimated number and rate of consultations with physicians for genital herpes infection increased from 29,560 in 1966 to 260,890 in 1979 (Fig. 11-1). The rate at which patients consulted fee-for-service office-based phy-

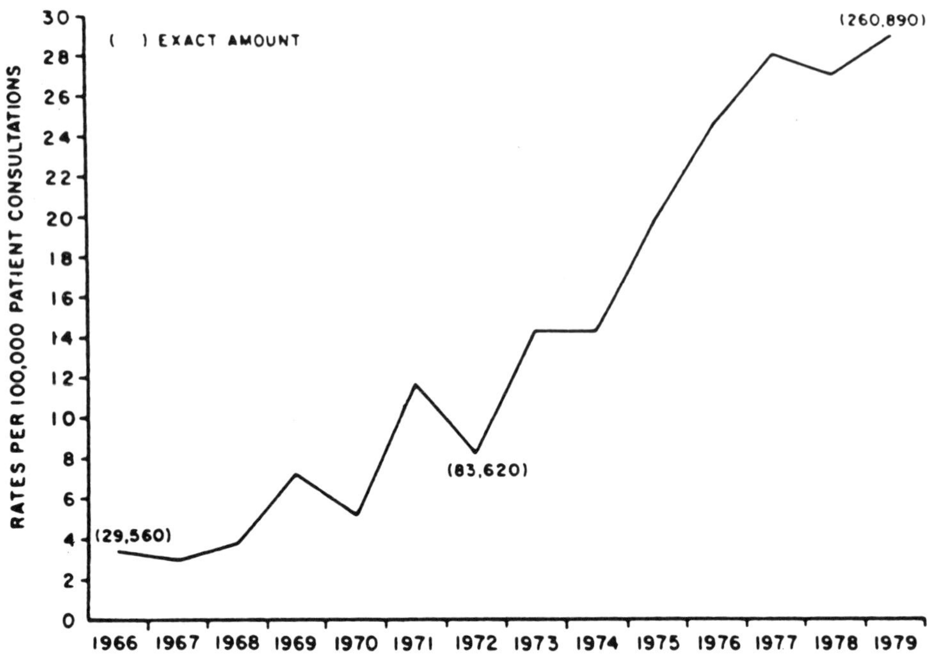

Fig. 11-1 Estimated rates of patient consultations for genital herpes infection. United States 1966–1979. (From Centers for Disease Control, National Disease and Therapeutic Index: MMWR 31:137, 1982)

sicians for genital herpes infection increased almost 9-fold from 3.4/100,000 consultation in 1966 to 29.2/100,000 in 1979.[1] Since patients with genital herpes seeking care in public health care facilities, hospital emergency rooms, prepaid practices, and outpatient clinics of community hospitals were not included in the survey; only the upward trend can be confirmed and not the total number of health care consultations for genital herpes.

Figures published by the CDC (1976–1977) showed that herpes genitalis accounted for 0.1 to 7.3% of venereal disease clinic visits (depending on clinic location), while gonorrhea accounted for 20.1 to 44.4% of visits.[2] Using this ratio and the 2.7 million cases of gonorrhea reported per year, it is estimated by the CDC that the number of new cases of herpes genitalis is approximately 300,000 per year.[3]

The 10:1 ratio, however, is disputed. A study at the University of California at Los Angeles Student Health Clinic showed the ratio of gonorrhea to herpes to be reversed. They concluded that in the middle and upper socioeconomic sectors of the community, where the prevalence of gonococcal infections may be less, genital herpes is a more significant problem.[4] If the above is now true, the incidence of new cases may approach 500,000 or more per year.

A population-based epidemiologic study of herpes genitalis was conducted in residents of Rochester, Minnesota for the 15-year period 1965 through 1979. A continuous increase in incidence was demonstrated throughout the study period, peaking at 128/100,000 population in 1979, the final year of the study.[5] Another author reviewing private practice gynecologic records (Houston, Texas, 1979) concluded that the incidence of herpes genitalis among private patients exceeded the combined incidence of all other major venereal diseases.[6] Similar studies show a sudden rise in herpes genitalis in England. Until 1971, herpes genitalis was not even recorded as a separate sexually transmitted disease by British public venereal disease (VD) clinics. In 1971 the recorded new cases were 12.2/100,000 population, doubling in 1976 to 24/100,000, and increasing again in 1978 to 28,8/100,000. Genital herpes in England is about twice as common as syphilis[7] and is increasing at a rate greater than that of other sexually transmitted diseases.[8]

Genital herpes is primarily a disease of the young adult population. Mean onset ranges in various studies from 22 to 26.9 years for women and 25 to 30 years for men.[9-11] Teenagers accounted for nearly half the patients seen with genital herpes in an Atlanta VD clinic.[12] The rapidly increasing incidence of this frequently recurring contagious entity in such a young population is epidemiologically alarming.

Various studies have attempted to depict the "typical" herpes patient, but when they are examined as a whole, it is evident that genital herpes affects all individuals regardless of sex, sexual preference, race, or socioeconomic status. Significant positive risk factors were young age at first intercourse and multiple sexual partners,[13] both of which obviously increase the chance of contact with the virus.

ETIOLOGY

Organism

The etiologic organism of genital herpes is herpes simplex virus 2 (HSV-2) and herpes simplex virus 1 (HSV-1) (previously known as herpesvirus hominus). Recent studies have proven erroneous the view that genital herpes is caused almost exclusively by HSV-2. Genital herpes was caused by HSV-1 in 37% of isolates from the Pennsylvania State University Health Service.[14] This high incidence of HSV-1 was attributed to the increasing popularity of orogenital sex among younger persons. When individuals were divided by age in another

study, HSV-1 was isolated from about a third of patients in the age group of 15 to 24 years and from only 7% of those 25 years of age or greater.[15] It is now assumed that herpesvirus does not discriminate as to body surface on which it sets up a new infection. Given a chance, the virus can infect any area of the body of a susceptible person.[16]

Determination of the HSV type of the genital herpes infection may have prognostic as well as epidemiologic value. During follow-up of first-episode genital herpes patients, it was found that only 14% of HSV-1 infections recurred, as compared with 60% of HSV-2 infections.[17] Whether HSV-1 is less likely than HSV-2 to produce latent infection of sacral dorsal-root ganglia after genital infection, or the two virus types behave differently after latent infection of the ganglia, remains to be determined. Another significant finding of this study was that primary first episodes were caused by HSV-1 much more often than nonprimary first episodes (15 vs 30%), indicating an apparent protective effect of prior HSV-1 labial infection.

Recently it has been shown that there exist different strains of each type. These intratypic differences can be found by analysis of the deoxyribonucleic acid (DNA) nucleotide sequences with restriction endonucleases, enzymes that recognize and cleave at specific sites within the DNA. Using this technique of "fingerprinting" different virus types and intratypic strains, it has been found that an individual can become exogenously infected in similar areas with more than one genetically different strain,[18] or more than one type.[19,20] Multiple-type viral-infected persons can continue to carry multiple types in latent form and experience periodic recurrences from each.[19,20] Presumably individuals can continue to carry different strains as well.[18] Whether transmission and reinfection of an individual with a different virus type or strain results in an increased recurrence rate, has not been proven, although theoretically it seems possible.

Not only is there no "protection" from exogenous reinfection, but one may even be autoinoculated with one's own virus at another site.[21] This technique was tried in the past as an autovaccination procedure, with little success, other than initiating a new infection site.[22]

Herpes simplex virus contains a double-stranded linear DNA. Its structure consists of a DNA core, a surrounding icosahedral protein capsid consisting of 162 subunits (capsomeres), a tegument composed of fibrillar material (protein), and an impermeable envelope, derived in part from the cell nuclear membrane, consisting of lipids, polyamines, and virus-specific glycoproteins[23] (Plate 11-1). The intact, enveloped particle is probably the epidemiologically important infectious unit.[24] The envelope contains the antigenic sites reactive with neutralizing antibodies.[23]

The two different serotypes (1 and 2) of herpes simplex virus can be differentiated by serologic, biologic (tissue culture plaque and neurotropic differences), and biochemical (DNA homology) means.[25]

Life Cycle

The human herpes simplex viruses develop a complex relationship with humans, their only natural host. They can interact in a number of ways to cause a productive infection, a latent infection, and possibly cell transformation[26] (Fig. 11-2).

The virus is first introduced into a susceptible host by direct mucocutaneous contact with infectious material, usually via sexual intercourse or orogenital sex in the case of herpes genitalis. Although herpesvirus isolated from patients with oral lesions were found to survive for as long as 3 hours on cloth and 4 hours on plastic,[27] fomites have yet to be documented as a significant source of genital herpes. Not enough information is presently available to determine the acquisition rate of genital herpes. In addition, the multiple variables involved (virus titer, virus type, prior serologic status, time of contact, site of contact) make determinations of the exact transmissibility of HSV extremely difficult.

After innoculation, a productive, usually symptomatic, phase of the infection develops, during which the virus engages in invasion of and replication in host cells, resulting in their eventual destruction. The replicative cycle consists of virus entry into the host cell by fusion of the viral envelope with the plasma membrane. The capsid is uncoated in the cytoplasm, and the core DNA enters the nucleus. Early transcription follows, utilizing host DNA-dependent RNA polymerase. The necessary virus-coded enzymes and structural proteins are synthesized and viral DNA replication occurs. Assembly of new herpesvirus occurs in the nucleus, with envelopment taking place at the inner lamella of the nuclear membranes.[28] The nature of the process by which the virus emerges from the infected cell is not clear, although in vitro experiments seem to indicate that the virus can spread both extracellularly and via an intracellular route.[29] This biosynthesis of infectious progeny results in cell death and lysis, with the entire process occurring within 5 to 6 hours of virus entry. Statistics of virus production in human cells are impressive, with approximately 80,000 to 120,000 copies of viral DNA being made per cell. Of these, however, only about 20% are encapsulated.

Studies in mice indicate that after epithelial inoculation, the virus spreads along sensory nerves to regional sensory ganglia. In the case of herpes genitalis, the spread is usually, but may not be exclusively, to the sacral ganglia, from which virus has been recovered.[30] It is believed that the virus reaches ganglia by retrograde intraaxonal transport. This spread from the infected epithelium to the ganglion begins about 24

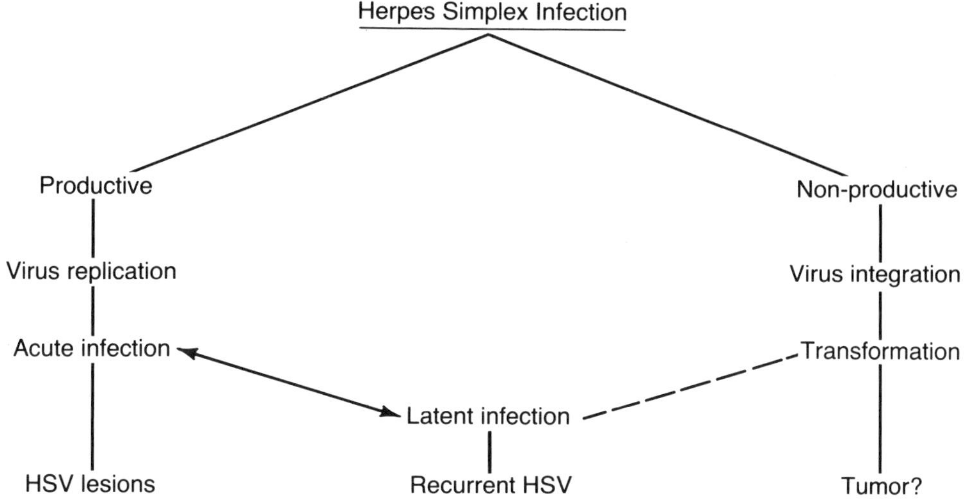

Fig. 11-2 Forms of herpes simplex virus infections.

hours after inoculation.[31] Once at the ganglion, a productive infection begins during which infectious virus can be demonstrated in cell-free ganglionic homogenates, and viral antigens can be detected by immunofluorescent staining. Once the acute infection has cleared (usually about 2 weeks), the latent stage of the ganglionic infection begins.[32] This stage is characterized by the absence of infectious virus in cell-free ganglionic homogenates and also by the absence of viral antigens detectable by immunofluorescence. However, the presence of the virus or virus genome can be demonstrated by explanation of ganglia to HSV-sensitive cell culture, in which infectious virus can be found in 4 to 6 days.[33]

The precise physical state of the latent viral genome and the controls over latency, subsequent reactivation, and possible cell transformation and oncogenicity have yet to be established. Recent advances have been made, however, in the delineating structure of the viral genome and the function of some of these genes. Three sets of viral genes, α, β, and γ, code in an orderly sequence for over 50 polypeptides that are produced by the viruses.[34] One of the five α genes is known to be required for viral replication. The functions of the other genes remain unknown. Functions associated with the β genes include death of the host cell, shutoff of α gene expression, and synthesis of viral enzymes such as DNA polymerase, thymidine kinase, and ribonucleotide reductase. The γ genes are associated with inhibition of expression of some β genes and synthesis of viral structural proteins (glycoproteins).[35] Genes that are responsible for transformation or oncogenicity appear to be associated with either the β or γ genes.[36] There are some indications that there may be two viral genes that are responsible for latency: one to establish latency and the other to maintain it. Two groups of mutants with lesions to prevent latent infections have been found, one with a lesion in the γ gene area, (not essential for viral replication), and the other lesion believed to be in the α group of genes.[37]

At the present time there are two main theories for the triggering of viral reactivation. The first is the "ganglionic trigger" theory that proposes that a stimulus (ganglionic manipulation, menses, fever, stress) acts on the latent infection in the ganglion, reactivating the virus, which then travels down the peripheral nerve to the epidermal cells, where it may lead to a skin lesion. The second is the "skin trigger" theory that proposes that the virus is continually produced in the ganglion and travels to the skin, establishing microfoci of infection that are eliminated by host defenses. However, occasional changes in the skin (trauma, heat, sunburn) allow these microfoci to become symptomatic either by enhancing virus replication or by temporary suppression of local defenses.[38] There is evidence supporting and contradicting both theories, and the issue is still being actively debated.

The final way in which the virus is thought to interact with the host is to cause cell transformation with possible subsequent oncogenesis. This possible interaction will be discussed in the section on Genital Herpes and Cancer.

IMMUNOLOGY

The response to herpes simplex infection is a complex interaction of humoral, cell-mediated, and nonimmune defense mechanisms. It is generally thought that humoral immunity is probably responsible for ameliorating the disease and may offer some protection against reinfection, whereas cellular immunity, mediated by T lymphocytes or by antibody-dependent lymphocyte cytotoxicity, is more important in recovery from infections.[39] Macrophages have also been implicated in playing a critical role in resistance to HSV[40]; a recent study implies that macrophage competence in mice is more important in resistance to primary herpes infections than is T-lymphocyte competence.[41] How macrophages function in this capacity is unknown, and, in view of the complex interactions of macrophages and lymphoid cells in immunologic phenomena, attempts to assign primary roles may be problematic.

With primary HSV infection—the very first exposure to HSV-1 or HSV-2—the production of neutralizing antibodies, cytotoxic antibodies, and complement-fixation antibodies occurs. Once these antibodies develop, levels remain high for several months.[42] The role of antibody in the pathogenesis of illness is not completely understood. Neutralizing antibody does not appear to fluctuate markedly between periods of reactivation, and in fact antibody levels tend to be slightly higher in those individuals with frequent episodes than in those with no history of recurrence.[43] This was confirmed in another study that found the probability of recurrence following primary HSV-2 infection was directly related to neutralizing antibody to HSV-2 in convalescent serum.[17] It is also known that individuals with selectively impaired humoral antibody responses do not suffer from more severe primary herpesvirus infections. A possible reason for this lack of neutralizing antibody importance may be the fact that virus may spread via an intercellular route, and thus be protected from the neutralizing antibody. Also, mouse models suggest that immunoglobulin G (IgG) may play a role as a blocking antibody, protecting virus-infected cells from immune surveillance.[44]

An intact cell-mediated immunity (CMI) is considered crucial in preventing severe local or widespread herpesvirus disease and in effecting recovery. Defects in CMI, either from disease or iatrogenic immune suppression, can result in persistent, locally destructive lesions, especially in the perianal and genital areas. The duration of viral excretion and clinical symptoms in HSV infection correlate better with the lymphocyte transformation index than with the titer of complement-fixing or complement-independent neutralizing antibody.[45] However, in otherwise normal patients with frequent recurrences, studies indicate that CMI, especially during attacks, is not defective, and its failure does not account for the recurrences.[46,47] It is possible, though, that there are some as yet undetected defects that await more refined techniques.

CLINICAL MANIFESTATIONS

The clinical manifestations of herpes genitalis can be divided into two broad categories, primary and recurrent (recrudescent). By definition, the term "primary" infection is reserved to denote an individual's first exposure to either HSV-1 or HSV-2. Thus, a person can have either a primary HSV-1 or HSV-2 infection, but not both. Also, some authors prefer to use "recurrent" to include symptomatic or asymptomatic viral reactivations, and use "recrudescent" to signify only clinically apparent infections.[26] "Recurrent" will be used in this discussion with the understanding that some may be asymptomatic.

Primary Infection

Clinical symptoms usually appear within 3 to 7 days following an adequate exposure to HSV-2 or HSV-1, although the incubation period may extend up to 20 days. In true "primary" adult genital herpes infections, the clinical lesions seen are usually extensive. In the female, lesions may involve the labia majora, labia minora, perianal skin, and vulva (most common site), as well as vaginal and ectocervical mucosa. Early in the disease, the patients may complain of mild paresthesias and burning before lesions become visible. Systemic symptoms of headache, generalized aching, and malaise, associated with low-grade fever, are not uncommon. Whether the systemic symptoms are related to viremia, to extension of virus to the central nervous system, or to toxic metabolic products of viral infection is not clear. The patients may also complain of inguinal pain as well as pelvic pain related to pronounced inguinal and pelvic lymphadenopathy. Urination may be exceedingly painful and may develop into urinary retention. With severe involvement of the cervix, a profuse, watery discharge is frequently present. As the disease develops, the classic grouped vesicles on an erythematous base may be seen over all or some of the aforementioned areas. In moist areas such as the labia minora, the vesicles erode within 24 to 48 hours (Plate 11-2), while in drier areas the vesicles may persist longer. Lesions may coalesce to form bullae and large erosions involving extensive areas of the vulva and perianal skin associated with severe vulvar pain and exquisite tenderness. Considerable erythema and edema, particularly of the labia minora and clitoris, may be present. Lesions on the cervic and vagina may present only as superficial erosions. Sometimes these lesions have a necrotic appearance. Rarely, a fungating, necrotic-appearing mass may be seen covering the cervix. A variant seen mostly in women is lumbosacral herpes simplex, in which lesions occur on the low back, buttocks, and posterior thighs. In such cases the clinician should also check the genitalia, since one form does not preclude the other.

The male may experience the same initial constitutional symptoms as the female. Extensive vesiculation and erosions of the penis and pubis may be seen, with considerable edema and erythema (Fig. 11-3). The lesions are found most frequently on the glans, prepuce, and shaft of the penis. A variant finding is herpetic infection of the anus and perianal area in homosexual men associated with severe anorectal pain, difficulty in urinating, sacral paresthesias or pain, and diffuse ulceration fo the distal rectal mucosa (proctitis).[48]

In both sexes, lesions last from 2 to 6 weeks and generally heal without scarring. If lesions persist longer, one must think of secondary infection, an associated venereal disease, or underlying immunosuppression.

Patients with nonprimary first episodes less often develop constitutional symptoms, have fewer complications, and have a shorter duration of disease than persons

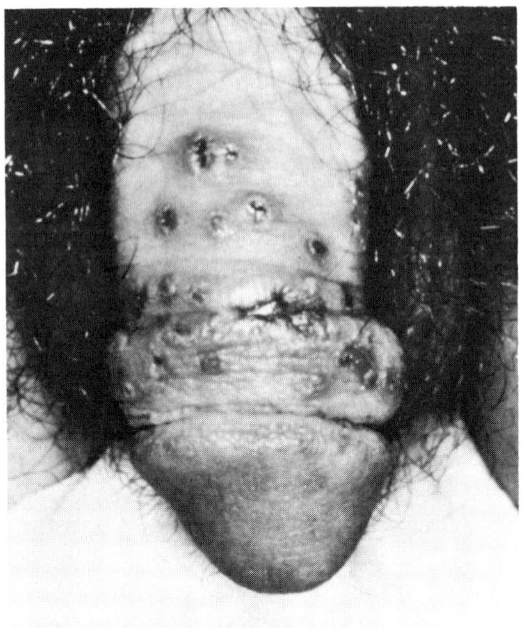

Fig. 11-3 Primary genital herpes infection in the male.

with true primary genital herpes. The rate of subsequent recurrences, however, is the same.[10]

Asymptomatic primary infections have also been documented. In a large series of patients, serologic evidence of past HSV-2 infection in acute phase sera was evident in 8% of patients with historic first episodes of genital herpes, suggesting previous asymptomatic acquisition of HSV-2 infection.[10] Other studies found virus in isolates from 7 of 30 asymptomatic female contacts of males with overt genital herpes,[49] as well as 4% of a routine asymptomatic obstetric population.[50] If the CDC estimate is correct, that 9 to 35% of the general population has had genital exposure to the virus,[51] then the number of asymptomatic carriers may be considerably higher than expected.

Recurrent Infection

Recurrent attacks occur in about two thirds of all cases during the year following the first episode. A statistical study showed little difference between men and women in the frequency of recurrences, with 53% reporting one or more per month, 33% every 2 to 4 months, and 14% less frequently than every 4 months.[9]

In general, recurrent lesions are much less severe, being restricted to smaller areas and usually occurring near the same site as the initial primary lesion. The classic clinical picture is that of grouped vesicles on an erythematous base in varying numbers and at times in separate patches (Plate 11-3. The vesicles rapidly become pustular crust and heal, usually without scarring, in a few days to 3 weeks.

As in the primary disease, lesions in moist areas (labia minora, introitus, and fourchette in women, and under the foreskin in men) show indistinct stages because of early maceration. Vesicular lesions (Fig. 11-4) are rarely seen because of rapid evolution to erosions. These moist lesions heal by gradual repithelialization from their peripheries. Thus, in these moist regions it is more difficult to define a healed stage, which in dry lesions is heralded by loss of crust. In general, these moist lesions take longer to heal.[9]

Many times the recurrent lesions are inconspicuous and difficult to identify, especially if they are minute and few in number. Also, if the lesions are on the cervix, with its hidden location and decreased number of sensory nerves, they may be asymptomatic and inapparent to the patient.

The academic issue of whether asymptomatic shedding of virus is a result only of inapparent lesions, or in fact occurs in the absence of lesions, remains problematic. The evidence in females seems to favor the occasional shedding of virus without lesions. In one study HSV-2 was isolated from the cervix of 5 of 50 women with a history of genital herpes during the preceding six months, but who, at the time of isolation, demonstrated no signs or symptoms of the illness.[52] Numerous similar studies confirm this finding by virus isolation[53–56]

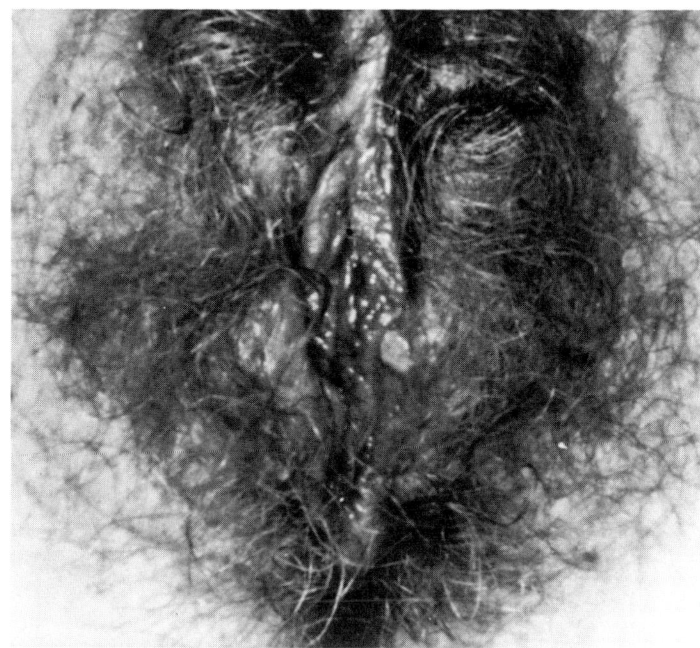

Fig. 11-4 Recurrent genital herpes infection in the female.

as well as cytologic means.[57] Only in one recent study was there found an absence (99.8% of cultures) of virus in the absence of active lesions.[58] Still unresolved is whether the decreased viral shedding (10–1,000 viral particles vs 1,000,000–10,000,000 particles/cc vesicular fluid)[42] during these asymptomatic periods causes significant transmission of genital or neonatal herpes.

The evidence for asymptomatic shedding in the male is less convincing. In a study of 190 randomly selected males, 15% showed incidence of HSV-2 in various genitourinary cultures from urethra, prostatic fluid, prostate, and vas deferens.[59] Yet, in another study no virus was isolated from 144 random vasectomy specimens.[60] Also, no virus was isolated from the semen, between recurrences, of 30 patients with a history of recurrent herpes genitalis.[61] The latter study would seem to be extremely significant, since semen is the most likely vehicle of transmission in the absence of overt cutaneous lesions. Another author[26] states that asymptomatic infections in males, pri-

marily urethral, seem to occur at an incidence of around 1%.

The basic control of reactivation of genital herpes is unknown. Clinically, there are numerous environmental or systemic "triggers" that patients report bring on recurrent lesions. Among those commonly reported are fever, menses, environmental heat, trauma, sexual intercourse, sunlight (lumbosacral herpes), fatigue, and emotional stress. Whether these are just coincidental or do, in fact, play a role is not known. A known trigger in humans is ganglionic manipulation, as demonstrated by a 60% recurrence rate in patients who had a history of herpes labialis and underwent microneurosurgical decompression of the trigeminal sensory root for treatment of trigeminal neuralgia.[62] In mice, reactivation of infection was caused by the trauma of stripping the skin with cellophane tape,[63] exposing it to ultraviolet light, and injecting prostglandin E_2.[64] The involvement of prostaglandins is an intriguing link between many of the preceding triggers.

A prodrome, in both men and women,

prior to a recurrence, is a common event. In one study 46% of patients experienced prodromal symptoms. These symptoms lasted more than 24 hours in 75% of the patients. Two thirds of those with prodromes had localized paresthesias consisting of itching, burning, or a hypersensitivity of the skin surface at the site of the subsequent lesion. Prodromal neuralgia (burning, aching) occurred in about 25% of the patients, was always ipsilateral, and subsided shortly after the appearance of lesions. The buttock and groin were the most common sites of neuralgia, but the thigh, calf, foot, and scrotum may also be involved.[9]

Another problem, as a result of involvement of sensory nerves is severe pruritus in some patients, which may not be limited to the lesions alone but can also involve contiguous areas of skin. The itching may be the only symptom, and it may precede the onset or follow the disappearance of the local lesions.[65]

Whether the preceding symptoms are a result of damage or destruction of nerve cells upon reactivation of latent virus is not known. Rare instances of neuropathy have been reported[66]; however, a study of latent infection in mouse dorsal root ganglia suggested that reactivation causes the destruction of the neuron in which the virus was latent.[67] That this neuronal destruction occurs in humans is difficult to believe in light of the numerous recurrences in some patients.

With time, the recurrent lesions generally tend to occur less frequently. Thus, the usual natural course of the disease is encouraging in many individuals, even though it may take several years for recurrences to diminish to a relatively insignificant frequency.[68,69]

COMPLICATIONS

Genital herpes is, in most cases, a benign and self-limited disease in the otherwise healthy individual. Significant complications can, however, occasionally arise.

Herpes pharyngitis is a common manifestation of primary genital herpes, occurring in about 10% of patients.[42] It usually follows orogenital contact and can result from HSV-1 or HSV-2. Patients present with sore throat, adenopathy, fever, malaise, and tonsillar exudate, often confused with streptococcal pharyngitis. Whether oral-labial HSV-2 recurs as frequently as oral-labial HSV-1 or genital HSV-2 is unknown.

HSV urethritis may occur as the sole symptomatic manifestation of genital herpes. In a study of women with the urethral syndrome (dysuria-frequency syndrome), HSV was isolated from the urethra or cervix in 5% of cases.[70] HSV has also been isolated from the urine of both men and women with dysuria or hematuria, and cystoscopic examination has shown mucosal ulcerations in some of these patients,[71] probably as a result of ascending infection from the urethra.

Aseptic meningitis, presenting with symptoms of stiff neck, headache, photophobia, and occasional fever, frequently (36% women, 13% men) accompanies primary genital herpes.[10] Herpes simplex virus has been isolated from the cerebrospinal fluid in a small percentage of patients,[72] and further examination of cerebrospinal fluid in patients with HSV-2 meningitis may show a slightly elevated opening pressure, leukocyte counts ranging from 5 to greater than $1,000/mm^3$ with a predominance of lymphocytes.[24] The cerebrospinal fluid glucose value is usually more than 50% of the blood sugar. With bed rest, analgesics, and intravenous fluids (if hospitalized), symptoms and signs gradually resolve, almost always without neurologic sequelae or recurrence.[10] The pathogenesis of herpes simplex virus meningitis is unclear.

Autonomic nervous system dysfunction with urinary retention and constipation[10] has been reported in women with primary genital herpes and has a high incidence in the herpes proctitis syndrome of homosexual men (described earlier). The usual course is slow recovery without sequelae.

Spread of lesions to extragenital sites such as the buttocks, groin, thighs, fingers, or, rarely, the eye may occur, probably by autoinoculation; therefore, strict hygiene should be observed during a primary infection.

Erythema multiforme can be seen in some individuals following a herpes simplex infection, and is known to recur sometimes periodically following recurrences of the herpes simplex infection. Cutaneous or visceral dissemination is always a possibility in the immunosuppressed.

One must also think of and rule out any additional venereal diseases. At a major university health center, 25.2% of episodes diagnosed as genital herpes were associated with another sexually transmitted disease of a different etiology.[4] Bacterial and/or fungal (candida) superinfection are other potential diagnostic considerations.

The more common complications of genital herpes[25] are the nonmedical, psychosocial and interpersonal problems associated with having a potentially contagious "incurable" venereal disease, which recurs unpredictably. The patient with genital herpes is usually young, sexually active, and healthy, this being in many cases their first experience with a chronic recurring entity beyond their control. The patient often feels a combination of embarrassment, guilt, anger, and hopelessness. Social isolation and withdrawal caused by fear of rejection by a "herpes-free" companion or fear of transmission of genital herpes unfortunately is not uncommon. These fears have been compounded by the generally irrational and sensationalistic media attention given to the subject, exposing and exaggerating the problems, while not offering constructive approaches to the treatment of the infections and prevention of subsequent problems. It is in this area that a knowledgeable, understanding and nonjudgmental physician can be of great assistance in educating the patient.

The two most feared and potentially serious complications of herpes genitalis are neonatal herpes simplex and the hypothetical relationship between cervical cancer and herpes genitalis.

Neonatal Herpes Simplex

If the epidemiologic statistics hold true, in the next decade there will be an enormous pool of young pregnant mothers with genital herpes. How herpesvirus affects the newborn and what can and should be done to prevent such often tragic neonatal infections will be discussed.

Herpes in the newborn is almost always acquired from the mother's infected birth canal, either as an ascending infection through ruptured membranes or during passage through the birth canal.[75] The exact risk of neonatal herpes simplex virus infection and subsequent clinical illness after vaginal delivery through a birth canal infected with herpes simplex has not been precisely ascertained, with estimates ranging from 5 to 50%.[76–77] Yearly incidence estimates range from 120 to 1,000 affected neonates. These statistics may be artificially low because of the difficulty in clinically distinguishing forms of the disease from other problems of the neonate, especially when premature,[71] and because of lack of reporting, or some yet to be understood protective variable. Possible determinants of whether infants will develop infection include virus titer in maternal secretions, duration of rupture of membranes, local environmental and immune factors, cellular immune responsiveness of the neonate, use of fetal monitoring devices,[79] and titer of maternal antibody in serum or amniotic fluid.[80] Occasionally an infant may become infected with HSV acquired postnatally. Sources of virus may be labial lesions in any person handling the newborn,[20] or, rarely, baby-to-baby transmission in the nursery, or breast milk.[81]

Cutaneous involvement is present in 50% of infected neonates. The lesions are similar to those seen in older children or adults, that is, grouped tense vesicles on an erythematous base. Frequently these lesions are misdiagnosed and treated as "impetigo" or "folliculitis."[82] Patients may also have an infection localized to the eye.[83] With dissemination of disease, as occurs in around 75% of cases, there are associated constitutional symptoms such as fever or hypothermia, poor feeding, irritability, lethargy, and vomiting. In infants who have died of disseminated disease, HSV has been cultured from vesicular fluid, eye, spinal cord, brain, spleen, kidney, pancreas, liver, gastrointestinal tract, bone marrow, cord blood, lung, and urine.[82] Although dissemination can manifest with multisystem involvement, it usually is accompanied by central nervous system manifestations and hepatomegaly and, less commonly, by respiratory disease, disseminated intravascular coagulation, and splenomegaly.[75] The statistical prognosis of infected neonates is poor. In an extensive series of 298 infants with neonatal herpes, 178 died, 54 survived with sequelae (most commonly neurologic and/or ocular), while only 66 survived without apparent sequelae.[84]

Some conclusions have come from the NIAID Collaborative Antiviral Study Group's extensive analysis (400 infants) of neonatal herpes simplex.[85] Approximately 75% of the virus isolates in neonatal herpes simplex were HSV-2; the remainder were HSV-1. No difference in outcome was found between the two types. Herpetic infection occurs four times more frequently in premature infants than in term infants. Transplacental antibodies do not appear to be protective to infants with local disease. Although infants with diseminated disease appear to be more likely to lack transplacental antibodies, there was little difference in outcome between those with or without such antibodies. Cesarean section performed over intact membranes or within four hours of ruptured membranes greatly decreased the risk of neonatal herpes simplex infection. In most of the infants delivered by cesarean section who became infected, an ascending route of infection most likely occurred. Transplacental infection is a very rare occurrence.[86] The intrauterine infections probably are secondary to maternal viremia during the course of a primary infection.

In light of the known danger to a fetus passing through an infected vaginal canal, the high incidence of neonatal infections caused by asymptomatic maternal infections (up to 70%),[87] the occurrence of viral shedding in asymptomatic pregnant women with a known history of genital herpes (3–12%)[54,88,89] and in a general obstetric population (4%),[50] and the known occurrence of asymptomatic primary infections, certain high-risk pregnancy groups should be screened. These high-risk groups are women with clinically suspect genital herpes infections, a prior history of genital infection, sexual partners with a history of genital infection, and a history of HSV infection below the waist, since they often have concomitant genital herpes.[90] In these individuals, monitoring by cervicovaginal cultures should be performed at 32, 34, and 36 weeks and weekly thereafter, so that information will be ready whenever the time of delivery arrives, which in many cases of maternal genital herpes is premature.[10,87,91] It is the general consensus that, if virus is present at or near the time of delivery, with the last culture positive, cesarean section should be performed, optimally before rupture of the membranes. If the membranes have been ruptured for more than 4 to 6 hours, the protection of cesarean section is probably lost, making this procedure no longer helpful or indicated.[92–94] In women with recurrent genital herpes who have active external lesions at the time of labor, the infants may not come in prolonged contact with infected genital secretions—until the late stages of labor. Thus, if no cervical involvement has been shown, cesarean delivery may be indicated irrespective of the duration of rupture of the membranes.[10]

Genital Herpes and Cancer

A very common malignant disease of women in the United States is carcinoma of the cervix. There are approximately 35,000 new cases of cervical carcinoma and 10,000 deaths reported annually.[95] The first evidence of an association between genital HSV infection and cervical neoplasia was the observation that women with cytologically detected herpes infections[96] or serologic evidence of previous HSV-2 infections[97] had a greater frequency of cervical neoplasia than women in the general population. Next, population studies showed retrospectively the frequency of cervical neoplasia in women with genital herpes between 1963 and 1979 was 18%, much higher than the frequency in the general population. Prospectively, a subpopulation of women (618) with cytologic, virologic, or serologic proof of HSV-2 infection was followed and compared with an epidemiologically similar group of women (400) with no evidence of a past history of genital herpes, no cervical neoplasia, and no serum HSV-2 antibodies. The rate of severe dysplasia, carcinoma in situ, and invasive carcinoma was four times higher in the herpes group than in the control group.[98]

Other evidence supporting the hypothesized oncogenic role of HSV in cervical cancer includes the common location of HSV infection on the cervix, often at the squamocolumnar junction where most cervical neoplasms arise,[26] the demonstration that the virus transforms cells in culture and is oncogenic in experimental animals,[99] the detection of HSV antigens, viral DNA, or RNA transcripts in human cervical carcinoma tissue by some workers;[100] and the finding of genes (β or γ) that appear to be involved in cell transformation and oncogenicity.[36] Furthermore, very little evidence has been presented to refute the likelihood that that HSV is involved in cervical cancer. The theory has yet to be scientifically discredited.[101]

Certainly, women with a history of primary or recurrent genital herpes should have yearly Papanicolaou smear tests, since cervical carcinoma is a curable disease if detected early. The five-year cure rate of carcinoma in situ, if treated surgically, approaches 100%.[102]

Recent evidence seems to implicate HSV in other malignancies or pseudomalignancies. Herpesvirus-induced antigens (HSV-2) were found to be associated in 9 of 10 cases examined with squamous cell carcinoma in situ of the vulva.[103] The epidemiologic finding of a higher incidence of HSV-2 neutralizing antibodies in patients with cancer of the urinary bladder and prostate,[104] as well as the virus itself in the prostate,[59] has prompted speculation of an etiologic role in these genitourinary cancers. Bowenoid papulosis of the genitalia, a lesion featuring aspects of squamous cell carcinoma in situ, was thought to be related in 10 of 28 such male patients with a history of genital herpes, 5 of whom has received photoinactivation therapy.[105]

It is evident that further work is necessary to determine the true oncogenic risk of herpes genitalis in both men and women, and the various possible contributing factors to this oncogenic risk (structural, hormonal, genetic, chemical, etc.).

DIAGNOSIS

The keys to adequate control and prevention of genital herpes and its complications are awareness of its prevalence and prompt diagnosis. A high index of suspicion and knowledge of the varied forms of herpes can first alert the physician to the diagnosis.

If culture facilities are available, recovery

of virus from genital lesions is the most definitive test. The optimal yield of virus is found in early vesicular fluid (10^9 viral units per vesicle).[26] Virus titers rapidly decline to very low levels in 3 to 5 days,[9,106] although viruses can occasionally still be found in crusted lesions. The virus demonstrates characteristic cytopathic effects in tissue culture within 1 to 3 days.[107]

Alternative, more available, but less sensitive to diagnostic methods are the Tzanck and Papanicolaou smears. The Tzanck smear is done by smearing scrapings of the base and margins of vesicles or erosions with immediate fixation for 1 minute in absolute alcohol, followed by Giemsa or Wright stainings for 3 minutes. A "quick" Tzanck smear has been described, using only air-dried material on a slide to which a 50/50 mixture of tap water and Giemsa stain is applied for 30–40 seconds.[108] HSV infection is detected by finding characteristic multinucleated giant cells in the Tzanck smear (Plate 11-4), and both multinucleated giant cells and intranuclear inclusions in the Papanicolaou smear. The Papanicolaou smear is particularly useful for asymptomatic herpetic cervicitis. The morphologic findings of the Papanicolaou smear have been found to be approximately two thirds as sensitive as viral cultures in detecting herpetic infection, while the Tzanck smear is about half as sensitive as the Papanicolaou smear because of its lesser ability to detect intranuclear inclusions.[23,26] The Tzanck smear will not differentiate cutaneous herpes simplex from herpes zoster, nor will routine histopathology. With these staining methods, a greater sensitivity (70 to 85%) was found in the vesicular stage, as compared to only 25 to 40% in the erosive stage.[109]

Histologic examination of biopsy sections from lesions (best fixed in Bouin's solution) shows characteristic viral intraepidermal vesicles featuring ballooning and reticular degeneration, as well as viral nuclear changes.[110]

Serologic diagnosis is useful in confirming a primary infection only if a fourfold rise in serum antibody can be demonstrated between acute (negative) and convalescent samples (two or more weeks later).[107] Otherwise, neutralizing antibody titers are of little use, since levels fluctuate without much relation to recurrences. Typing of HSV isolates can be done by various techniques but very rarely is clinically indicated or necessary, since the approach to treatment is the same whether the etiology is HSV-1 or HSV-2.

The use of electron microscopy is very attractive because results can be available rapidly. The results, however, are not specific because members of the herpes virus group cannot be distinguished and the sensitivity is low. Other tests requiring further investigation are the enzyme-linked immunosorbent assay and the radioimmunoassay.[111] Monoclonal antibodies to HSV-1 and HSV-2 are presently being tested and may soon be a powerful tool for the rapid diagnosis and simultaneous typing of HSV infections.[112,113]

Differential Diagnosis

There is considerable overlap in the clinical manifestations of genital herpes simplex virus infection and those of other types of genital ulcerations—syphilis, chancroid, lymphogranuloma venereum, and granuloma inguinale.

Information from the history and examination pointing toward a diagnosis of genital herpes include a history of vesicles preceding the genital ulcerations (only seen with herpes), a history of recurrences of similar lesions at or near the same location, a history of sexual exposure to the herpes virus, and characteristic small, painful, superficial lesions. In all such cases cultures should be obtained that, if positive, confirm the diagnosis of herpes genitalis.

Primary syphilis chancres classically are

nontender and indurated. Darkfield microscopic examination should be performed on all such suspicious lesions. Occasional dual infection has been reported.[119]

Chancroid also causes painful genital ulcerations; however, they usually are more indurated and accompanied by fluctuant suppurative adenopathy. Cultures for *Haemophilus ducreyi* should be obtained in suspicious cases.

Lymphogranuloma venereum rarely presents with genital ulcers, which are usually healed at the time of fluctuant tender adenopathy. The lesions of granuloma inguinale are usually chronic and progressive, with gradual expansion.

Other possible diagnoses include noninfectious causes of genital ulcerations such as those associated with Behçet's or Crohn's disease, trauma, scabies, or pyoderma.

TREATMENT

Is it true that genital herpes is an "incurable" disease? One has to say that, at the present time, there is no consistently proved therapy that will eradicate a latent infection once established, and although multiple topical remedies may in fact eradicate some surface virus and possibly shorten the course of an infection, they still do not alter the frequency of future recurrences.

It is best to divide treatment into three major categories: preventive, symptomatic, and therapeutic.

Preventive

As discussed previously, part of the problem of herpes genitalis is the unpredictability of recurrences and the possibility of asymptomatic recurrences with viral shedding. Even though virus cannot be isolated between recurrences from the cutaneous

sites of infection (even by cocultivation of explants),[115] the female pattern of asymptomatic cervical recurrences and the possibility of asymptomatic urethral infections in the male make precautions desirable. What can an individual do to be protected from either spreading or contracting genital herpes?

At the present time there are two commonly available theoretical barriers to the genital transmission of HSV. Spermicidal foams have been shown to be potent viricidal agents in vitro.[115–117] Also, condoms can provide a barrier to viral penetration.[118,119] Using these modalities, one can advise, for maximum protection, the use of a spermicidal foam by the woman and the concurrent use of a condom by the man. Just as with contraception, we are dealing with decreasing risk, not 100% assurance.

Current prophylactic recommendations are as follows: If active lesions are present: abstinence from sexual contact; for women with a history of recurrent genital herpes: maximum protection as described above; and for men with a history of recurrent genital herpes: use of a condom by the man and/or foam by the woman. The reason for the difference in prophylaxis for men and women is that there is stronger evidence for asymptomatic shedding in women. When pregnancy is desired, one has to go with the old guideline of avoidance when active lesions are known to be present. Although the preceding recommendations may be esthetically unappealing, the alternatives— abstinence, anxiety due to uncertainty, or herpes genitalis—are to most people even more unappealing.

A second approach to prevention is the possible development of a prophylactic vaccine. Herpes vaccines appear to work on the principle that induced antibody to herpes simplex virus will protect against subsequent infection; nevertheless, naturally acquired antibody to herpes simplex virus does not protect against the subsequent development of genital herpes, though it may modify the course of the infection. These vaccines will probably not prevent genital herpes, but they may alter its clinical course.[120]

Various kinds of vaccines are being considered, developed, and tested. These can be categorized as viable (live) or nonviable (killed). The killed virus vaccines consist of whole virus inactivated by various techniques (formalin, ultraviolet light, heat) rendering the virus nonviable yet still antigenic, or structural components such as proteins or glycoproteins, which would be immunogenic without the additional risk of the potentially oncogenic viral genome. With the rapid development of genetic engineering techniques, consideration is being given to an attenuated live virus with the gene for latency, or even oncogenic transformation, deleted or deprogrammed.[36]

The most extensively tested vaccines in humans are the heat-inactivated HSV-1 (Lupidon-H) and HSV-2 (Lupidon-G), manufactured in Germany. Since 1971 the type 2 vaccine has been in clinical use, and when given for extended periods, clinical improvement was claimed in 60 to 100% of cases.[12] The question that arises is this: since the vaccine was used for periods of months to years, was the improvement a result of the vaccine or merely the natural course of the disease?

Numerous subunit vaccines are presently being evaluated: an inactivated HSV-2 glycoprotein vaccine,[122] an inactivated HSV-1 protein subunit vaccine,[123] a specific glycoprotein vaccine (glycoprotein D, believed to be critical to the ability of the viruses to invade cells), and a specific early-appearing HSV-1 protein vaccine (thought to be vital to invasion and replication in the host cell.)[124] A genetically reengineered smallpox vaccine containing genes from HSV-1 and HSV-2 is also presently awaiting testing.[124]

Finally, avoidance of any possible individual triggers known by the patient to be exacerbating may be of some help in preventing numerous recurrences.

Symptomatic

Adequate analgesia during a primary attack is indicated. Aspirin is preferred because, in addition to its analgesic effect, its antiprostaglandin effect may have a role in preventing viral spread.[125] Moisture and excessive heat are to be avoided by wearing loose clothing and air-drying when possible in a cool, ambient temperature. Topical application of antiseptic drying agents, such as povidone-iodine, may decrease the slight risk of secondary infection, may have a beneficial drying effect, and may, according to some studies, shorten healing time.[126,127] Whether early destruction of the vesicle is beneficial is debatable, as is the use of occlusive antibiotic ointments.

Therapeutic

Therapy of genital herpes simplex infections has been one of the most frustrating and challenging tasks facing medical researchers. Herpes simplex virus is sensitive in vitro to a long list of agents. The difficulty, however, lies not with the destruction of free surface virus, but rather with the blocking of intracellular viral replication and the establishment of latency in primary episodes, or with the destruction of the latent viral reservoir, or at least the blocking of viral reactivation in recurrent genital herpes.

The problem with evaluation of therapy for genital herpes under uncontrolled conditions is that recurrences normally resolve without therapy and can be of variable duration and frequency, both of which usually decrease with time. Almost anything that does no harm probably will help (and seemingly has been reported), especially when the placebo factor is included. None of these "cures," however, have consistently proved effective when evaluated under double-blind controlled conditions.

Some of the better known and more widely used therapies that have been disproved include ether,[128] smallpox vaccines,[129] photoinactivation,[130,131] (potentially oncogenic),[132] Bacillus Calmette-Guérin (BCG),[133] levamisole,[134] vidarabine cream,[135] idoxuridine cream,[136] L-lysine,[137] and nonoxynol-9.[138]

A study showed that the topical use of 2-deoxy-D-glucose (2DG) resulted in a marked difference between placebo and 2DG-treated groups, as well as significantly decreasing the recurrence rate in the treated group.[139] Doubts were expressed, however, concerning the mechanics of the study and the fact that, even though there was a difference between the healing time in placebo and treated groups, neither healed faster than has been shown for untreated lesions.[140] 2DG has since been shown ineffective in a small double-blind controlled study.[141]

Though not available in the United States, 5% and 20% idoxuridine (IDU) and 20% IDU in dimethylsulfoxide (DMSO) has been reported of value in reducing the duration of infections,[142] while the 30% IDU paradoxically showed no clinical effect.[143]

Interferon was used in a study to try to inhibit the development of herpes simplex labialis after trigeminal nerve root surgery in patients with a history of HSV infection. Interferon given during, and for five days after, surgery resulted in a reduction in the number of patients developing lesions. (5/19 interferon vs 10/18 placebo).[144]

Prostaglandins may possibly be the common denominator between many of the presumed triggers such as fever, trauma, ultraviolet light, and menses. Whether antiinflammatory, antipyretic, antiprostaglandin drugs, such as aspirin or indomethacin, are effective in suppressing or reducing recurrences is currently under study, although in vitro these drugs have been shown to be potent inhibitors of viral replication.[145]

ACYCLOVIR

The development of acyclovir (9-(2-hydroxyethoxymethyl)guanine; Zovirax), with its unique mechanism of action, represents a major breakthrough in antiviral therapy. It is emerging as the first antiviral drug with demonstrable efficacy in the treatment of genital herpes simplex infections.

Acyclovir is a selective substrate for viral thymidine kinase, thus making the drug specific for herpesvirus-infected cells. Herpesvirus specified thymidine kinase concentrates acyclovir in the herpes-infected cell by phosphorylating it to the monophosphate derivative. Cellular kinase then converts the monophosphate derivative to acyclovir triphosphate, which is the active form of the drug.[146] The triphosphate derivative is both a competitive inhibitor of the viral DNA polymerase and a DNA chain terminator, thus inhibiting viral DNA synthesis (Fig. 11-5). Acyclovir triphosphate is much more active against viral DNA polymerase (about 30-fold lower inhibition) than cellular DNA polymerase.[147] In summary, acyclovir is much less toxic for normal uninfected cells because less is taken up, less is converted to the active form, and cellular DNA polymerase is less sensitive to the effects of the active form. Acyclovir has been manufactured in topical (5% ointment), oral, and intravenous forms. The topical and intravenous forms have been approved by the FDA and made available for use by the medical community.

Intravenous acyclovir has been found to affect the parameters by which clinical benefit is evaluated in genital herpes, that is, to significantly decrease the duration of viral shedding, new lesion formation, and local and systemic symptoms, while accelerating the healing rate of lesions.[148,149] Topical acyclovir has also been shown to have marked effectiveness in the treatment of first episodes of primary genital herpes.[150–152] The earlier the therapy was

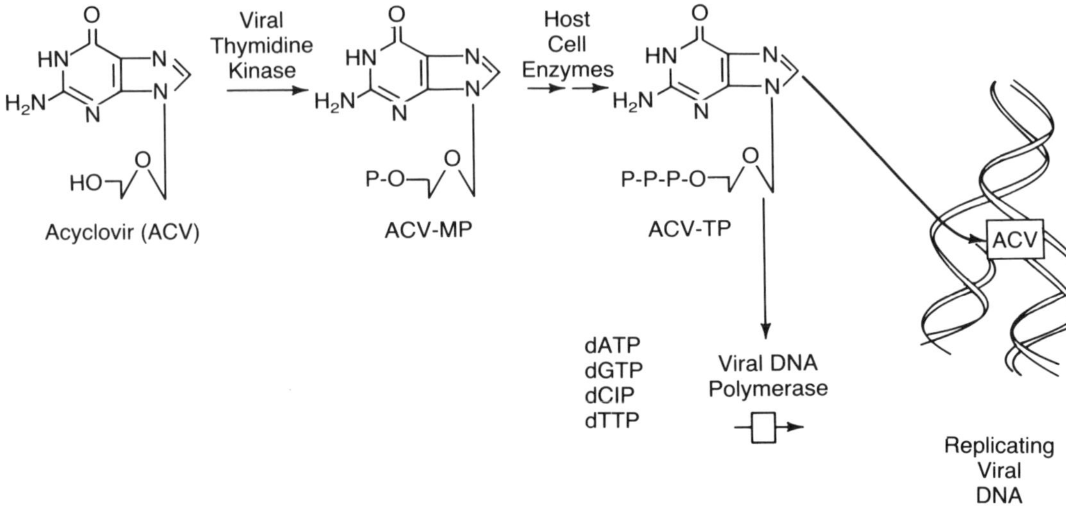

Fig. 11-5 Mechanism of activation and action of acyclovir.

started the better the results that were obtained. In recurrent genital herpes, however, it produced little clinical benefit.[150,153] Oral acyclovir has shown significant clinical benefit in both primary and recurrent genital herpes.[154,155] Although acyclovir has shown efficacy in treating the signs and symptoms of genital herpes, in no setting has it reduced the time to subsequent recurrences or frequency of subsequent recurrences, that is, prevented or effected latency.

A note of caution is urged in the use of topical acyclovir.[156] Resistant viruses have been reported in vitro and in vivo,[157] although their clinical significance remains to be determined. Topical acyclovir should therefore be used only for its established indications. It should not be used indiscriminantly if no clinical benefit is gained just because of the lack of alternatives.

The development of acyclovir has been a great biomedical scientific achievement and holds much promise for the future of antiviral therapy. Even if latent herpes simplex virus cannot be eradicated, prevention of recurrent disease with earlier or chronic suppressive treatment, resulting in probable reduction of disease transmission, are worthy goals. Studies of earlier administration of oral and topical acyclovir are now in progress. It is hoped that the development of acyclovir derivatives or other nucleoside analogs[124] will negate the possible problem of acyclovir-resistant herpesviruses. A new exciting age of antiviral therapy has begun that holds much promise for the control, if not the cure, of herpesvirus infections.

COUNSELING THE HERPES PATIENT

It is hoped that the preceding discussion has presented the facts, as presently understood, necessary to dispel some of the myths of the "herpes hysteria," and put it into perspective for the patient and his or her loved ones. An explanation of the virus and its life cycle should be presented, stressing that, although herpes is usually recurrent, the majority of the time the patient is disease-free and can engage in normal sexual activities while taking the precautions outlined. with these prophylactic measures ("a new contraception") and a knowledge of the disease pattern and prodromes, a sense of renewed control can be obtained. Female patients should be advised that childbearing can proceed with minimal complications if the proper precautions are taken. Cervical cancer still occurs in only a minority of women with genital herpes, although the incidence is increased, and can be detected at an early curable stage with regular yearly Papaniculaou smears. Restricted personal relationships, with only other herpes patients, is not necessary,[158] since from a medical point of view the same prophylactic measures should be taken if one or both members of a couple have genital herpes, because of the possibility of exogenous reinfection with a different type or strain. The "herpes hysteria" unfortunately has created an environment where understanding and nonjudgmental companionship is many times more easily obtained from other herpes patients than an uneducated public.

As can be seen, diagnosis is only the first step; adequate counseling is equally necessary. As previously stated, it is hoped that with a broader understanding of the problem by the patient, his or her loved ones, and the public, much of the exaggerated fear of genital herpes can be allayed, and it will not serve as an impedance to a healthy, happy, "normal" life.

REFERENCES

1. Centers for Disease Control, National Disease and Therapeutic Index: MMWR. 31:137, 1982
2. Centers for Disease Control: Non-reported sexually transmissible diseases. United States. MMWR. 28:61, 1979
3. Centers for Disease Control: Herpes genital infection. Publication 00-2939, 1980
4. Suimeya CV, Marx J, Ullis K: Genital infections with herpes simplex virus in a university student population. Sex Transm Dis 7:16, 1980
5. Chuang T, Su WPD, Perry HO, et al: Incidence and trend of herpes progenitalis: A 15-year population study. Mayo Clin Proc 58:436, 1983
6. Gardner HL: Herpes genitalis: Our most important venereal disease. Am J Obstet Gynecol 135:553, 1979
7. Editorial: Genital herpes. Br Med J 2:1335, 1980
8. Sexually Transmitted Disease Surveillance 1979: Br Med J 282:155, 1981
9. Brown AZ, Kern ER, Spruance SL, et al: Clinical and virologic course of herpes simplex genitalis. West J Med 130:414, 1979
10. Corey L, Adams HG, Brown ZA, et al: Genital herpes simplex virus infections: Clinical manifestations, course, and complications. Ann Intern Med 98:958, 1983
11. Knox RS, Corey L, Blough HA, et al: Historical findings in subjects from a high socioeconomic group who have genital infections with herpes simplex virus. Sex Transm Dis 9(1):15, 1982
12. Nahmias AT, Dowdle WR, Naib ZM, et al: Genital infection with type 2 herpes virus hominus, a commonly occurring venereal disease. Br J Vener Dis 45:294, 1969
13. Stavraky KM, Rawls WE, Chiavetta J, et al: Sexual and socioeconomic factors affecting the risk of past infections with herpes simplex virus type 2. Am J Epidemiol 118(1):109, 1983
14. Kalinyak JE, Fleagle G, Docherty J: Incidence and distribution of herpes simplex virus types 1 and 2 from genital lesions in college women. J Med Virol 1:175, 1977
15. Wolontis J, Jeansson S: Correlation of herpes simplex virus types 1 and 2 with clinical features of infection. J Infect Dis 135:28, 1977
16. Change TW: Genital herpes and type 1 herpes virus hominis. JAMA 238:155, 1977
17. Reeves WE, Corey L, Adams HG: Risk of recurrence after first episodes of genital herpes: Relation to HSV type and antibody response. N Engl J Med 305(6):315, 1981
18. Buchman TG, Roizman B, Nahmias AJ: Demonstration of exogenous genital reinfection with herpes simplex virus type 2 by restriction endonuclease fingerprinting of viral DNA. J Infect Dis 140:295, 1979
19. Fife KH, Schmidt O, Remington M, et al: Primary and recurrent concomitant genital infection with herpes simplex virus types 1 and 2. J Infect Dis 147:163, 1983
20. Kit S, Trkula D, Qaui H, et al: Sequential genital infections by herpes simplex viruses

types 1 and 2: Restriction nuclease analysis of viruses from recurrent infections. Sex Transm Dis 10(2):67, 1983

21. Blank H, Haines H: Experimental human reinfection with herpes simplex virus. J Invest Dermatol 61:223, 1973

22. Lazar MP: Vaccination for recurrent herpes simplex infection: Initiation of a new disease site following the use of unmodified material containing the live virus. Arch Dermatol 73:70, 1956

23. Nahmias AJ, Roizman B: Infection with herpes simplex viruses 1 and 2. N Engl J Med 289:667, 1973

24. Roizman B: The herpes viruses—A biochemical definition of the group. Curr Top Microbiol Immunol 419:1, 1969

25. Nahmias A, Dowdle W: Antigenic and biologic differences in herpes virus hominus. Prog Med Virol 10:110, 1968

26. Nahmias AJ, Norrold B: HSV 1 and 2, basic and clinical aspects. DM 25:4, 1979

27. Turner R, Shehab Z, Osborne K: Shedding and survival of herpes simplex virus from "fever blisters." Pediatrics 70(4):547, 1982

28. Rosenthal CS: Replication of herpes viruses and latency. Can J Microbiol 25:239, 1979

29. Babick LA, Rouse BT: Immune control of herpes virus latency. Can J Microbiol 25:268, 1979

30. Baringer JR: Recovery of herpes simplex virus from human sacral ganglions. N Engl J Med 291:878, 1974

31. Cook ML, Stevens JG: Pathogenesis of herpetic neuritis and ganglionitis in mice: Evidence of intraaxonal transport of infection. Infect Immun 7:272, 1973

32. Openshaw H, Puga A, Notlcins A: Herpes simplex virus infection in sensory ganglia: Immune control, latency and reactivation. Fed Proc 38:2660, 1979

33. Stevens JG, Cook ML: Latent herpes simplex virus in spinal ganglia of mice. Science 173:843, 1971

34. Honess RW, Roizman B: Regulation of herpes virus macromolecular synthesis. I. Cascade regulation of the synthesis of three groups of viral proteins. J Virol 14:8, 1974

35. NIAID: Summary of a workshop on antiviral agents for genital herpes virus infections. J Infect Dis 145(5):774, 1982

36. NIAID: Concept review of genital herpes vaccines. J Infect Dis 145(3):413, 1982

37. Watson K, Steven JG, Cook ML, et al: Latency competence of thirteen HSV-1 temperature sensitive mutants. J Gen Virol 49:149, 1980

38. Hill TJ, Blyth WA: An alternative theory of herpes-simplex recurrence and a possible role for prostaglandins. Lancet 1:397, 1976

39. Rouse BT, Babick LA: Mechanisms of recovery from herpes virus infections. A review. Can J Comp Med 42:414, 1978

40. Morahan PS, Morse SS, McGeorge MB: Macrophage extrinsic antiviral activity during herpes simplex infection. J Gen Virol 46:291, 1980

41. Schlabach AJ, Martinez D, Field AK, et al: Resistance of C58 mice to primary systemic herpes virus infection: Macrophage dependence and T-cell independence. Infect Immun 26:615, 1979

42. Corey L: The diagnosis and treatment of genital herpes. JAMA 248(9):1041, 1982

43. Lopez C, O'Reilly RJ: Cell mediated immune responses in recurrent herpes virus infections. I. Lymphocyte proliferation assay. J Immunol 118:895, 1977

44. Lehner T, Wilton JMA, Shillitoe EJ: Immunological basis for latency, recurrences, and putative oncogenicity of herpes simplex virus. Lancet 2:60, 1975

45. Corey L, Reeves WC, Holmes KK: Cellular immune response in genital herpes simplex virus infection. N Engl J Med 299:986, 1978

46. Shillitoe EJ, Wilton JMA, Lehner T: Sequential changes in cell-mediated immune responses to herpes simplex virus after recurrent herpetic infection in humans. Infect Immun 18:130, 1977

47. Rasmussen L, Merigan TC: Role of T lymphocytes in cellular immune reponses during herpes simplex virus infection in humans. Proc Natl Acad Sci USA 75:3957, 1978

48. Goodell SE, Quinn TC, Mkrtichian E, et al: Herpes simplex proctitis in homosexual men: Clinical, sigmodoscopic, and histopathological features. N Engl J Med 308(13):868, 1983

49. Rawls WE, Gardner HC, Flanders RW, et

al: Genital herpes in two social groups. Am J Obstet Gynecol 110:682, 1971

50. Scher J, Bottone E, Desmond E, et al: The incidence and outcome of asymptomatic herpes genitalis in an obstetric population. Am J Obstet Gynecol 144(8):906, 1982

51. Centers for Disease Control: Herpes genital infection. Publication 00-2939, 1980

52, Adam E, Kaufman RH, Mirkourc RR, et al: Persistence of virus shedding in asymptomatic women after recovery from herpes genitalis. Obstet Gynecol 54:171, 1979

53. Rahray MC, Corey L, Reeves WC, et al: Recurrent genital herpes among women: Symptomatic vs. asymptomatic viral shedding. Br J Vener Dis 54:262, 1978

54. Vontver LA, Hickok HE, Brown Z, et al: Recurrent genital herpes simplex virus in pregnancy: Infant outcome and frequency of asymptomatic recurrences. Am J Obstet Gynecol 143(1):75, 1982

55. Adam E, Dreesman GF, Kaufman RH, et al: Asymptomatic virus shedding after herpes genitalis. Am J Obstet Gynecol 137(7):341, 1978

56. Willmott FE, Mair HJ: Genital herpes virus infection in women attending a venereal diseases clinic. Br J Vener Dis 54:341, 1978

57. Ng ABP, Reagan JW, Yen SSC: Herpes genitalis, clinical and cytopathologic experience with 256 patients. Obstet Gynecol 30:645, 1970

58. Guinan ME, MacCalman J, Kern ER, et al: The course of untreated recurrent genital herpes simplex infection in 27 women. N Engl J Med 304(13):763, 1981

59. Centifanto YM, Drylie DM, Deardourff SL, et al: Herpes type 2 in the male genitourinary tract. Science 178:318, 1971

60. Traub RG, Madden DL, Fuccillo DA, et al: The male as a reservoir of infection with cytomegalovirus, herpes, and mycoplasma. N Engl J Med 289:697, 1973

61. Detare FA, Drylie DM, Kaufman HE, et al: Herpes virus type 2: Study of semen in male subjects with recurrent infections. J Urol 120:449, 1978

62. Pozin GJ, Ho M, Jannetta PJ: Reactivation of herpes simplex virus after decompression of the trigeminal nerve root. J Infect Dis 138:405, 1978

63. Hill TJ, Blyth WA, Harbour PA: Trauma to the skin causes recurrence of herpes simplex in the mouse. J Gen Virol 39:21, 1978

64. Blyth WA, Hill TJ, Field HJ, et al: Reactivation of herpes simplex virus infection by ultraviolet light and possible involvement of prostaglandins. J Gen Virol 33:547, 1976

65. Chang TW, Fumara WJ, Weinstein L: Genital herpes. Some clinical and laboratory observations. JAMA 229:544, 1974

66. Krohel GB, Richardson JR, Farrell DF: Herpes simplex neuropathy. Neurology 26:496, 1976

67. McLennan JL, Darby G: Latent herpes simplex in dorsal root sensory ganglia. In Abstracts of International Conference on Human Herpes Viruses. Emory University, Atlanta, GA, March 17, 1980

68. Blank H: Herpetism. Arch Dermatol 115:1440, 1979

69. Bierman SM: A retrospective study of 375 patients with genital herpes simplex infections seen between 1973 and 1980. Cutis 31:548, 1983

70. Stamm WE, Wagner KF, Amsel R, et al: Causes of the acute urethral syndrome in women. N Engl J Med 303:409, 1980

71. Person DA, Kaufman RH, Gardner HL, et al: Herpes virus type 2 in genitourinary tract infection. Am J Obstet Gynecol 116:993, 1973

72. Skoldenberg B, Jeansson S, Wolontis S: Herpes simplex virus type 2 and acute septic meningitis. Clinical features of cases with isolation of herpes simplex virus from cerebrospinal fluids. Scand J Infect Dis 7:227, 1975

73. Riehle RA, Williams JJ: Transient neuropathic bladder following herpes simplex genitalis. J Urol 122:263, 1979

74. Caplan LR, Kleman FJ, Berg S: Urinary retention probably secondary to herpes genitalis. N Engl J Med 297:920, 1977

75. Hanshaw JB: Herpes virus hominus infections in the fetus and the newborn. Am J Dis Child 126:546, 1973

76. Monif GRG, Hardt NS: Management of herpetic vulvovaginitis in pregnancy. Semin Perinatol 7(1):16, 1983

77. Nahmias AJ, Visintine M: Herpes simplex virus. p. 156. In Remington JJ, Kelin JD (eds): Infectious Diseases of the Fetus and Newborn. Saunders, Philadelphia, 1976

78. Jenista JA: Perinatal herpes virus infections. Semin Perinatol 7(1):9, 1983

79. Parvey LS, Chien LT: Neonatal herpes simplex virus infection introduced by fetal monitor scalp electrodes. Pediatrics 65:1150, 1980

80. Yeager AS, Arvin AM, Urbani LJ, et al: Relationship of antibody to outcome in neonatal herpes simplex virus infections. Infect Immun 66:489, 1980

81. Light IJ: Postnatal acquisition of herpes simplex virus by the newborn infant: A review of the literature. Pediatrics 63:480, 1979

82. Honig PJ, Holzwanger J, Leyden JJ: Congenital herpes simplex virus infections. Arch Dermatol 115:1329, 1979

83. Berkovich S, Ressel M: Neonatal herpes keratitis. J Pediatr 69:652, 1966

84. Nahmias AJ, Visintine AM, Reimer CB, et al: Herpes simplex virus infection of the fetus and newborn. Prog Clin Biol Res 13:63, 1975

85. Visintine AM, Nahmias AJ, Whitley R, et al: The natural history and epidemiology of neonatal herpes simplex infection. In Abstracts of International Conference on Hinman Herpes Viruses. Emory University, Atlanta, GA, March 17, 1980

86. Komorous JM, Wheeler CE, Briggaman RA, et al: Intrauterine herpes simplex infections. Arch Dermatol 113:918, 1977

87. Whitley RJ, Nahmias AJ, Visintine AM: The natural history of herpes simplex virus infection of mother and newborn. Pediatrics 66(4):489, 1980

88. Harger JH, Pazin GJ, Armstrong JA: Characteristics and management of pregnancy in women with genital herpes simplex infection. Am J Obstet Gynecol 145(7):704, 1983

89. Grossman JH, Wallen WC, Sever JL: Management of genital herpes simplex infection during pregnancy. Obstet Gynecol 58(1):1, 1981

90. Visintine AM, Nahmias AJ, Josey WE: Genital herpes. Perinat Care 2:32, 1978

91. Nahmias AJ, Josey WE, Naib AM, et al: Perinatal risk associated with maternal genital herpes simplex virus infection. Am J Obstet Gynecol 129:159, 1977

92. Amstey MS: Management of pregnancy complicated by genital herpes virus infection. Obstet Gynecol 37:515, 1971

93. Light IJ, Linnemann CC Jr: Neonatal herpes simplex infection following delivery by cesarean section. Obstet Gynecol 44:496, 1974

94. Committee on Fetus and Newborn, Committee on Infectious Disease: Perinatal herpes simplex infections. Pediatrics 66:147, 1980

95. Goldberg RJ, Gravell M: A search for herpes simplex virus type 2 markers in cervical carcinoma. Cancer Res 36:795, 1976

96. Naib ZM, Nahmias AJ, Josey WE, et al: Genital herpetic infection: Association with cervical dysplasia and carcinoma. Cancer 23:940, 1969

97. Rawls W, Tompkins WA, Melnick JL: The association of herpes virus type 2 and carcinoma of the uterine cervix. Am J Epidemiol 89:547, 1969

98. Adelusi B, Naib J, Muther J, et al: Epidemiological studies relating genital herpes simplex virus infection with cervical neoplasia. An update. In Abstracts of International Conference on Human Herpes Viruses. Emory University, Atlanta, GA, March 17, 1980.

99. Rapp F, Reed C: Experimental evidence for the oncogenic potential of herpes simplex virus. Cancer Res 36:800, 1976.

100. Nahmias A, Sawanobori S: The genital herpes cervical cancer hypothesis—10 years later. p. 117. In Ito Y (ed): Viral Oncogenesis. Karger, Basel, 1978

101. Smith JW: Herpes simplex virus, an expanding relationship to human cancer. J Reprod Med 28(2):116, 1983

102. Rudolp J: Cancer of the uterine cervix. p. 217. In Rubin P (ed): Clinical Oncology. American Cancer Society, New York, 1974

103. Kaufman RH, Dreesman GR, Burek J, et al: Herpes virus-induced antigens in squamous-cell carcinoma in situ of the vulva. N Engl J Med 305(9):483, 1983

104. Luleci G, Sakizli M, Gunlap A, et al: Herpes simplex type 2 neutralization antibodies in patients with cancers of urinary bladder, prostate, and cervix. J Surg Oncol 16:327, 1981

105. Wade TR, Kopf AW, Ackerman AB: Bowenoid papulosis of the genitalia. Arch Dermatol 115:306, 1979

106. August MJ, Nordlund JJ, Hsiung GD: Persistence of herpes simplex virus types 1 and 2 in infected individuals. Arch Dermatol 115:30, 1979
107. Lennartz H: Diagnosis of herpes simplex. Adv Ophthalmol 38:17, 1979
108. Wheeland RG, Burgdorf WHC, Hoshow RA: A quick Tzanck smear. J Am Acad Dermatol 8(2):258, 1983
109. Brown ST, Jaffe HW, Zaidi A, et al: Sensitivity and specificity of diagnostic tests for genital infection with herpes virus hominus. Sex Transm Dis 6:10, 1979
110. Lever WF, Schaumberg-Lever G: p. 361. In Histopathology of the Skin. Lippincott, Philadelphia, 1983
111. Sever JL, Jacob AJ: Laboratory diagnosis of herpes virus infections. Semin Perinatol 7(1):57, 1983
112. Volpi A, Lakeman AD, Pereira L, et al: Monoclonal antibodies for rapid diagnosis and typing of genital herpes infections during pregnancy. Am J Obstet Gynecol 146(7):813, 1983
113. Goldstein LC, Corey L, McDougall JK, et al: Monoclonal antibodies to herpes simplex viruses: Use in antigenic typing and rapid diagnosis. J Infect Dis 147(5):829, 1983
114. Frumara NJ, Schmidt-Ulirck B, Comite H: Primary herpes simplex and primary syphilis: A description of seven cases. Sex Transm Dis 7:130, 1980
115. Smith EB, McLaren LC: Attempts to recover herpes simplex virus from skin sites of recurrent infection. J Gen Virol 47(1):705, 1980
116. Singh B, Postic, Cutler J: Viricidal effect of certain contraceptives on type 2 herpes virus. Am J Obstet Gynecol 12 6:422, 1976
117. Postic B, Singh B, Squeglia NL, et al: Inactivation of clinical isolates of herpes virus hominis, types 1 and 2 by chemical contraceptives. Sex Transm Dis 5:22, 1978
118. Smith L Jr, Oleske J, Cooper R, et al: Efficacy of condoms as barriers to HSV-2 and gonorrhea: An in vitro model. In Program and Abstracts of the First Sexually Transmitted Diseases World Congress. San Juan, Puerto Rico, 1981
119. Kish SC, McMahon JT, Bergfeld WF, et al: An ancient method and a modern scourge: The condom as a barrier against herpes. J Am Acad Dermatol 9(3):769, 1983
120. Adler MW, Mindel A: Genital herpes: Hype or Hope? Br Med J 286:1767, 1983
121. Nasemann TH, Wassilew SW: Vaccination for herpes simplex genitalis. Br J Vener Dis 55:121, 1979
122. Hilleman MR, Larson VM, Lehman ED, et al: Subunit herpes simplex 2 vaccine. p. 503. In Nahmias AJ, Dowdle WR, and Schinazi RF (eds): The Human Herpes Viruses. Elsevier, New York, 1981
123. Skinner GRB, Woodman CBS, Hortley LE, et al: Preparation and immunogenicity of vaccine AC NFU 1 (5-) MRC towards the prevention of herpes genitalis. Br J Vener Dis 58:381, 1982
124. Genital Herpes Research: Many aim to tame maverick virus. Medical New. JAMA 250(18):2417, 1983
125. Harbour DA, Blyth WA, Hill TJ: Prostaglandins enhance spread of herpes simplex virus in cell cultures. J Gen Virol 41:87, 1978
126. Friedrich EG, Masukawa T: Effect of povidone-iodine on herpes genitalis. Obstet Gynecol 45:337, 1974
127. Woodbridge P: The use of betadine antiseptic paint in the treatment of herpes simplex and herpes zoster. J Int Med Res 5:378, 1977
128. Corey L, Reeves WC, Chang WT, et al: The effectiveness of topical ether for the treatment of genital herpes simplex infection. N Engl J Med 299:237, 1978
129. Kern AB, Schiff BL: Smallpox vaccinations in the management of recurrent herpes simplex: A controlled evaluation. J Invest Dermatol 33:99, 1959
130. Myers MG, Oxman MN, Clark JE, et al: Failure of neutral red photodynamic inactivation in recurrent herpes simplex virus infections. N Engl J Med 293:945, 1975
131. Felbee TD, Smith EB, Knox JM, et al: Photodynamic inactivation of herpes simplex: Report of a clinical trial. JAMA 223:289, 1973
132. Li SHL, Jerkofsky MA, Rupp E: Demonstration of oncogenic potential of mammalian cells transformed by DNA-containing viruses following photodynamic inactivation. Int J Cancer 15:190, 1975

133. Beerman SM: BCG immunoprophylaxis of recurrent herpes progenitalis. Arch Dermatol 112:1410, 1976

134. Beerman JM: Double-blind cross-over study of levamisole as immunoprophylaxis for recurrent herpes progenitalis. Cutis 21:352, 1978

135. Adams HG, Benson EA, Alexander ER, et al: Genital herpetic infection in men and women: Clinical course and effect to topical application of adenine arabinoside. J Infect Dis 133:151, 1976

136. Burnett JW, Katz SL: A study of the use of 5-iodo-2-deoxyuridine in cutaneous herpes simplex. J Invest Dermatol 40:7, 1962

137. Scheibel M, Jessen O: Lysine prophylaxis in recurrent herpes simplex labialis: A double-blind controlled cross over study. Acta Derm Venereol (Stockh) 60:895, 1979

138. Vontver LA, Reeves NC, Rattray M, et al: Clinical course and diagnosis of genital herpes simplex virus infection and evaluation of topical surfactant therapy. Am J Obstet Gynecol 133:548, 1979

139. Blough HA, Giuntoli RL: Successful treatment of human genital herpes infections with 2-deoxy-d-glucose. JAMA 241:2798, 1979

140. Corey L, Holmes KK: The use of 2-deoxy-d-glucose for genital herpes. JAMA 243:29, 1980

141. McCray MK, Zugerman C: 2-deoxy-d-glucose for herpes simplex. J Am Acad Dermatol 6(4):550, 1982

142. Parker JD: A double-blind trial of idoxuridine in recurrent genital herpes. J Antimicrob Chemother 3(Suppl A):131, 1977

143. Silvestri DC, Corey L, Holmes KK: Ineffectiveness of topical idoxuridine in dimethyl sulfoxide for genital herpes. JAMA 248:953, 1982

144. Pazin GJ, Armstrong JA, Lam MTR, et al: Prevention of reactivated herpes simplex infection by human leukocyte interferon after operation on the trigeminal root. N Engl J Med 301:225, 1979

145. Newton AA: Inhibitors of prostaglandin synthesis as inhibitors of herpes simplex virus replication. Adv Ophthalmol 38:;58, 1979

146. Elson GB, Furman PA, Fyfe JA, et al: Selectivity of action of an antiherpetic agent. 9-(2-Hydroxyethoxymethyl)guanine. Proc Natl Acad Sci USA 74(12):2716, 1977

147. Furman PA, St. Clair MH, Fyfe JA, et al: Inhibition of herpes simplex virus induced DNA polymerase activity and viral DNA replication by 9-(2-hydroxyethoxymethyl)guanine and its triphosphate. J Virol 32(1):72, 1979

148. Mindel A, Adler MW, Sutherland S, et al: Intravenous acyclovir treatment for primary genital herpes. Lancet 1:697, 1982

149. Corey L, Fifek H, Benedetti JK, et al: Intravenous acyclovir for the treatment of primary genital herpes. Ann Intern Med 98:958, 1983

150. Corey L, Nahmias AJ, Guinan ME, et al: A trial of topical acyclovir in genital herpes simplex infections. N Engl J Med 306:1313, 1983

151. Corey L, Benedetti JK, Critchlow CW, et al: Double-blind controlled trial of topical acyclovir in genital herpes simplex virus infections. Am J Med 73:326, 1982

152. Thin RN, Nabarro JM, Parker JD, et al: Topical acyclovir in the treatment of initial genital herpes. Br J Vener Dis 59:116, 1983

153. Reichman RC, Badger GJ, Guinan ME et al: Topically administered acyclovir in the treatment of recurrent herpes simplex genitalis: A controlled trial. J Infect Dis 147(2):336, 1983

154. Nilsen AD, Aasen T, Halsos AM, et al: Efficacy of oral acyclovir in the treatment of initial and recurrent genital herpes. Lancet 2:571, 1982

155. Bryson YJ, Dillon M, Covett M, et al: Treatment of first episodes of genital herpes simplex virus infection with oral acyclovir. N Engl J Med 308(16):916, 1983

156. Raab B, Lorincz AL: Topical acyclovir caution. J Am Acad Dermatol 8(1):124, 8(5):756, 1983

157. Balfour HH: Resistance of herpes simplex to acyclovir. Ann Intern Med 98(3):404, 1983

12

Condylomata Acuminata and Genital Molluscum Contagiosum

J. D. Oriel

CONDYLOMATA ACUMINATA

History

Genital warts were known to physicians in the ancient world, who called them "figs" or condylomas.[1] Since then, they have been variously described as fig warts, venereal vegetations, gonorrheal warts, venereal warts, and condylomata acuminata; the last of these terms, which means "pointed condyloma," is modern. In the eighteenth and nineteenth centuries the lesions were attributed first to syphilis, then to gonorrhea, and later to irritation by genital secretions "disordered through venery."[2] Toward the end of the nineteenth century it was realized that condylomata acuminata were related to common cutaneous warts: there were histologic similarities, and in a few experiments inoculation of material from genital condylomas into nongenital sites had been followed by the appearance of common warts.[2]

This evidence suggested that condylomata acuminata were a type of wart. The viral etiology of common cutaneous warts was finally confirmed in 1949, when virus particles were seen by electron microscopy in extracts of common warts[3] and twenty years later particles of similar appearance were seen in low concentration in extracts of genital warts.[4,5] Although inability to propagate the viruses in the laboratory meant that Koch's postulates could not be satisfied, it was generally agreed that both cutaneous and genital warts had a viral etiology. At this time it had not been shown that "cutaneous" and "genital" wart viruses were identical, but it was assumed that they were, and a "unitary theory" was proposed and generally accepted. According to this, all kinds of human wart, including condylomata acuminata, were caused by the same virus, the morphology of the wart depending only on the kind of epithelium the virus infected. Sexual contact was regarded as one of the many ways in which this virus could reach the genital area.

It is now known that this opinion was erroneous, as there are many different wart viruses, of which some are apparently present only in condylomata acuminata. Moreover, there is substantial evidence that condylomata acuminata are a sexually transmitted disease.

153

Etiology

Basophilic nuclear inclusions can be seen in vacuolated cells in the stratum granulosum of all kinds of wart, and electron microscopy reveals that these inclusions are composed of aggregates of virus particles.[4-6] The particles are spherical and unenveloped, 45–55 nm in diameter, and they show cubic symmetry in the arrangement of their subunits. The genome is a single molecule of double-stranded DNA.[7] The morphology of virions recovered from different clinical varieties of wart is identical, but their concentration shows marked variation, being highest in plantar warts and lowest in condylomata acuminata.

Wart viruses belong to the papovavirus family; the genus is called papillomavirus. They have not yet been propagated in cell culture, so human papillomaviruses (HPV) cannot be studied by the procedures of classical virology. In recent years it has been possible to characterize virus extracted from individual warts by immune electron microscopy, DNA mapping by restriction endonuclease cleavage, molecular hybridization, and gel electrophoresis. From these studies it is clear that there are multiple strains of human papillomavirus, and that many of these are specifically associated with a particular clinical type of wart. HPV-6 has been recovered only from condylomata acuminata, and HPV-11 from some condylomata acuminata, many flat condylomas of the cervix and recurrent laryngeal papillomas of infants, and some biopsy specimens from cervical epithelial neoplasia; neither HPV-6 nor HPV-11 have been found in cutaneous warts.[8-10] Anal warts have also

Table 12-1. Human Papilloviruses with Corresponding Lesions and Possibility of Malignant Transformation

Virus	Lesions	Possibility of Malignancy
HPV-1	Palmar and plantar warts	−
HPV-2	Common warts	−
HPV-3	Plane warts Epidermodysplasia verruciformis	−
HPV-4	Common warts	
HPV-5	Epidermodysplasia verruciformis	+
HPV-6	Condylomata acuminata	? +
HPV-7	Common warts	−
HPV-8	Epidermodysplasia verruciformis	+
HPV-9	Epidermodysplasia verruciformis	+
HPV-10	Epidermodysplasia verruciformis	? +
HPV-11	Condylomata acuminata Flat condylomas Laryngeal condylomas of infants	? +
HPV-12	Epidermodysplasia verruciforms	+
HPV-13	Epithelial hyperplasia of mouth	?
HPV-14	Epidermodysplasia verruciformis	+
HPV-15	Epidermodysplasia verruciformis	+
HPV-16	Cervical carcinoma (some)	+

From Jablonska S, Orth G: Human papovaviruses. p 8. In Rook AJ, Maibach HI (eds): Recent Advances in Dermatology. 6th Ed. Churchill Livingstone, Edinburgh, London, New York, 1983, with permission.

been studied, but less thoroughly than genital warts. When hybridization analysis was performed under stringent conditions, one anal wart was found to contain genomic sequences related to the cutaneous papillomavirus HPV-1, but in 10 other anal wart tissue samples homology to HPV-1 or HPV-2 was not found.[8] It is not yet known whether these lesions contain HPV-6 or HPV-11.

Immunology

Study of the immunology of warts has been greatly hampered by inability to propagate papillomaviruses in the laboratory, which means that the only virus available is that which can be extracted from individual lesions. In patients with cutaneous warts, circulating antibodies can be identified by complement fixation tests, immunodiffusion gels, and immune electron microscopy.[11,12] IgM antibody is the commonest, but IgG antibody also occurs, particularly when the warts are regressing.[13,14] Immunologic studies are even more difficult with anogenital warts because they contain so little viral antigen. Circulating viral antibodies have been detected in patients with this disease, but their significance is unknown.[15]

It is believed that cell-mediated immunity (CMI) is important in the resolution of warts, and it is known that regressing warts often show infiltration with macrophages and lymphocytes.[16] The release of papillomavirus particles from warts as they disrupt could be the explanation of the raised levels of circulating antibodies which have been observed. The incidence of warts, including genital warts, is increased during immunosuppressive treatment, and in patients with defective cell-mediated immunity.[17,18]

Epidemiology

The peak age of onset of genital warts is between 19 and 22 years.[2] In England, where genital warts are reportable from clinics for sexually transmitted diseases, the number of patients with the condition in 1971 was 8,916 men and 4,814 women, but in 1980 the number had risen to 16,760 men and 9,384 women.[19,20]

Although there had previously been a vague belief that genital warts might be infectious, it was not until 1954 that data indicating sexual transmission became available.[21] Since then several studies have confirmed that this is a sexually transmissible disease.[2,22,23] Contact tracing has shown that over 60% of individuals sexually exposed to genital warts subsequently develop the disease; the incubation period is between three weeks and several months.[2]

The infectivity of genital warts has two consequences. First, sex partners should be examined because they may be infected. Second, one sexually transmitted disease suggests the possibility of others, and many patients with genital warts have other concomitant infections, such as gonorrhea, nongonococcal urethritis, trichomoniasis, and syphilis.[2] Careful screening of patients with genital warts for other infections is clearly advisable.

Human papillomavirus affects the cervix in women, with or without associated vulval condylomas. The resulting disease (flat or papilliferous condylomas) is described below. The great majority (88%) of women with cervical human papillomavirus infection are under the age of 40, more than half are under 25, and 22% are under 20 years of age.[24] It has been shown that, in comparison with age-matched women without genital infection, women with cervical condylomas have an earlier age of onset of sex activity, more sex partners (including casual contacts), and more often given a history of other sexually transmitted diseases.[25] The male partners of women with cervical human papillomavirus infection often have penile or distal urethral condylomas.[26] The epidemiology of condylomas of the cervix apparently resembles that of vulval and penile condylomas in most important respects.

Condylomata acuminata can occur in the mouth. This was recorded many years ago in two prostitutes who had performed "coitus illegitimus,"[27] and is probably commoner than the scanty references in the literature might suggest.[28,29]

In young children vulval condylomas are not unusual, but penile and anal condylomas are rare.[30,31] The origin of these vulval lesions is not always clear. They may be due to child abuse,[32] but they can probably originate from infection during delivery, because the mothers of some of these babies have genital warts themselves.[33] A related pediatric condition is multiple papillomata of the larynx. For a long time the origin of these tumors, which histologically resemble condylomata acuminata, was unclear, but a link with maternal genital condylomas has now been shown.[34] Mature papillomavirus particles have not been identified in laryngeal papillomas, but HPV-11 has been found in 50% of a series of the tumors.[10] It seems probable that in babies with the disease infection of the larynx from the mother occurs during delivery, but the risk of the disease developing in infants exposed to human papillomavirus at this time is unknown.

The epidemiology of anal warts differs in the two sexes. In women, they are usually associated with vulval lesions. In men, anal warts sometimes accompany or follow penile warts, but more often they appear alone. In both sexes, 80% of patients with condylomas restricted to the anus given a history of anal coitus.[35] It has not hitherto been possible to establish a clear relationship between anal warts and the presence of penile warts in the "active" partner; furthermore, in male homosexuals anal warts are up to seven times as common as penile warts.[35,36] The explanation of this phenomenon may lie in a predilection of human papillomavirus for anal epithelium, together with the casual nature of many male homosexual contacts. Anal warts contain human papillomavirus in low concentration, but this has not yet been characterized.[8] Men with these lesions show a high incidence of associated infections, notably syphilis and gonorrhea,[35] and therefore need careful screening before treatment.

There is no evidence of any close epidemiologic relationship between genital and cutaneous warts.[2,25] Nevertheless, a small number of patients with common cutaneous warts develop penile, vulval, or perianal lesions of similar appearance. It is likely that in these patients the same virus has caused the warts at each site, having been accidentally transferred to the genitals by the hands. The virus in this form of genital wart has not yet been typed.

Pathology

Several different varieties of cutaneous wart are recognized in dermatology. Common warts (verruca vulgaris) are raised, circumscribed hyperkeratotic lesions, a few millimeters in diameter, which can be found on most areas but which are commonest on the hands. Plantar warts are up to 10 mm in diameter, partly buried in the epidermis and markedly hyperkeratotic. Plane warts are small and flat-topped, and appear mostly on the face and backs of the hands. Filiform warts are narrow and pedunculated, and occur on the neck and face. Epidermodysplasia verruciformis is a rare autosomal recessive disease in which there are extensive and persistent eruptions of plane warts, many of which become malignant. Lastly, condylomata acuminata are soft fleshy tumors which appear on moist areas, chiefly but not exclusively the anogenital region.

All warts share some histologic features.[37] There is elongation of the dermal papillae. The stratum germinativum is intact and the stratum spinosum hyperplastic (acanthosis). The stratum granulosum is well developed, and the stratum corneum is often hyperkeratotic. Large vacuolated

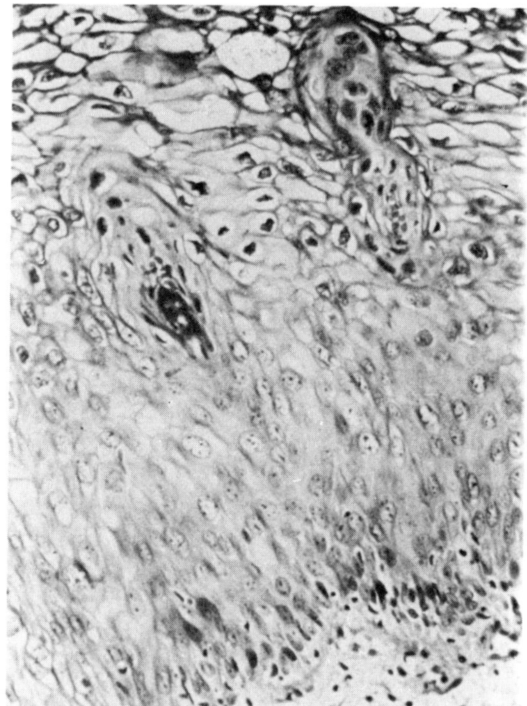

Fig. 12-1 Condyloma acuminatum. Penile lesion. The sections shows acanthosis, papillomatosis, and superficial vaculolated cells. ×40

cells are present in the stratum granulosum; some of these contain eosinophilic cytoplasmic inclusions that are composed of abnormal keratin, and basophilic nuclear inclusions that are composed of aggregated papillomavirus particles. Virus particles are also found in the stratum corneum, but not in the stratum spinosum.

The preponderance of these histologic features varies with the type of wart. Thus hyperkeratosis is a constant feature of common and plantar warts, and vacuolated epithelial cells numerous in plane warts. In genital warts (Fig. 12-1) acanthosis is very marked, forming the bulk of the tumors, and multiple mitotic figures are present; hyperkeratosis is unusual, but may develop as the lesions age or are unsuccessfully treated.

Viral antigen can be demonstrated in the nuclei of cells in the stratum granulosum of genital warts by several techniques, including the peroxidase-antiperoxidase test,[38] indirect immunofluorescence,[39] and an indirect immunoalkaline phosphatase reaction.[40]

Clinical Features

Genital warts are polymorphic. Verruca vulgaris can develop on the shaft of the penis (Fig. 12-2), but the commonest variety is condyloma acuminatum (Fig. 12-3). These lesions are soft, fleshy, and vascular; initially very small, they may enlarge rapidly, particularly on moist areas, and coalesce to form large masses. The commonest sites affected are the frenum, coronal sulcus, and inner lining of the prepuce.[2] Urethral condylomas are quite common. They appear first at the urinary meatus, but can spread to affect any part of the urethra.[41] They can be identified by urethroscopy, but can also be demonstrated radiologically by voiding cystourethrography, which avoids urethral instrumentation.[42] Warts have been described in the bladder, but are rare at this site.[43]

Anal warts appear first on the perianal area (Fig. 12-4), but in 50% of cases they also affect the anal canal below the pectinate line (Fig. 12-5), so anoscopy is mandatory. Anal warts can reach a considerable size.

In women, verruca vulgaris is sometimes seen on the labia majora, but condylomata acuminata are much commoner. They usually appear first at the fourchette and adjacent areas, then spread to affect other parts of the vulva (Fig. 12-6); in 20% of patients they involve the perineum and anus. The vagina is affected in some patients; although in some only the lower and upper third are involved, condylomas can occasionally fill the whole vagina.

The existence of cervical condylomas has been acknowledged for many years, but until recently they were regarded as rare.[44] Condyloma acuminatum of the cervix (ex-

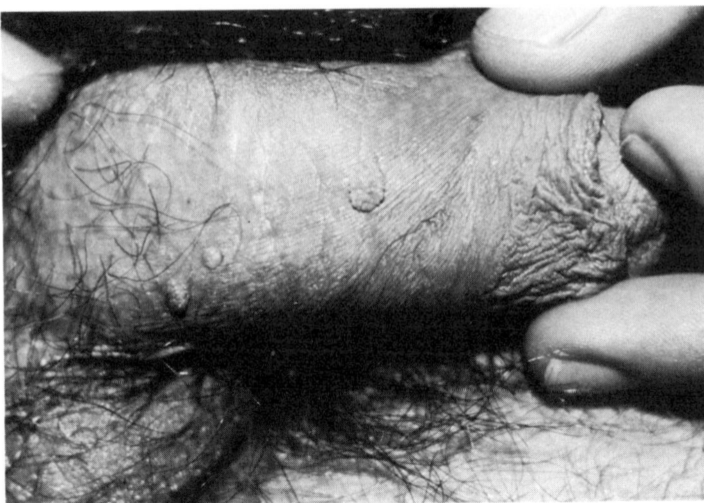

Fig. 12-2 Common warts (verruca vulgaris) of shaft of penis.

ophytic condyloma, Fig. 12-7) is associated with a characteristic cytologic picture of koilocytosis and dyskeratosis,[45] but several studies have shown that these changes are present in smears from some cervices without exophytic condylomas, these cytologic changes being present in 1–1.5% of routine cervical smears.[24,46] Although in these cases no cervical abnormality is visible to the naked eye, colposcopy reveals cervical lesions (Fig. 12-8). There are patches of flat or very slightly raised epithelium, which appears rough and shiny white after the ap-

plication of acetic acid. Although there may be regularly spaced capillary loops of the kind seen in condylomata acuminata, most colposcopically abnormal areas show only nonspecific punctate vascular atypia.[46] These abnormalities affect the transition zone, but can extend beyond the squamo-columnar junction. Lesions of this kind have been called "flat condylomas",[47] but some workers prefer the term "noncondylomatous wart virus infection."[46] There seems to be no doubt that they are viral. Histology of biopsy specimens shows a

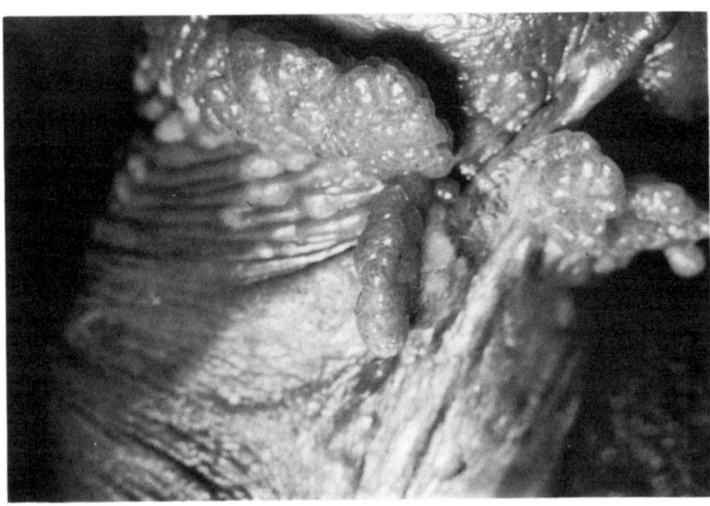

Fig. 12-3 Condylomata acuminata of penis.

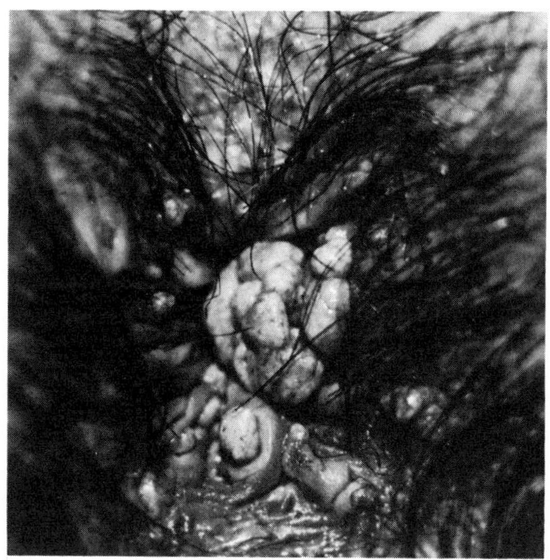

Fig. 12-4 Perianal condylomata acuminata.

wartlike structure,[24] immunohistochemical techniques indicate the presence of HPV antigen,[40] electron microscopy of koilocytotic cells from the lesions has demonstrated the presence of papillomavirus particles,[48] and HPV type 6 DNA has been found in the lesions by DNA-DNA hybridization.[49]

It may be concluded that human papillomavirus infection of the cervix can be expressed either as exophytic condylomas or as noncondylomatous wart virus infection. In the past the latter was often misdiagnosed as cervical dysplasia. The true diagnosis is revealed by histology and cytology, but some workers believe that "flat condylomas" are sufficiently distinctive to be accurately diagnosed by colposcopy[40,46]; this claim is not accepted by others.[50] Be this as it may, cytologic and histologic studies indicate that flat condylomas are often *associated* with cervical dysplasia,[24,51–53] a fact that may be of great significance.

Genital warts are influenced by host factors. They often enlarge in conditions in which cell-mediated immunity is depressed. Extensive condylomas occur in some patients with Hodgkin's disease, and are not uncommon in immunosuppressed patients, for example, those who have received renal transplants.[54] They also enlarge during pregnancy, when a temporary depression of

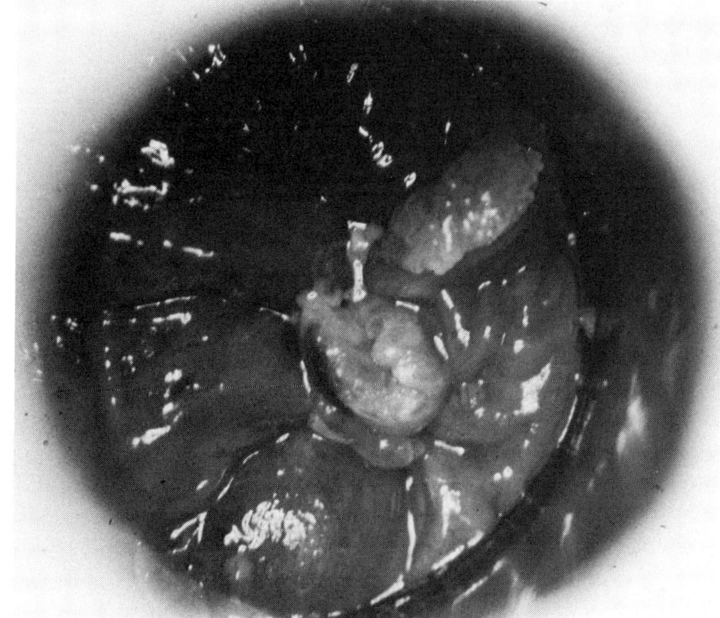

Fig. 12-5 Condylomata in anal canal.

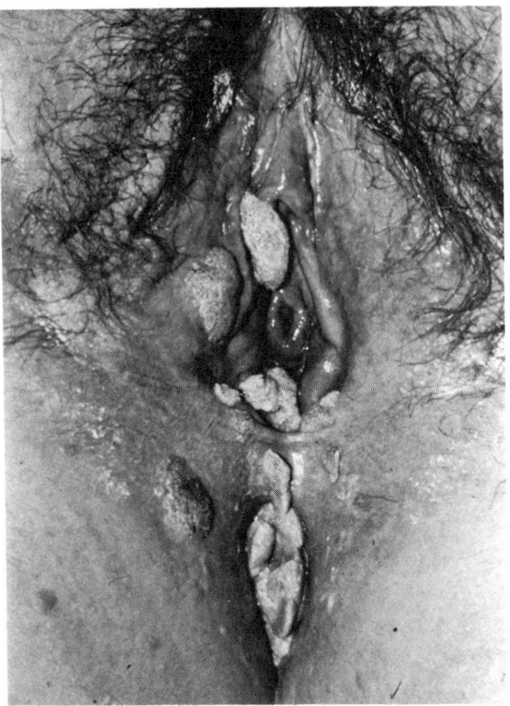

Fig. 12-6 Condylomata acuminata of vulva.

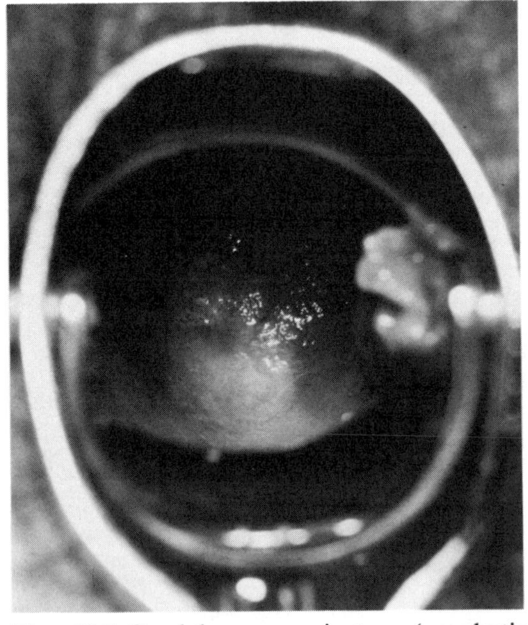

Fig. 12-7 Condyloma acuminatum (exophytic condyloma) of cervix.

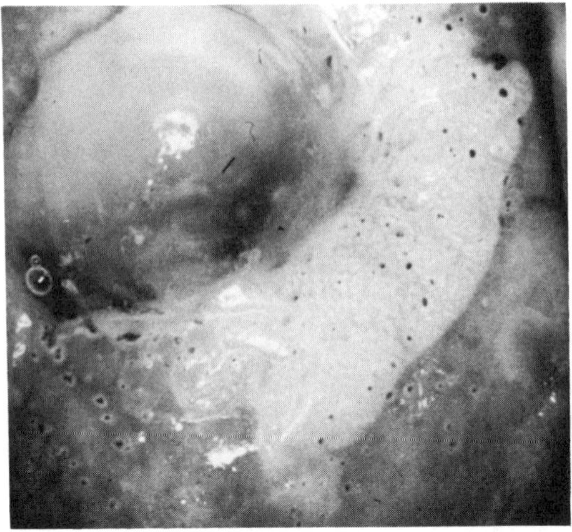

Fig. 12-8 Flat condyloma of cervix. This condition is also called noncondylomatous wart virus infection.

cell-mediated immunity occurs; after delivery they regress, or even disappear completely.[2]

Complications

Both genital and anal condylomata acuminata may reach a large size and be unpleasant for the patient through secondary infection and occasional hemorrhage. In pregnancy, large condylomas can cause real problems during labor because of obstruction of delivery, hemorrhage, and the difficulty in suturing condylomatous tissue; cesarean section has sometimes been necessary.[55]

Giant condyloma is a rare complication of condylomata acuminata, particularly on the penis, but sometimes on the vulva or anus. It was first described by Buschke and Loewenstein.[56] Initially a wart develops, usually in the coronal sulcus; relentless enlargement then occurs and large areas of the penis are destroyed, with the formation of multiple fistulae. Clinically, although metastasis does not occur it resembles a florid carcinoma, but histologically it is benign and has the features of condyloma acuminatum.[57] DNA of HPV-6 and HPV-11 has been recovered from giant condylomas.[58] The reason for the aggressive behavior of this histologically benign tumor is not known.

Giant condyloma can progress to malignancy[59,60]; in addition, however, a long series of reports have described malignant transformation of classical condylomata acuminata affecting the penis, vulva and anus.[61–65] Both intraepithelial and squamous cell carcinoma have been described in association with these lesions. Some of the bowenoid lesions of the genital area are now believed to be related to HPV infection.[66]

The possible connection between human papillomavirus and cervical neoplasia has been the subject of much recent discussion. Cervical condylomatous lesions are associated with cervical dysplasia of all degrees of severity.[45,46,67,68] Is this association causal or just a coincidence? There is certainly circumstantial evidence that human papillomavirus may play a role in cervical carcinoma: (1) Papillomaviruses are known oncogens in animals, inducing, among other diseases, skin cancers in rabbits[69] and (in association with an environmental agent) gastrointestinal cancers in cattle.[70] (2) Chronic persistent lesions of epidermodysplasia verruciformis and chronic laryngeal papillomas can both undergo malignant transformation[71,72]; cervical human papillomavirus infection too is often subclinical and can persist for many years,[73] and malignant transformation of long-standing condylomas has often been observed.[74,75] (3) The key epidemiologic markers of women with genital warts (and other sexually transmitted diseases) and of women with cervical carcinoma are the same, namely, early age of first intercourse and multiple and/or casual sex partners.[25,76]

This evidence does not prove that human papillomavirus is involved in the pathogenesis of cervical carcinoma, but it is consistent with the idea, which receives further support from recent virologic studies. There is now evidence that a part of the HPV genome is present in cervical cancer cells. DNA of HPV type 16 was present in 11 of 18 cervical cancer samples from German women and in 8 of 23 cancer biopsy specimens from Brazil and Kenya. HPV-16 was found in 2 of 33 condylomata acuminata, but both positive specimens contained HPV-6 or HPV-11 as well.[77] These results suggest that progression of condylomatous lesions to malignancy may depend, among other factors, on the viral type that is present.

It is too soon to make a judgment on the complicated issue of the natural history and oncogenicity of human papillomavirus in the genital tract. It has been suggested that a combination of HPV and an "initiating event" is needed for the development of cancer. This concept receives support from studies of viral papillomas in animals: the Shope papilloma of rabbits progresses to carcinoma following the application of tar,[69] and bovine viral papillomas of the esophagus become malignant if the animal is fed with bracken.[70] It has been suggested that the action of herpes simplex virus in cervical cells which are chronically infected with HPV may provide such an "event," and lead to carcinoma.[78] The truth of the matter will no doubt emerge as current research proceeds.

Diagnosis

The diagnosis of condylomata acuminata is usually clinical. Penile warts need to be distinguished from other papular lesions of the area. A minor condition which is sometimes confused with warts is "hirsutes papillaris penis" in which parallel rows of threadlike lesions appear on the corona. Histologically these are hypertrophic papillae,[79] and they do not need treatment. The characteristic umbilicated lesions of molluscum contagiosum are easily distinguished from warts. Among other infective diseases the most important are the skin lesions of secondary syphilis, both papular eruptions and condylomata lata; darkfield microscopy for *Treponema pallidum* and serologic tests will ensure the correct diagnosis. In the tropics, granuloma inguinale (donovanosis) may resemble condylomata acuminata, but the demonstration of Donovan bodies in impression smears stained with Giemsa is diagnostic. Carcinoma of the penis, particularly of the papillary "cauliflower" type, may give difficulty in the differential diagnosis, particularly since it may arise from condylomata acuminata. Hardness and fixity of the tumor and inguinal gland enlargement suggest carcinoma, but these are late signs and if there is the slightest doubt early biopsy is advisable.

Vulval warts must be distinguished from fibroepithelial polyps, molluscum contagiosum, and, in older women, seborrheic keratosis. Several benign neoplasms occur on the vulva, such as fibroma, lipoma, hidradenoma, adenoma, and endometrioma, which are usually diagnosed only after biopsy. The lesions of secondary syphilis affect the vulva, and again any possibility of carcinoma necessitates early biopsy.

In the differential diagnosis of anal warts, fibroepithelial polyps, the anal lesions of syphilis, and rare diseases such as granuloma inguinale and epithelioma of the anus must be considered. Of these, the distinction from condylomata lata is the most important; the two diseases can coexist.[80]

The only laboratory procedures that are of value in the diagnosis of HPV-induced lesions is histology of excised specimens and, in the case of lesions of the cervix, examination of Papanicolaou-stained smears. Biopsied material is best stained with hematoxylin and eosin; there is no advantage in using special stains for DNA. The histology of condyloma acuminatum has already been described, the essential features being papillomatosis, acanthosis, and the presence of vacuolated cells in the superficial epidermal layers. The histology of warts is altered if they have been treated with podophyllin; the nuclei of the acanthotic cells first become pale and swollen and later become pyknotic and necrotic.[81]

The routine Papanicolaou-stained cervical smear is invaluable for the detection of condylomatous lesions of the cervix. The cellular pattern comprises three types of cell: koilocytotic cells, dyskeratotic cells, and hyperkeratotic cells. These changes may coexist with those of cervical intraepithelial neoplasia.[24,46]

Treatment

The clinical behavior of warts is unpredictable, their response to treatment is variable, and spontaneous remission may occur. This last phenomenon is familiar to clinicians, although not well documented. Cervical condylomata have been observed to regress; they may also remain unchanged for many months, or progress to more advanced lesions.[24] The causes of the regression of warts is unclear; it may be determined immunologically.[14] The effect of therapy should be judged against this background, but unfortunately few controlled treatment studies have been undertaken.

The treatments used for anogenital warts are either cytotoxic or directly destructive. The best known cytotoxic agent is podophyllin, which has been used for the treatment of condylomata acuminata for the last 40 years. Podophyllum resin is extracted from the rhizomes of *Podophyllum peltatum* or *P. emodi*. Destruction of the condylomas is caused by the lignans podophyllotoxin, 4'-demethylpodophyllotoxin, α-peltatin and β-peltatin, of which podophyllotoxin is the most active in impeding cellular mitosis.[82] A 20 or 25% solution of podophyllin in ethanol or benzoin tincture is carefully applied to the lesions, allowed to dry and dusted with talc; initially, it is washed off after 4 hours, but this interval is lengthened to 24 hours with successive applications. Treatment is continued once or twice weekly until the warts have disappeared. Follow-up should continue for at least four weeks after apparent resolution, in case of recurrence.

Podophyllin has several disadvantages. Its composition is variable, and since it is not a pure product cannot be standardized. It is irritating to normal skin, which means that it must be applied by medical or paramedical staff rather than by the patient. Moreover, it is potentially toxic. The application of small quantities is well tolerated, but liberal applications to extensive condylomas has been followed by absorption and systemic effects ranging from dizziness and vomiting to peripheral neuropathy, coma, and death.[83] These complications if they occur during pregnancy have been disastrous for both mother and baby.[84] Further there is a possibility that in some circumstances podophyllin may be oncogenic; dysplasia has followed its repeated application to vulval warts, and podophyllin-induced cervical dysplasia may even resemble carcinoma in situ.[85]

The risk of toxic effects and oncogenesis is small, but it exists, and podophyllin should be used carefully. Not more than 0.5 ml of 25% solution should be applied at a time, prolonged courses of treatment should be avoided, and podophyllin should not be used for the treatment of cervical condylomas or during pregnancy.

5-Fluorouracil has been considered as an alternative to podophyllin. This is a fluorinated pyrimidine that inhibits DNA synthesis. Intraurethral condylomas have been successfully treated with an 8-day course of 5% 5-fluorouracil cream applied after each urination,[86] and this preparation has also been considered for use, under careful supervision, for the treatment of confluent vaginal condylomas, which present great therapeutic problems. A 1% solution of 5-fluorouracil in ethanol has been recommended for the treatment of condylomata acuminata which are refractory to podophyllin.[87]

Of the destructive methods of treatment, cryosurgery or liquid nitrogen is the easiest to use because no anesthetic is required. They are reasonably effective against lesions up to 5 mm in diameter. An electric cautery can be used for small keratinized warts on the shaft of the penis or labia majora, where a local anesthetic such as 2% lignocaine can be injected; cautery is also sometimes used for the treatment of condylomata in the terminal urethra after the application of a surface acting anesthetic (lignocaine gel 1%). For extensive condylomas diathermy, with its bigger capacity for work, is preferable, but a general anesthetic is necessary. This form of treatment must be used cautiously for extensive perianal warts because of the risk of postoperative anal stenosis; a scissor excision procedure has been described which gives good results and avoids this complication.[88] A carbon dioxide laser can be used for the vaporization of genital warts, and has the advantage of precision in use followed by rapid healing.[89] It is possible to treat extensive condylomas with staged laser applications, but general anesthesia may be necessary.

An autogenous vaccine has been recommended for the treatment of genital warts.[90] Anxiety about the oncogenic potential of papillomaviruses has limited the use of this procedure. Its efficacy in any case seems to be doubtful because one controlled trial showed no difference in the clinical responses of patients receiving vaccine or placebo injections.[91]

To summarize, penile, vulval, and anal condylomata acuminata are best treated initially with once- or twice-weekly applications of podophyllin as described above. If there has been no response after four weeks therapy an alternative treatment—cautery, cryotherapy or carbon dioxide laser (if available)—should be used. Keratinized warts do not respond well to podophyllin, and are best treated with these destructive procedures in the first instance. Extensive genital or anal condylomas will require surgery. Lesions in the terminal urethra should be treated with cautery, cryotherapy, or possibly applications of 5% 5-fluorouracil.

Patients with clinical or cytologic evidence of HPV infection of the cervix should not be treated with podophyllin. Both exophytic condylomas and flat condylomas require colposcopically directed treatment with cryosurgery or carbon dioxide laser; if there is cytologic evidence of cervical intraepithelial neoplasia, biopsy before treatment will be necessary. Finally, since cervical intraepithelial neoplasia often accompanies or follows vulval warts, it is advisable that all women who have been treated for vulval or cervical condylomas are followed with annual cervical cytology indefinitely.

MOLLUSCUM CONTAGIOSUM

Molluscum contagiosum is a benign viral cutaneous infection that occurs in children and young adults. Its viral etiology was decided many years ago when the disease was transmitted by the inoculation of filtrates of molluscum contagiosum material,[92,93] and there is now good evidence that the disease is sexually transmitted.

Etiology

The virus of molluscum contagiosum is a member of the family Poxviridae. Its structure has been established by electron microscopy.[7] It is a brick-shaped particle, measuring $300 \times 200 \times 100$ nm, and the outer tubular structures are arranged spirally, giving a "ball of yarn" appearance. The genome is double-stranded DNA.[94] Like other poxviruses, the virus of mollus-

cum contagiosum replicates in the cytoplasm of infected cells, where it produces inclusions.

Detailed study of the virus has been hampered by the inability to grow the organism in vitro. Although several workers have been able to passage the cytopathic effects induced by the virus, an actual increase in the number of virions has not been demonstrated.[95] However, the growth cycle of molluscum contagiosum virus is probably similar to those of other poxviruses. After a short eclipse period, lysis of the viral envelope and extrusion of the viral core has been observed for molluscum contagiosum virus.[96] Subsequent release of viral DNA has not been seen for this virus in vitro, but in vivo there is evidence that it probably occurs.[97] Viral DNA and protein synthesis is followed by the development of membranes which enclose areas of viroplasm, and the particle then undergoes several changes in shape before reaching its mature form.

Pathology

The pathology of the molluscum contagiosum lesion has been well described by Blank and Rake.[98] The complete series of changes can be seen in one histologic section (Fig. 12-9). The base of the papule is composed of lobules of acanthotic prickle cells. As the epithelial cells move toward the core of the lesion they undergo increasing distortion. The cytoplasm of the cell enlarges, and virus particles can now be identified by electron microscopy. The nucleus is forced to the margin of the cell by the developing cytoplasmic contents, and eventually disappears completely. The process culminates in a large structure, the "molluscum contagiosum body," which is little more than a sack of virus particles; these bodies stain intensely with hematoxylin and eosin and with stains for DNA such as toluidine blue. The central core of the mol-

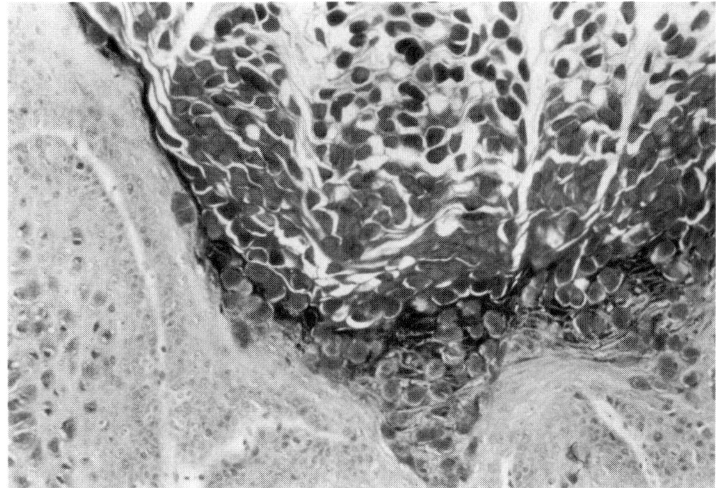

Fig. 12-9 Molluscum contagiosum. Vulval lesion. The section shows acanthosis and numerous amorphous molluscum bodies. ×40.

luscum contagiosum lesion is composed of these bodies, together with cell debris.

Molluscum contagiosum lesions may become inflamed, the lobules then being surrounded and infiltrated by histiocytes and lymphocytes. These inflamed lesions may become ulcerated, with inflammatory cells densely infiltrating the necrotic area.

Immunology

Circulating antibodies to molluscum contagiosum virus can be detected by complement fixation, neutralization, immunofluorescence techniques, and immunodiffusion, but standardization and comparison of these methods have not been thoroughly performed.[95] The role of these antibodies in the spontaneous cure of the disease is not known. It has been suggested that the release of virus or other antigenic material into the dermis, either spontaneously or through trauma, may provoke a cell-mediated immune response.[99] Such a response might explain the eczematous reaction which can be seen in many patients with molluscum contagiosum,[100] and the observation that many lesions are cured by simple pinprick trauma.

Epidemiology

Molluscum contagiosum occurs throughout the world.[99] It appears to affect for the most part two groups, children and young adults. In children, lesions appear on the face, trunk, and limbs, and transmission is believed to be by direct contact or possibly fomites. In young adults the disease affects the genitals, and infection probably occurs during sexual intercourse. There is a relationship between the age of the patient and the location of the disease[101]; lesions have been identified in sex partners of affected individuals[102,103]; other sexually transmitted diseases are often present in patients will molluscum contagiosum.[103] All these observations indicate that in young adults molluscum contagiosum is a sexually transmitted disease.

In England there has been a steady increase in the number of cases reported from clinics for sexually transmitted diseases. In 1971, 371 cases in men and 143 in women were reported; the corresponding figures for 1980 were 644 in men and 377 in women. In 1980 one case of molluscum contagiosum was reported for every 55 cases of gonorrhea.[19,20]

In selected clinics in the United States molluscum contagiosum was identified once for every 42 cases of gonorrhea during the period 1976–1980.[95] The greatest incidence of genital molluscum contagiosum has been found in the age groups of 20 to 24 years and 25 to 29 years, and the majority of infections in men are in heterosexuals; the incidence of the disease in men appears to be increasing.[100]

Clinical Features

The incubation period of molluscum contagiosum is between two and six weeks.[104] The lesion is typically papular, with a pit or dimple at its summit (Fig. 12-10). At first, lesions are small and inconspicuous, but they grow slowly to reach a usual size of 2–5 mm; single lesions as large as 15 mm have been reported.[102] They are pear- or flesh-colored, and if they are squeezed a milky material appears. The number of lesions is usually between 1 and 20; in adults they appear on the lower abdomen, pubis, genitalia, and inner surface of the thighs. Very numerous lesions can appear in patients with atopy or impaired immunity.[105] Molluscum contagiosum, like genital warts, can become more extensive during pregnancy, when cell-mediated immunity is depressed.[103]

In most people genital molluscum contagiosum causes no symptoms, and the condition is noticed by chance. In a small number of cases the papules are painful or itchy, and in about 10% there are surrounding eczematous changes[106]; this is presumed to be caused by an immune reaction, which can also sometimes lead to ulceration of the lesions.

Spontaneous resolution of the disease may occur in a few months, but conversely in many patients the lesions persist for years. The fact that many sex partners of patients with molluscum contagiosum do not develop the disease suggests that natural immunity can occur.

Diagnosis

The presence of small umbilicated papules on the genitals of sexually active adults suggests the diagnosis of molluscum contagiosum, but if necessary this can be confirmed in the laboratory. A lesion is biopsied and a section examined after staining with hematoxylin and eosin: molluscum bodies can easily be identified. Alternatively, molluscum bodies can be demonstrated by scraping out the core of a papule with a small curette and mixing the material

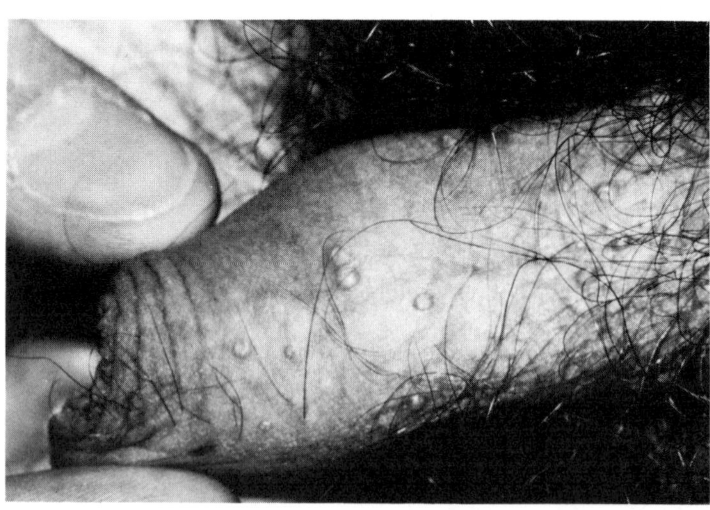

Fig. 12-10 Molluscum contagiosum of shaft of penis and prepuce.

with a drop of 10% potassium hydroxide solution on a slide; at magnification × 400 the molluscum bodies appear as irregular masses, approximately 35 μm in length. There is a large amount of virus in the lesions, so that although it cannot be cultured it can be readily identified by electron microscopy with the negative staining technique.

Molluscum contagiosum lesions are sometimes wrongly diagnosed as warts, but the central umbilication should help to differentiate the two diseases. Isolated molluscum lesions in adults may resemble nonpigmented naevi, syringomas, keratoacanthoma, sebaceous adenoma, and basal cell carcinoma; if necessary, biopsy will establish the diagnosis. Secondarily infected molluscum lesions may resemble pyoderma, and the rare giant lesions may mimic furuncles. Ulcerated molluscum lesions will need differentiation from other causes of genital ulceration.

Treatment

This is a self-limiting condition, but treatment will shorten its duration, and thereby reduce autoinoculation and infectivity to others. It is important that therapy should be painless and leave no scars. The simplest treatment is to introduce pure phenol into the substance of the lesion on the point of a sharpened orange stick. Alternatively, it may be removed with a sharp curette under local anesthesia. Cryotherapy with liquid nitrogen or by similar means is also satisfactory. Whichever method is used, it is advisable to review the patient four weeks after treatment to ensure that no further lesions have developed.

Since genital molluscum contagiosum is a sexually transmitted disease it is important to exclude the presence of other infections by appropriate laboratory tests; as a minimum, a culture for *Neisseria gonorrhoeae* and syphilis serology should be performed. Sex partners may also have molluscum contagiosum, and should be examined if possible.

REFERENCES

1. Bafverstedt B: Condylomata acuminata—past and present. Acta Derm Venereol (Stockh) 47:376, 1967
2. Oriel JD: Natural history of genital warts. Br J Vener Dis 47:1, 1971
3. Strauss MJ, Shaw EW, Bunting H, Melnick JL: "Crystalline" virus-like particles from skin papillomas characterized by intranuclear inclusion bodies. Proc Soc Exp Biol Med 72:46, 1949
4. Dunn AEG, Ogilvie MM: Intranuclear virus particles in human genital wart tissue: Observations on the ultrastructure of the epidermal layer. J Ultrastruct Res 22:282, 1968
5. Oriel JD, Almeida JD: Demonstration of virus particles in human genital warts. Br J Vener Dis 46:37, 1970
6. Almeida JD, Howatson AF, Williams MG: Electron microscope study of human wart: Sites of virus production and nature of the inclusion bodies. J Invest Dermatol 38:337, 1962
7. Andrewes C, Pereira HG, Wildy P: Viruses of Vertebrates. 4th Ed. Ballière Tindall, London, 1978
8. Krzyzek RA, Watts, SL, Anderson DL, et al: Anogenital warts contain several distinct species of human papillomavirus. J Virol 36:236, 1980
9. Zur Hausen H, de Villiers EM, Gissmann L: Papillomavirus infections and human genital cancer. Gynecol Oncol 12:124, 1981
10. Gissmann L, Wolnik L, Ikenberg H, et al: Human papillomavirus types 6 and 11 DNA sequences in genital and laryngeal papillomas and in some cervical cancers. Proc Natl Acad Sci USA 80:560, 1983
11. Almeida JD, Goffe AP: Antibody to wart virus in human sera demonstrated by electron microscopy and precipitin tests. Lancet 2:1205, 1965
12. Pyrhonen S, Penttinen K: Wart virus antibodies and the prognosis of wart disease. Lancet 2:1330, 1972

13. Matthews RS, Shirodamia PV: Study of regressing warts by immunofluorescence. Lancet 1:689, 1973
14. Pyrhonen S, Johansson E: Regression of warts. An immunological study. Lancet 1:592, 1975
15. Almeida JD, Oriel JD, Stannard LM: Characterization of the virus found in human genital warts. Microbios 3:225, 1969
16. Oguchi M, Komura J, Tagami H, et al: Ultrastructural studies of spontaneously regressing plane warts. Arch Dermatol Res 270:403, 1981
17. Lee AKY, Eisinger M: Cell-mediated immunity (CMI) to human wart virus and wart-associated tissue antigens. Clin Exp Immunol 26:419, 1976
18. Von Krogh G: Warts: Immunologic factors of prognostic significance. Int J Dermatol 18:195, 1979
19. Chief Medical Officer: Sexually transmitted diseases: Extract from annual report of the Chief Medical Officer to the Department of Health and Social Security for the year 1971. Br J Vener Dis 49:89, 1973
20. Chief Medical Officer: Sexually transmitted diseases: Extract from annual report of the Chief Medical Officer to the Department of Health and Social Security for the year 1980. Br J Vener Dis 59:134, 1983
21. Barrett TJ, Silbar JD, McGinley JP: Genital warts—a venereal disease. JAMA 154:333, 1954
22. Teokharov BA: Non-gonococcal infections of the female genitalia. Br J Vener Dis 45:334, 1969
23. Von Krogh G: Localisation, manner of transmission and treatment of condylomata acuminata. Sartryck Lakartid 72:2167, 1975
24. Meisels A, Morin C, Casas-Cordero M: Human papillomavirus infection of the cervix. Int J Gynecol Pathol 1:75, 1982
25. Syrjanen K, Vayrynen M, Castren O, et al: Sexual behavior of females with human papillomavirus lesions in the uterine cervix. Br J Vener Dis 60:243, 1985
26. Levine RU, Crum CP, Herman E, Richart RM: Cervical papillomavirus infection and intraepithelial neoplasia: a study of male sexual partners. Obstet Gynecol 64:16, 1984
27. Heidingsfeld ML: Condylomata acuminata linguae (venereal warts of the tongue). J Cutan Dis Genitourin Dis 19:226, 1901
28. Oriel JD: Genital warts. Sex Transm Dis 4:153, 1977
29. Judson FN: Condvloma acuminatum of the oral cavity: A case report. Sex Transm Dis 8:218, 1981
30. Eftaiha MS, Amshiel AL, Shonberg IL: Condylomata acuminata in an infant and a mother: Report of a case. Dis Colon Rectum 21:369, 1978
31. Hajek EF: Contribution to the etiology of laryngeal papilloma in children. J Laryngol Otol 70:166, 1956
32. Storrs FJ: Spread of condylomata acuminata to infants and children. Arch Dermatol 113:1294, 1977
33. Patel R, Groff DB: Condylomata acuminata in childhood. Pediatrics 50:152, 1972
34. Cook TA, Cohn AM, Brunschwig JP, et al: Laryngeal papilloma: Etiologic and therapeutic considerations. Ann Otol 82:649, 1973
35. Oriel JD: Anal warts and anal coitus. Br J Vener Dis 47:373, 1971
36. Carr G, William DC: Anal warts in a population of gay men in New York City. Sex Transm Dis 4:56, 1977
37. Lever WF: Histopathology of the Skin. 4th Ed. Pitman, London, 1967
38. Woodruff JD, Braun L, Calavieri R, et al: Immunologic identification of papillomavirus antigen in condyloma tissues from the female genital tract. Obstet Gynecol 56:727, 1980
39. Dunn J, Weinstein L, Droegemueller W, Meinke W: Immunologic detection of condylomata acuminata-specific antigen. Obstet Gynecol 57:351, 1981
40. Walker PG, Singer A, Dyson JL, et al: Colposcopy in the diagnosis of papillomavirus infection of the uterine cervix. Br J Obstet Gynecol 90:1082, 1983
41. Gartman E: Intraurethral verruca acuminata in men. J Urol 75:717, 1956
42. Pollack HM, de Bebenictis TJ, Marmar JL, et al: Urethrographic manifestations of venereal warts (condylomata acuminata). Radiology 126:643, 1978
43. Pettersson S, Hansson G, Blohme I: Condyloma acuminatum of the bladder. J Urol 115:535, 1976

44. Marsh MR: Papilloma of the cervix. Am J Obstet Gynecol 64:281, 1952

45. Meisels A, Fortin R: Condylomatous lesions of the cervix and vagina. I. Cytologic patterns. Acta Cytol 20:509, 1976

46. Reid R, Laverty CR, Coppleson M, et al: Noncondylomatous cervical wart virus infection. Obstet Gynecol 55:476, 1980

47. Meisels A, Fortin R, Roy M: Condylomatous lesions of the cervix and vagina. II. Cytologic colposcopic and histopathologic study. Acta Cytol 21:379, 1977

48. Hills E, Laverty CR: Electron microscopic detection of papillomavirus particles in selected koilocytotic cells in a routine cervical smear. Acta Cytol 23:53, 1979

49. McCance DJ, Walker PG, Dyson JL, et al: Presence of human papillomavirus DNA sequences in cervical intraepithelial neoplasia. Br Med J 287:784, 1983

50. Kirkup W, Evans AS, Brough AK, et al: Cervical intraepithelial neoplasia and "warty" atypia: A Study of colposcopic, histological and cytological characteristics. Br J Obstet Gynaecol 89:571, 1982

51. Syrjanen KJ, Heinonen U-M, Kauraniemi T: Cytologic evidence of the association of condylomatous lesions with dysplastic and neoplastic changes in the uterine cervix. Acta Cytol 25:17, 1981

52. Purola E, Savia E: Cytology of gynecologic condyloma acuminatum. Acta Cytol 21:26, 1977

53. Walker PG, Colley NV, Grubb C, et al: Abnormalities of the uterine cervix in women with vulval warts: A preliminary communication. Br J Vener Dis 59:120, 1983

54. Pass F: Progress towards a new wart biology. J Invest Dermatol 70:109, 1979

55. Wilson J: Extensive vulval condylomata acuminata necessitating caesarean section. Aust NZ J Obstet Gynaecol 13:121, 1973

56. Buschke A, Loewenstein L: Über die Beziehungen von Spitzen Kondylomen zu Karzinomen des Penis. Dtsch Med Wochenschr 58:809, 1932

57. Chakravarth I, Kalyanam KA: Buschke-Loewenstein tumour. J R Coll Surg Edinb 18:191, 1973

58. Gissmann L, de Villiers E-M, Zur Hausen H: Analysis of human genital warts (condyloma acuminatum) and other genital tumors for human papillomavirus type 6 DNA. Int J Cancer 29:143, 1982

59. Dawson DF, Duckworth JK, Bernhardt H, Young JM: Giant condyloma and verrucous carcinoma of the genital area. Arch Pathol 79:225, 1965

60. Litvak AS, Melnick J, Lieberman PR: Giant condyloma acuminatum associated with carcinoma. J Med Soc NJ 63:165, 1966

61. Gardner HC, Kaufman RH: Condylomata acuminata. Clin Obstet Gynecol 8:938, 1965

62. Charlewood GP, Shippel S: Vulval condyloma acuminata as a premalignant lesion in the Bantu. S Afr Med J 27:149, 1953

63. Rhatigan RM, Jimenez S, Chopskie EJ: Condyloma acuminatum and carcinoma of the penis. South Med J 65:423, 1972

64. Friedberg MJ, Serlin O: Condyloma acuminatum: Its association with malignancy. Dis Colon Rectum 6:352, 1963

65. Burns FJ, van Goidsenhoven: Condylomata acuminata of the rectum with associated malignancy. Proc R Soc Med 63:119, 1970

66. Ridley CM: The Vulva. Saunders, London, 1975

67. Syrjanen KJ: Condylomatous epithelial changes in the uterine cervix and their relationship to cervical carcinogenesis. Int J Gynecol Obstet 17:415, 1980

68. Reid R, Stanhope R, Herschman BR, et al: Genital warts and cervical cancer: 1. Evidence of an association between subclinical papillomavirus infection and malignancy. Cancer 50:377, 1982

69. Kidd JG, Rous P: Cancers deriving from the virus papillomas of wild rabbits under natural conditions. J Exp Med 71:469, 1940

70. Jarrett WFH: Transformation of warts to malignancy in alimentary carcinoma in cattle. Bull Cancer 65:191, 1978

71. Ostrow RS, Bender M, Niimura M, et al: Human papillomavirus DNA in cutaneous primary and metastasized squamous cell carcinomas from patients with epidermodysplasia verruciformis. Proc Natl Acad Sci USA 79:1634, 1982

72. Olotsson J, Bjelkenkrantz K, Grontoff O: Malignant degeneration of a juvenile laryngeal papilloma: A follow-up study. J Otolaryngol 9:329, 1980

73. Laverty CR, Russell P, Hills E, Booth N: The significance of noncondylomatous wart virus infection of the cervical transformation zone: A review with discussion of two cases. Acta Cytol 22:195, 1978

74. Josey WE, Nahmias AJ, Naib ZM: Viruses and cancer of the lower genital tract. Cancer 38:526, 1976

75. Zur Hausen H: Human papillomaviruses and their possible role in squamous cell carcinomas. Curr Top Microbiol Immunol 78:1, 1977

76. Rotkin ID; A comparison review of key epidemiological studies in cervical cancer related to current searches for transmissible agents. Cancer Res 33:1353, 1973

77. Durst M, Gissmann L, Ikenberg H, Zur Hausen H: A papillomavirus DNA from a cervical carcinoma and its prevalence in cancer biopsy samples from different geographic regions. Proc Natl Acad Sci USA 80:3812, 1983

78. Zur Hausen H: Human genital cancer: Synergism between two virus infections or synergism between a virus infection and initiating events. Lancet 2:1372, 1982

79. Wigley JEM, Haber H: Hirsutes papillaris penis. Br J Dermatol 61:427, 1949

80. Dexter HLT, Rockwell EM: Simultaneous condylomata acuminata and condylomata lata: Report of a case. Arch Dermatol Syphilol 64:205, 1951

81. Sullivan M, King L: Effects of resin of podophyllin on normal skin, condylomata acuminata and verruca vulgaris. Arch Dermatol Syphilol 56:30, 1957

82. Von Krogh G: Podophyllotoxin dor condylomata acuminata. Acta Derm Venereol (Stockh) Suppl 98, 1981

83. Montaldi DH, Giambrone JP, Courey NG, et al: Podophyllin poisoning associated with the treatment of condyloma acuminatum: A case report. Am J Obstet Gynecol 119:1130, 1974

84. Chamberlain MJ, Reynolds AL, Yeoman WB: Toxic effect of podophyllum in pregnancy. Br Med J 3:391, 1972

85. Saphir O, Leventhal ML, Kline TS: Podophyllin-induced dysplasia of the cervix uteri: Its histologic resemblance to carcinoma in situ. Am J Clin Pathol 32:446, 1959

86. Dretler SP, Klein CA: The eradication of intraurethral condylomata acuminata with 5 percent 5-fluorouracil cream. J Urol 113:195, 1975

87. Von Krogh G: The beneficial effect of 1 percent 5-fluorouracil in 70 percent ethanol on therapeutically refractive condylomas in the preputial cavity. Sex Transm Dis 5:137, 1978

88. Thomson JPS, Grace RH: The treatment of perianal and anal condylomata acuminata: A new operative technique. J R Soc Med 71:180, 1978

89. Hahn GA: Carbon dioxide laser surgery in the treatment of condyloma. Am J Obstet Gynecol 141:1000, 1981

90. Powell LC: Condyloma acuminatum: Recent advances in development, carcinogenesis and treatment. Clin Obstet Gynecol 21:1061, 1978

91. Malison MD, Morris R, Jones LW: Autogenous vaccine therapy for condyloma acuminatum—a double blind controlled study. Br J Vener Dis 58:62, 1982

92. Juliusberg M: Zur Kenntnis des Virus des Molluscum Contagiosum. Dtsch Med Wochenschr 31:1598, 1905

93. Wile UJ, Kingery LB: Etiology of molluscum contagiosum. J Cutan Dis 37:431, 1919

94. Parr RP, Bennett JW, Garon CF: Structural characterization of the molluscum contagiosum virus genome. Virology 81:247, 1977

95. Brown ST, Nalley JF, Kraus SJ: Molluscum contagiosum. Sex Transm Dis 8:227, 1981

96. McFadden G, Pace WE, Purres J, Dales S: Biogenesis of poxviruses: Transitory expression of molluscum contagiosum early functions. Virology 94:297, 1979

97. Epstein WL, Fukayama K: Maturation of molluscum contagiosum virus in vivo: Quantitative electron microscopic autoradiography. J Invest Dermatol 60:73, 1973

98. Blank H, Rake H: Viral and Rickettsial Diseases of the Skin, Eye and Mucous Membranes. Churchill, London, 1955

99. Postlethwaite R: Molluscum contagiosum. Arch Environ Health 21:432, 1970

100. Felman YM, Nikitas JA: Sexually transmitted molluscum contagiosum. Dermatol Clin 1:103, 1983

101. Cobbold RJC, MacDonald A: Molluscum

contagiosum as a sexually transmitted disease. Practitioner 204:416, 1970
102. Brown ST, Weinberger J: Molluscum contagiosum. Sexually transmitted disease in 17 cases. J Am Vener Dis Assoc 1:35, 1974
103. Wilkin JK: Molluscum contagiosum venereum in a women's out-patient clinic. A venereally transmitted disease. Am J Obstet Gynecol 128:531, 1977
104. Felman YM, Nikitas JA: Genital molluscum contagiosum. Cutis 26:28, 1980
105. Pauly CR, Artis WM, Jones HE: Atopic dermatitis, impaired cellular immunity and molluscum contagiosum. Arch Dermatol 114:391, 1978
106. De Oreo GA, Johnson HH, Brinkley GW: An eczematous reaction associated with molluscum contagiosum. Arch Dermatol 74:344, 1956

13

Evolving Views of Scabies and Pediculosis Pubis

Milton Orkin
Howard I. Maibach

SCABIES

Bonomo's discovery in 1687 of the itch mite (*Sarcoptes scabiei*) marked scabies as the first disease in humans with a known cause. Von Hebra, in the nineteenth century, delineated much of our basic knowledge about scabies. He noted the relative unimportance of fomites in its transmission; however, this concept was not generally accepted until a century later, when reintroduced by Mellanby,[1] as a result of studies of experimentally induced scabies in volunteers during World War II. At the same time, Heilesen[2] wrote a monograph on scabies. This work is another rich source of information.

Etiology

The adult female itch mite has a rounded body, four pairs of legs and measures 400μm in length. She walks rapidly on human skin, covering 2.5 cm/min.[3] When she finds a suitable location, she burrows into the horny layer to the boundary of the stratum granulosum. The burrow provides a home for the duration of her life, approximately 30 days. Within hours of burrowing, she begins laying enormous eggs (two or three a day). These eggs progress through larval and nymphal states to form adult mites in 10 days. The average number of adult female mites on an infested patient is 11.

The mites concentrate in special sites, two thirds on the hands and wrists. Because the eruption may be caused in part by immature stages of the mite and by sensitization, the distribution of adult female mites does not parallel that of the typical scabies lesions. In primary infestation, itching or eruption does not occur for several weeks, the time required for sensitization.

Epidemiology

Epidemics of scabies tend to occur in 30-year cycles with a 15-year gap between the end of one epidemic and the beginning of the next. The epidemics usually last about 15 years; however, the current pandemic is extending beyond the 15-year period. The reason for this is not clear. Many factors, such as poverty, poor hygiene, sexual promiscuity, misdiagnosis, increased travel, and demographic and ecologic considerations promote the development of scabies.[4] Increasing information suggests that immunologic factors are important, probably a combination of humoral and cell-mediated elements.[5]

The socioeconomic characteristics of patients with this infestation are representative of those of the general population. The frequency of scabies in black Americans is significantly lower than in white Americans and some other racial groups.[6]

Although it is unwise to be dogmatic about the way in which a particular patient contracted scabies, close personal contact is usually involved.[7] In the majority of patients, the source is a sexual partner. Scabies is one of the few sexually transmitted diseases (STDs) also commonly transmitted nonsexually in households to individuals of all ages. Scabies is usually transmitted to children by nonsexual, close, personal contact (e.g., sharing a bed in a crowded dwelling); however, one should not exclude transmission by sexual abuse or misuse, which are not uncommon with other STDs.

The long incubation period, usual in persons infested for the first time, may make it difficult to trace the source. If one member of the household becomes infested, other members may eventually be affected unless specific treatment is instituted. When several members of a family or group complain of a pruritic eruption, scabies is a likely diagnosis. In two thirds of families of patients with scabies, there was no transmission to other family members; in one third of families, two or more members became infested.[8]

As with most STDs, scabies is common in sexually active young adults (15 to 40 years of age), and is more common in men than in women.[9,10] Although syphilis and gonorrhea are frequently transmitted by brief sexual contact, scabies is more likely to be transmitted when the partners spend the night together.

The greater the parasitic load in an individual, the greater the likelihood of transmission. The important role of those few individuals who have large numbers of parasites, such as patients with crusted scabies, in transmitting scabies is obvious. Immature mites are capable of causing infestation, although the usual cause is probably the newly fertilized adult female.

Scabies is frequent in school-aged children but is unlikely to be transmitted in schools.[11] Outbreaks are not uncommon in nursing homes, hospitals, and other institutions. Nosocomial outbreaks of scabies occur.

Control

A high index of suspicion on the part of the clinician is important. Attempting to prove the diagnosis by demonstrating the organism helps prevent overdiagnosis. Early diagnosis and treatment with an effective scabicide, for the patient as well as for selected members of the household (see the section on Treatment) and sexual contacts of infested persons, are the keys to prevention.

Scabies outbreaks in nursing homes and other institutions are widespread and difficult to manage and eradicate; Juranek and coworkers[12] presented strategies for prevention and control of scabies in institutions.

Clinical Diagnosis

Patients with suspected scabies should be completely disrobed and examined thoroughly with good lighting; if this is not done, then signs (sometimes subtle), unreported by the patients, will be missed.

CLASSIC SCABIES

In the current cycle, classic scabies is seen less frequently than in previous cycles. Itching is frequently severe and may manifest by vigorous excoriations; it is characteristically nocturnal, producing much loss of sleep. Lesions are roughly symmetrical.[13] The hands are often the first areas involved; lesions (frequently eczematous) occur mainly on the fingerwebs and the sides of the digits. The flexor surfaces of the wrist are commonly involved, as are the extensor surfaces of the elbows (lesions may be nodular, but more frequently are dry and eczematous) and the anterior axillary folds. The breasts may have eczematous lesions resembling those of Paget's disease. Papular lesions are usually present on the abdomen, particularly around the umbilicus, in a spokelike arrangement. Penile involvement is characteristic, and nodules may dominate. Chancriform changes or pyoderma may be present. The disease may affect the lower portion of the buttocks in the crease where they join the upper part of the thighs; impetiginous crusting on the buttocks should make the physician suspicious of scabies. In adults, the upper back, center of the chest, neck, face, scalp, palms, and soles are seldom involved.

In neglected cases, or under conditions in which treatment is difficult (prisoners of war, members of ships' crews on long voyages, etc.) the eruption may be extensive, may appear anywhere on the skin surface, and usually has secondary bacterial infection.[14]

The pathognomonic burrow is a short, wavy, dirty-appearing line that often crosses skin lines; it is most common on the fingerwebs, volar wrists, elbows, and penis. Most burrows are ripped away by the patient's incessant scratching.

At most sites, small, erythematous, often excoriated papules are encountered; many of these may be larval papules, which are important morphologic components of the current cycle. Secondary eczematization and infection may overshadow other features, making diagnosis more difficult. Many dermatoses present with monomorphous lesions; scabies is usually a polymorphous disease.

SPECIAL FORMS OF SCABIES

Scabies has many guises that may be difficult to diagnose. Physicians should be alert to the special forms the disease may take.[15]

Scabies in the Clean Patient

There is a definite increase in the incidence of scabies in clean persons, in whom the disease is easily misdiagnosed because lesions may be barely observable and burrows difficult to find,[16] but even in these individuals one or two sites of predilection are affected. The person presumably removes many mites with frequent bathing. Larval papules may be notable. Meticulous physical examination suggests the diagnosis, which is confirmed by mite identification.

Scabies Incognito

Administration of corticosteroids (topical or systemic) may ameliorate symptoms and signs of scabies, while the infestation and transmissibility persist. This frequently results in unusual clinical presentations such as atypical distribution and unusual extent of involvement, in some instances closely simulating other entities.[16] It will be of interest to see if scabies incognito occurs after use of the recently released over-the-counter preparations of 0.5% hydrocortisone.

Scabies may be superimposed on other conditions, for example, mycosis fungoides, psoriasis, systemic lupus erythematosus, South American pemphigus foliaceus, elastosis perforans serpiginosa, and epidermolysis bullosa hereditaria dystrophica.[15]

Scabies superimposed on systemic lupus erythematosus (SLE) tends to be more generalized (including lesions on the face and ears) and severe, and there is a propensity to develop crusted scabies[17]; delayed diagnosis is common, and inappropriate treatment can lead to unfortunate complications. The scabies tends to be atypical but the presence of pruritus, uncommon in the rash of SLE, suggests the diagnosis of scabies. The florid expression of scabies in SLE probably has an immunologic basis; it may occur without the patient's having been on systemic steroids or other immunosuppressive agents.

Herpes simplex infections (particularly HSV-2) may be innoculated on a scabietic infestation by scratching; this combination presents management problems.[18]

Nodular Scabies

In nodular scabies, the nodules are reddish-brown and pruritic and occur in covered parts, most frequently male genitalia, groin, and axillary regions. Mites are seldom identified in nodules. The disease frequently remains misdiagnosed for long periods; histiocytosis X and lymphoma may be considered clinically. The histologic features are similar to those of lymphoma (especially Hodgkin's disease) and arthropod bites. Diagnosis is facilitated by the overlapping occurrence or recent history of more typical scabies (usually responding to scabicides). The nodules probably develop as a hypersensitivity reaction.

Scabies in Infants and Young Children

Misdiagnosis is frequent in infants and young children because of low index of suspicion, secondary eczematous changes (possibly widespread) suggesting other conditions, and atypical distribution to include head, neck, palms, and soles. Itching is most severe at night and at naptime; it is often so severe that infants refuse feedings.[19] Vesicles are common. Secondary bacterial infection, manifest as pustules, bullous impetigo, severe crusting, or ecthyma, is frequent. Poor feeding and failure to gain weight appropriately are characteristic features in scabies contracted during the neonatal period.[20]

Children recently adopted from foreign countries, especially Korea and Vietnam, have a high frequency of scabies, which often appears after the children arrive at their destinations.[16]

DYSHIDROSIFORM SCABIID. Bjornberg and Friis[21]; reported a characteristic syndrome in children recently adopted into Scandinavian homes from Asia. The children arrived having typical scabies; treatment wth scabicides cleared most of the eruption of the children and all of the eruption of any infested members of the adopted families. Some of the adopted children had recurrent crops of vesicles and pustules (despite repeated scabicidal therapy) on the hands and feet (occasionally elsewhere) which gradually cleared after several months to more than one year. Mites could not be demonstrated in these persistent lesions.

We have observed 12 such small children in recent years; most (not all) had recently arrived from Asia. Most had an atopic personal or family history. The eruption was dyshidrosiform or resembled a recalcitrant pustular eruption. Skin scrapings were negative and cutaneous biopsies were nonspecific. The eruption gradually cleared after three to four months, sometimes improving with the use of 3% sulfur in calamine lotion.

Scabies in the Elderly

In the elderly, the reaction to the mite is muted, but the patient itches severely.[22] The vivid inflammatory reactions seen in younger people are usually absent. Scabies is frequently not recognized and instead the itching is attributed to dry skin, anxiety, or old age. For elderly patients in nursing homes and other extended care facilities, particularly when bedridden for lengthy periods, there may be involvement of the back (unique for adults with scabies), which has converted into an intertriginous area (Plate 13-1).

Animal-Transmitted Scabies

No other permanent parasitic mite has such a large variety of hosts as does *S. scabiei.*[23] This mite produces scabies in 40 different hosts belonging to 17 families in 7 orders of mammals.

Animal-transmitted scabies is not uncommon; although persons may be infested with mites from various animals, dogs (usually puppies) are the major source. Animal mites do not differ morphologically from human mites, but differ biologically. Human beings are infested inadvertently by direct or indirect contact. The condition often goes undiagnosed.

The frequency of scabies in dogs has increased. The external surface of the ears is the most frequent site of predilection, corresponding to the high frequency of involvement of the hands in human scabies.

Canine-transmitted scabies in human beings differs from human scabies; the former has greater ease of transmission, different distribution patterns, absence of burrows, and a shorter incubation period.

Crusted Scabies (Norwegian Scabies)

Crusted scabies (formerly called Norwegian scabies) is a rare condition, and is highly contagious, even on casual contact, because of myriads of mites present in exfoliating scales. Local or regional epidemics of more typical forms of scabies frequently result, usually in hospitals or other insti-tutions. Crusted scabies is a psoriasiform dermatosis of the hands and feet, with dystrophy of the nails and a variable erythematous, scaling eruption that may become generalized; it usually takes months for this morphology to become fixed. Pruritus is minimal. There is frequently an associated superficial lymphadenopathy. Eosinophilia may be present.

The disease shows a predilection for the mentally retarded, physically debilitated, or immunologically deficient (from congenital or iatrogenic cause). Immunosuppressive drugs may convert ordinary scabies into the crusted form. Crusted scabies is a rare complication in immunosuppressed renal transplant patients.

An abortive papular form of scabies, probably due to infestation with immature forms (without adult females), has been noted in fellow patients and particularly in medical, nursing, and supportive staff exposed to patients with crusted scabies. This eruption consists of erythematous papules, similar to papular urticaria, on the arms, legs, and anterior trunk.

Scabies Occurring with Other Sexually Transmitted Diseases

Scabies is seen frequently at venereal disease clinics and may coexist with gonorrhea, syphilis, pediculosis pubis, genital herpes, and other sexually transmitted diseases. The diseases may have been contracted during the same, a prior, or a subsequent exposure.[24] Often the signs or symptoms of one disease bring the patient to medical attention, at which time the other disease(s) are discovered; sexual partners may contract more than one of these diseases.

A diagnosis of scabies, particularly when genital lesions are present, should prompt search for coexisting sexually transmitted diseases, beginning with the culture for *Neisseria gonorrhoeae* and a serologic test for syphilis. The frequence of asymptomatic gonorrhea is high in young women with scabies. The chancre of syphilis is sometimes seen in cutaneous lesion of scabies (chancre galeuse).

Acquired Immunodeficiency Syndrome (AIDS) and Scabies

The association of atypical scabies—for example, crusted scabies or scabies incognito—with *Pneumocystis carinii* pneumonia (a disease primarily of immunocompromised hosts) in a previously healthy, heterosexual, non-drug-abusing woman with no apparent underlying disease or demonstrable immunodeficiency, is of great interest.[25] Crusted scabies and scabies incognito can occur in immunocompromised patients. *Pneuomcystis carinii* pneumonia is an established part of AIDS.

We believe that this association of atypical scabies with *Pneumocystis carinii* pneumonia suggests that the medical community will soon begin to document the association of atypical scabies as another opportunistic infection of AIDS.[26]

Urticarial and Vasculitic Forms

Uncommonly, widespread urticaria overshadows inconspicuous lesions of scabies; the patients are usually treated for urticaria.[26,27]

Evidence of vasculitis is frequent histopathologically in the dermis in a variety of inflammatory scabies lesions, particularly in nodular scabies. Immunopathologically, a cutaneous vasculitis-like pattern may be found.[26,28] Uncommonly, patients have clinical vasculitis, particularly on the lower extremities (Plate 13-2), but it may be generalized, overshadowing the elements of scabies; the patients are commonly treated for vasculitis.

In the uncommon urticarial form, and in the vasculitis form, the diagnosis is suspected by the history of contact cases of scabies (family, sexual contacts, or close associates), and inconspicuous findings of scabies such as burrows, papules, and so on; the diagnosis is proved by isolating the mites on skin scrapings or other techniques (including skin biopsy). The eruption clears with the use of scabicides.

Localized Scabies

In occasional patients scabies may be limited to localized or solitary locations, such as one axilla[29] or the buttocks.[30] Because this is a difficult diagnosis, it is important to maintain a high index of suspicion and try to demonstrate the mite. Examine close household members and sexual contacts; treat proven cases and selected close contacts.

Secondary Infections and Their Complications

Secondary bacterial infections may complicate scabies. Nephritogenic streptococcal strains may colonize scabietic lesions and lead to acute glomerulonephritis. This has been reported mainly in tropical areas; its potential is universal.

Differential Diagnosis

Differential diagnosis includes nearly all pruritic dermatoses, including atopic dermatitis, contact dermatitis, prurigo, papular urticaria, pyoderma, pruritus due to systemic disease, pruritic dermatoses of pregnancy, infectious eczematoid dermatitis, insect bites, cheyletiella dermatitis, excoriations, lichen planus, dermatitis herpetiformis, mastocytosis, urticaria, and pediculosis, as well as syphilis, keratosis follicularis, and vasculitis.

There is a relationship in some patients between scabies and atopic dermatitis: difficulty in differentiating scabies from variations of atopic dermatitis (especially papular urticaria), a significant number of patients in whom scabies seems combined with atopic dermatitis, with the latter persisting (frequently nummular in character) after the scabies clears, and a high incidence of scabietic hypersensitivity sequelae (nodular scabies, dyidrosiform scabiid) in patients with an atopic background.[31]

Laboratory Diagnosis

SKIN SCRAPINGS.[32]   Burrows, if present, or recently developed unexcoriated papules are located with the help of a hand lens or head loupe; the most successful sites are (in descending order) the fingerwebs, wrists, and elbows. Mineral oil, placed on a No. 15 blade of a sterile scalpel and allowed to flow onto these lesions, facilitates visibility. Vigorous scrapings with the blade removes the top of the burrows or papules. The oil and scraped material are transferred to a glass slide, a coverslip is applied, and the *entire* specimen examined under low power of the microscope. Diagnosis is confirmed by the presence of any stage of the mite (adult, egg or egg casing, larva, nymph, *or* the typical fecal pellets, which outnumber the living organisms). Care should be taken with an infant, small child, or an anxious or uncooperative patient.

EPIDERMAL SHAVE BIOPSY.[32,33]   Locate a suspicious papule or burrow, elevate the papule between the thumb and forefinger, and gently saw off the top of the lesion with a No. 15 scalpel blade held parallel to the skin surface. The biopsy is so superficial that bleeding should not occur; nor should local anesthesia be necessary. The biopsy material is placed on a glass slide and examined under a light microscope. Care

should be taken with a small child or an anxious or uncooperative patient.

CURETTAGE (DERMAL CURET).[32]   Superficially curet the long axis of a burrow or across the summit of a papule, and deposit the material on a clean slide. Then, place one to two drops of mineral oil on the material and cover with a coverslip. This technique is particularly valuable in infants, small children, or anxious or uncooperative patients.

SEWING NEEDLE OR PIN.[32]   Use a sewing needle or a pin to pick out mite from undamaged burrows. The needle is used to perforate the burrow at the dark point (site of mite) except in a black patient, on whom it is a white point; the needle is moved tangential to the skin from side to side. The mite will grip the end of the needle, after which it is transferred to the slide.

GLUE STRIPPING.[32,34]   A drop of methacrylate glue is applied to a glass slide which is pushed down firmly over a lesion (preferably a burrow), allowed to set until adhered (30 seconds or longer), and then stripped off quickly. Repeat the stripping twice so as to retrieve the organisms and bottom of the burrow; apply more glue to the specimens on the slide, apply a coverslip, and study microscopically.

BURROW INK TEST (BIT).[32,35]   Gently rub the scabietic papule with the underside of an inexpensive fountain pen, covering it with ink; immediately wipe off the surface ink from the lesion with an alcohol pad. In the BIT-positive lesion the ink tracks down the burrow created by the mite and forms a characteristic, dark zigzag line running across and away from the papule. The Burrow Ink Test is painless and more useful in the child or uncooperative patient; however, it may yield false-negative results. Some prefer the Burrow Ink Test to identify suspicious lesions followed by a superficial shave biopsy.

TOPICAL TETRACYCLINE TO SUSPECTED BURROWS.[32,34] A liquid tetracycline preparation, such as Topicycline, is applied generously to suspected burrows. After 5 minutes of drying, the patient is instructed to wipe these areas vigorously with isopropyl alcohol, largely removing the background tetracycline fluorescence. The tetracycline penetrates areas of stratum corneum disruption. Illumination with Wood's light fluoresces the burrows, which appear as linear, yellow-green lesions, from which the mite or its products can be demonstrated by any of the above techniques.

SKIN SWAB TECHNIQUE WITH CLEAR CELLOPHANE ADHESIVE TAPE.[32] Clean the skin with ether; then apply cellophane tape to the lesion and remove with brisk movement. Strips of adhesive tape are stuck on the slide (six strips of the same lesion on one slide), which is examined microscopically.

PUNCH BIOPSY.[32] If the mites or their products cannot be demonstrated by the above techniques in a patient with highly suspected scabies, then a punch biopsy (usually No. 2 mm) can be taken from an unexcoriated lesion. Instruct the laboratory to do serial sections; every section should be thoroughly studied for the mite or its products, which may be found in the cornified layer.[36]

We demonstrate the organism in 60% of patients in whom we highly suspect scabies.[31] We mainly use the skin scraping technique, at times combined with epidermal shave biopsy; curettage is used in infants, small children, and uncooperative patients.

The main reasons for not finding the organism are (1) taking the material from an excoriated lesion (organism gone) or secondary lesion (crust, pyoderma, etc.) instead of from a burrow (almost 100% positive) or unexcoriated papule, and (2) taking insufficient material for microscopic examination.

TREATMENT

Principles

Careful explanation, answering of all patient or family questions and reassurance are vital. Patients frequently receive the diagnosis with inordinate concern, guilt, and sometimes skepticism.

The choice of a drug for treatment of scabies must take into account efficacy and potential toxicity.[37] There have been few comparative, controlled efficacy trials of scabicides.

Treatment may be preceded by a tepid (avoid hot bath or shower) bath to remove previous medications. Patients tend to apply the drugs more frequently and over longer periods than prescribed. Limiting the quantity prescribed prevents dermatitis caused by overtreatment, which the patient may mistake for persistence of the scabies, and minimizes percutaneous penetration. Approximately 30 mg (1 oz) of a topical preparation covers adequately the trunk and extremities of an average adult; proportionately less is needed for children and infants. The scabicide should be applied thinly but thoroughly from the neck downward to all areas, with special attention to the hands, feet, and intertriginous areas. In infants and small children, the scalp and head (except do not apply close to the eye) should be included. Treatment is more effectively done by an attendant or family member, since the patient may miss some portions of the body.

Selective treatment of other household members (symptomatic or asymptomatic) at high risk for acquiring the infestation from a confirmed case may be appropriate.[38] One must exercise good judgment; for example, if the patient (adult or child) routinely shares a bed with another person, the probability is high that transmission to that person has already occurred, and therefore treatment of the asymptomatic bed partner is justified. Similarly, infested mothers caring for their children or infants have a good chance for exposing their children through daily activities. Sexual contacts of infested patients should also be treated simultaneously. It is less significant to treat those with minimal skin-to-skin contact with an infested household member. We have recently been more insistent on examining family and other contacts (especially those with a history of seizures or atopic eczema) before treating them prophylactically.

At the conclusion of therapy, intimate articles of clothing (underwear and pajamas), bed linen (sheets and pillowcases), and towels should be machine washed and dried using the hot cycle of each machine. It is not necessary to clean outerwear or furniture, since the mites survive only briefly away from the human host.

An exception is the patient with crusted scabies. With crusted scabies prophylactic treatment of persons exposed to fomites should be considered. Bed linen and clothing in contact with such a patient should be placed in a plastic bag for transport to the laundry to avoid exposure to others, and floors, curtains, and furniture should be vacuumed.

Twenty-four hours after effective therapy, the patient may no longer transmit the disease. However, symptoms and signs may not clear for several weeks because the state of hypersensitivity, particularly in atopic individuals, does not cease immediately upon mite destruction. The patient should be alerted to this possibility so that he or she knows what to expect.

If itching persists beyond two weeks, carefully inspect the patient for active scabies, do skin scrapings (or equivalent), check source of reinfestation; then, if any

Table 13-1. Failure to Cure Scabies

1. Failure to diagnose—under or over
   a) Suspect scabies in any patient with chronic itch
   b) Attempt to identify mite in *all* suspected cases
2. Failure to treat *entire* skin
3. Failure to treat close contacts simultaneously
4. Failure to stop scabicide therapy
5. Resistance to scabicide?

Modified from Shelley WB, Shelley ED: Common causes of treatment failure in scabies. Illinois Med J 163(2):112, 1983, with permission.

of the above are positive, retreat; choice of agent and individuals to be retreated will depend upon circumstances.

Failure to cure scabies can be due to one or a combination of factors (Table 13-1); once the diagnosis is made and proper therapy is given, a common cause of failure is lack of patient compliance. Reinfestation from an outside source does not occur commonly except with sexual transmission. Dermatitis, generally from too frequent use of a scabicide, is usually irritant in nature.

RESISTANCE

Resistance to modern scabicides has been suggested.[39,40] Scabicide resistance can only be proved by finding new inflammatory papules or burrows, and demonstrating live mites, after proper therapy has been applied or closely supervised by the investigator, and infestation from another person has been ruled out.[41] In such circumstances one would expect to see clusters or outbreaks of resistant scabies, which is not, as yet, reported. The patients studied should be immunocompetent, otherwise other criteria for adequate therapy would obtain.

DELUSIONS OF PARASITOSIS

Delusions of parasitosis (acarophobia when relating to scabies) is an uncommon syndrome in which individuals, typically

Table 13-2. Treatment of Scabies

Medication*	Dosage
Lindane lotion 1% (Kwell, Kwellada, Scabene)	Apply one thin layer to entire trunk and extremities and leave on for 8 hr. At the end of 8 hr, shower or bathe to remove medication thoroughly. Change imtimate apparel and bed linen.
Crotamiton cream 10% (*N*-ethyl-*o*-crotonotoluide Eurax)	Massage medication into skin from neck downward nightly for 2 nights. Twenty-four hours after second application, wash off medication thoroughly. Change intimate apparel and bed linen.
Precipitated sulfur 6%	Apply preparation to trunk and extremities nightly for 3 nights. Twenty-four hours after last application, bathe to thoroughly remove medication. Change intimate apparel and bed linen.

* Physician should provide the patient with a non-refillable prescription for only the amount needed.

From Orkin M, Maibach HI: Scabies: A current pandemic. Postgrad Med 66:52, 1979.

women over the age of 50, are unrelenting in the conviction that their intense pruritus is caused by an infestation.[42] This may follow real or alleged infestation. Cutaneous findings are absent or manifest by a variety of traumatic lesions (scratches, gouged out pits and ulcers, admixed with scars), which are asymmetric and generalized or localized. Patients provide "specimens" in boxes or bottles, which usually contain bits of skin or debris; these should always be studied microscopically, since unfortunate mistakes can be made in which the patient really does have an infestation. The condition may represent a monosymptomatic hypochondriac psychosis.[43]

SPECIFIC AGENTS

Commonly used scabicides and instructions for their uses are presented in Table 13-2.[5,44]

Lindane is the most frequently used scabicide and the most thoroughly studied. Lindane lotion or cream (we prefer lotion for ease of application) is easy to use and effective. Allergic contact dermatitis caused by this medication has not been documented; irritant contact dermatitis from too frequent use is not uncommon. Ten percent of lindane applied to the skin can be observed in the urine[45]; this cutaneous absorption has been verified in scabietic and normal children.[46] Studies of acute toxicity have revealed toxicity of the central nervous system. Careful studies to determine the presence or absence of subclinical central nervous system toxicity have not been performed, nor has such toxicity from appropriately used topical therapy been proved. Clinical central nervous system toxicity has occurred only with misuse.[47]

We prefer not to use lindane in infants and young children (less than 10 years of age), because of the potential for misuse and the decreased safety ratios at these ages. We do not use lindane in pregnancy, nor in nursing mothers. We do not use lindane in patients with seizure disorders or other neurologic disease. In older children and nonpregnant adults, an application of the lotion is left on for 8 hours and washed off thoroughly; the lotion should be kept away from the eyes and mucous membranes. A second application is appropriate when there is evidence of failure of compliance (the family should be instructed again), a reinfestation, or apparent resistance.

Crotamiton is a satisfactory scabicide. Sensitization occurs rarely but not in scabies therapy. In the treatment of infants and young children with scabies, five daily applications may be better than the two currently recommended.[48] The five-day schedule should be studied further in all age groups.

Sulfur, used for centuries, is generally prescribed as precipitated sulfur (6%) in petrolatum. Patients find it less acceptable than modern scabicides because of odor, messiness, and staining. It occasionally produces an irritant dermatitis.

We prefer precipitated sulfur in infants and pregnant and lactating women and sulfur or crotamiton in older children and patients with seizure disorders or other neurologic diseases. Lindane and crotamiton are the treatment of choice in adults, with the aforementioned exceptions. It is not uncommon for us to use different preparations for different age groups in the same family, for example, lindane or crotamiton in adults and sulfur in young children.

TREATMENT OF SOME SPECIAL FORMS

NODULAR SCABIES. The pruritic hypersensitivity nodules called nodular scabies do not respond to scabicides; they clear spontaneously but may persist for months to more than a year. The nodules frequently subside with nightly application of tar gel (Estar Gel, Psori Gel) for 2 to 3 weeks. They also may improve or clear with intralesional injections of corticosteroid (5 mg/ml of triamcinalone acetonide).

SCABIES IN THE ELDERLY (PARTICULARLY IN NURSING HOMES). Scabies in nursing home patients (particularly the elderly) is difficult to eradicate both in the individual and in the institution. The itching is particularly severe, and the organisms may find refuge and protection from treatment under the free edge of the nail plate. In addition to the usual regimen it may help to keep the fingernails trimmed very short and to brush the scabicide under the free edge of the nails for several consecutive days.[49]

ANIMAL-TRANSMITTED SCABIES. Scabies transmitted by an animal is self-limited (several weeks) if the animal is cured or separated from the humans. The animal should be treated by a veterinarian skilled in veterinary dermatology. Symptomatic family members may be treated with supportive measures; scabicides are not needed. It is unnecessary to treat asymptomatic members of the household or sexual contacts outside the household because the condition is usually not contagious between humans.

CRUSTED SCABIES. Therapy for crusted scabies is similar to that for the more common types, although the former responds more slowly and may require sequential use of lindane, sulfur, and crotamiton, sometimes facilitated by keratolytic agents used prior to the scabicide.

POSTTREATMENT MANAGEMENT

An oral antipruritic medication, such as an antihistamine or salicylate, may be used simultaneously with the scabicide. For the pruritus that characteristically lingers after adequate antiscabietic therapy, a topical hydrocortisone preparation may provide symptomatic relief in adults, and a lubricating agent or emollient may be helpful in infants and small children.

Most patients with secondarily infected scabies do not require systemic antibacterial therapy; the bacterial aspect clears with scabicidal therapy. When bacterial infection is extensive, we sometimes use an oral antibacterial agent, particularly oral erythromycin.

In the rare instance of incapacitating posttreatment itching in an adult, a short course of systemic corticosteroid therapy, such as a 7- to 10-day course of prednisone at an initial dosage of 40 mg/day, gives prompt, dramatic relief.

PEDICULOSIS PUBIS

Lice infestations have been known since biblical times.[50] Francesco Redi described *Pediculus pubis* in 1668. For many years the louse was confused with the scabies mite. In Erasmus Wilson's textbook in 1842, lice and pediculosis were described in contemporary terms.

Etiology

Lice are wingless insects that are obligate parasites. Two species are parasitic for humans, *Phthirus pubis* and *Pediculus humanus*; the latter is divided into two distinct populations, *P. humanus capitis,* the head louse, and *P. humanus corporis,* the body louse. The pubic or crab louse is broader than it is long; the adult ranges in length from 0.8 to 1.2 mm. The second and third pairs of legs are equipped with powerful claws, which permit the louse to hold firmly to the pubic hair and also serve for locomotion. The life cycle of the pubic louse, egg to egg, is about 25 days.

The louse inserts its mouthparts into a cutaneous capillary of the human host and sucks blood at frequent intervals. The ensuing itching is immunologic. There is an approximately 30-day incubation period from exposure to onset of pruritus.

Epidemiology

There has been a sharp increase in the frequency of pediculosis pubis,[51] without restriction to lower socioeconomic groups. Pediculosis capitis is far more common in white American children than in black children. There is no racial difference in the distribution of pediculosis pubis in American adults.

Patients with pediculosis pubis are seen more commonly at venereal disease clinics, at student health services, and by family physicians than in dermatologists' offices.[52] The sexual revolution plays a vital role in this epidemic, particularly in young persons, because the condition is predominantly transmitted by sexual contact.[53] About one third of patients with pediculosis pubis have other currently untreated sexually transmitted diseases, especially gonorrhea, nongonococcal urethritis, and trichomoniasis.[54] As with most STDs, pediculosis pubis is most common in patients aged 15 to 40 years. As with gonorrhea, pediculosis pubis is more common in women aged 15 to 19 years than in men; the sex distribution is reversed[55] in patients over the age of 20.

Control

Early diagnosis and treatment with an effective pediculicide, for the patient as well as his or her sexual contacts, are vital to prevention. In addition, because about one third of these patients are currently infected with another sexually transmitted disease, all patients with pediculosis pubis should be evaluated for gonorrhea, syphilis, and other sexually transmitted infections.

Clinical Diagnosis

The most common site affected is the pubic region.[56] Although the organisms do not move far from the initial site of contact, involvement may occur, especially in hairy individuals, on the short hairs of the thighs and trunk and occasionally on the beard and mustache. Involvement of the eyelashes and periphery of the scalp occurs mainly in children, to whom transmission probably occurs through close contact with an infested mother. However, infestation of the scalp can occur rarely in adults of all ages. Pruritus, which may be severe, is the common symptom. Excoriations may lead to pyoderma, which may mask the parasites. This is probably less common in developed countries, where the discomfort frequently leads to early diagnosis and effective therapy.

Characteristic, but not common, are the maculae caeruleae (sky-blue spots): unique, asymptomatic, bluish, or slate-colored macules located on the trunk and thighs. These fade within a short time. They are probably caused by altered blood pigments of the infested patient or by an excretion from the louse's salivary gland.

When pediculosis pubis involves portions of the body other than the pubic region, the diagnosis may be difficult. This infestation should be suspected in any pruritic eruption of a hairy area. At times, diagnosis may be established more easily by examination of the axillae and other locations other than the pubic region because the patient may have already eradicated the public infestation by self-medication prior to consulting the physician but will be less likely to treat other sites.

Administration of a corticosteroid (topical or systemic) may reduce pruritus but potentiate the undiagnosed infestation and allow it to become generalized.

Infestation of the eyelashes is particularly difficult to diagnose because it may simulate seborrheic or infectious eczematous blepharitis; careful examination reveals that the crusts consist of parasitic organisms.

Differential diagnosis includes impetigo, pyoderma, infectious eczema, neurodermatitis, seborrheic dermatitis, psoriasis, and contact dermatitis.

Laboratory Diagnosis

Pediculosis pubis is one of the few STDs that can be diagnosed by physical examination alone; the less numerous adult lice can be identified with the aid of a magnifying lens or loupe. The parasites are more discernible after a blood meal, when they become rust-colored. Flecks of rust-colored excreta are sometimes observed at sites of infestation. Most commonly, however, the diagnosis is made by identifying the more numerous nits attached by a cementing substance to the pubic hair, initially at the hair's junction with the skin. Because the ova grow out with the hair, the approximate duration of the infestation can be judged by the distance of the ova from the cutaneous surface. Although the nits can be seen with the naked eye, they can be confused with kinks and knots in the hair or flakes of seborrheic dermatitis (which can be brushed off). The diagnosis should be confirmed by plucking the hair, placing it on a slide, and observing the nit under the microscope.

Treatment

Careful explanation, answering of all patient or family questions and reassurance are vital. Patients frequently receive the diagnosis with inordinate concern, guilt, and sometimes skepticism.

The physician should estimate and prescribe the specific amount to be used with no refills.[57] The medication is applied to the infested and adjacent hairy areas with particular attention to the pubic mons and perianal region. In hairy individuals the thighs, trunk, and axillary regions should also be treated because of the frequent involvement of these sites. A common cause of treatment failure in hairy individuals is treatment of only the pubic area. Sexual contacts should be treated simultaneously to prevent reinfestation. Other uninfested household members need not be treated. At the conclusion of therapy, infested individuals and their sexual partners should use clean underclothing, nightclothes, sheets, and pillow cases. They should be told to machine-wash and -dry the old items using the hot cycle.

Lindane lotion (Kwell, Kwellada, Scabene) is used extensively. A thin layer of lindane lotion is applied to the infested and adjacent hairy areas. The lotion is left on for 12 hours and is removed by thorough washing. The remaining nits may be removed with a fine-toothed comb or forceps. One application is usually sufficient; a second application is repeated in one week if viable eggs persist or new eggs appear at junctions of hair and skin. Many physicians prefer lindane shampoo (rather than lindane lotion) lathered into affected sites for four minutes, followed by thorough rinsing and towel-drying.

Synergized pyrethrins (RID and others) are over-the-counter products effective in the treatment of lice infestations.[58] They are applied undiluted until the infested areas are entirely wet and allowed to remain in place for 10 minutes; then the areas are washed thoroughly with warm water and soap and dried. A fine-toothed comb, provided in some trade packages, permits removal of dead lice and eggs. One application is usually sufficient; a second application is repeated in one week if viable eggs persist or new eggs appear at junctions of hair and skin.

Although extensive comparative studies of pediculicides have not been done, a study comparing lindane and synergized pyrethrins produced similar results in patients with pubic lice.[59]

Treatment for involvement of the eyelashes consists of thick applications of petrolatum twice a day for eight days and then mechanical removal of any remaining nits. Formerly, yellow oxide of mercury or anticholinesterase preparations were used.

No resistance of pubic lice to insecticides has been noted. Therapeutic inefficiency is usually a result of patients' failure to follow instructions completely, failure to treat sexual contacts, or reinfestation. Persistent itching may be caused by irritation from the pediculicide (usually from too-frequent use) or the patient's anxiety. Parasitophobia is not uncommon and is difficult to treat.

Allergic contact dermatitis from lindane has not been documented; irritant contact dermatitis from too-frequent use is not uncommon. Ten percent of lindane applied to the skin is absorbed.[60] Lindane has the potential to cause toxicity of the central nervous system and there have been reports of seizures following its use. These have occurred mainly in young children treated for scabies and, almost exclusively, the product has been misused. Because pediculosis pubis does not commonly occur in the groin and adjacent areas in prepubertal individuals, we have less concern about the use of lindane for pubic lice except in pregnant women or nursing mothers. In all circumstances we would apply the material thinly and observe precautions.

Synergized pyrethrins should not be used near the eyes or on mucous membranes. Although the pyrethrins are related to the Compositae (potentially potent plant allergens), the former have not been identified as allergens in pediculosis therapy.[52]

Posttreatment Management

Itching often persists for a short time after the lice have been removed, in part because hypersensitivity may take time to recede.[61] Reassurance of patients is helpful. Although usually not needed, an oral antipruritic medication such as an antihistamine or salicylate may help, as may a topical hydrocortisone preparation.

If there is a suggestion of reinfestation or apparent resistance, check for viable eggs by plucking hairs for examination under the microscope; empty nits require no further therapy.

REFERENCES

1. Mellanby K: Scabies. 2nd Ed. Classey, London, 1972
2. Heilesen B: Studies on Acarus scabiei and scabies. Acta Derm Venereol [Suppl] (Stockh) 26, 1946
3. Mellanby K: Biology of the parasite. In Orkin M, et al (eds): Scabies and Pediculosis. Lippincott, Philadelphia, 1977
4. Orkin M: Resurgence of scabies. JAMA 217:593, 1971
5. Orkin M, Maibach HI: Scabies. In Holmes K, et al (eds): Sexually Transmitted Disease. McGraw-Hill, New York, 1984
6. Alexander AM: Role of race in scabies infestation. Arch Dermatol 114:627, 1978
7. Mellanby K: Epidemiology of scabies. In

Orkin M, et al (eds): Scabies and Pediculosis. Lippincott, Philadelphia, 1977

8. Palicka P: The incidence and mode of scabies transmission in a district of Czechoslovakia (1961–1979). Folia Parastitol (Praha) 29:51, 1982

9. Felman YM, Nikitas JA: Scabies. Cutis 25:32, 1980

10. Schroeter AL: Scabies-a venereal disease. In Orkin M, et al (eds): Scabies and Pediculosis. Lippincott, Philadelphia, 1977

11. Juranek DD, Schultz MG: Epidemiologic investigation of scabies in the United States. In Orkin M, et al (eds): Scabies and Pediculosis. Lippincott, Philadelphia, 1977

12. Juranek DD, Currier RW, Millikan LE: Scabies control in institutions. In Orkin M, Maibach HI (eds): Cutaneous Infestations and Insect Bites. Marcel Dekker, New York, 1984

13. Epstein E Sr, Orkin M: Scabies: Clinical aspects. In Orkin M, et al (eds): Scabies and Pediculosis. Lippincott, Philadelphia, 1977

14. Moschella SL: Parasitology and tropical dermatology. In Moschella SL, Pillsbury DM, Hurley HJ Jr (eds): Dermatology. Saunders, Philadelphia, 1975

15. Orkin M: Special forms of scabies. In Orkin M, Maibach HI (eds): Cutaneous Infestations and Insect Bites. Marcel Dekker, New York, 1984

16. Orkin M: Today's scabies. JAMA 233:882, 1975

17. Ting HD, Wang F: Scabies and systemic lupus erythematosus. Int J Dermatol 22:473, 1983

18. Fiumara NJ: Scabies and genital herpes; a problem in management. Am Fam Physicians 25:125, 1982

19. Ginsburg CM: Scabies in infants and children: A pediatrician's view. Proceedings of symposium on the management of scabies and pediculosis. Cutis Suppl p 10, Sept 1981

20. Burns BR, et al: Neonatal scabies. Am J Dis Child 133:1031, 1979

21. Bjornberg A, Friis B: Persistent pustulosis in children adopted from Asia: A sequela of scabies? Int J Dermatol 17:69, 1978

22. Kligman AM: Round table discussion: Treatment of the elderly. Proceedings of symposium on the management of scabies and pediculosis. Cutis Suppl p 29, Sept 1981

23. Fain A: Epidemiological problems of scabies. Int J Dermatol 17:20, 1978

24. Fiumara NJ, Calhoun J: Multiple sexually transmitted diseases. Sex Transm Dis 9:98, 1982

25. Kobayashi M, Miyoshi I, Sonobe H, et al: Association of pneumocystis carinii pneumonia and scabies. JAMA 248:1973, 1982

26. Orkin M, Maibach HI: Current views of scabies and pediculosis pubis. Cutis 33:85, 1984

27. Chapel TA, Krugel KL, Chapel J, et al: Scabies presenting as urticaria. JAMA 246;440, 1981

28. Hoefling KK, Schroeder AL: Dermatoimmunopathology of scabies. J Am Acad Dermatol 3:237, 1980

29. Fiumara NJ, Mason S: Scabies in a solitary location. J Am Coll Health 31:103, 1982

30. Shelley WB, Shelley ED: Common causes of treatment failure in scabies. Illinois Med J 163(2):112, 1983

31. Orkin M, Maibach HI: Modern aspects of scabies. Curr Probl Dermatol (Recent Dev Clin Res) 13:109, 1985

32. Orkin M, Maibach HI: Ectoparasites. In Judson FN, Wentworth BB (eds): Laboratory Methods for the Diagnosis of Sexually Transmitted Diseases. American Public Health Association, Washington, DC, 1984

33. Martin WE, Wheeler CE Jr: Diagnosis of human scabies in epidermal shave biopsy. J Am Acad Dermatol 1:335, 1979

34. Estes S: The diagnosis and Management of Scabies. p 10. Reed and Carnrick, Piscataway, NJ, 1981

35. Woodley D, Saurat JH: The burrow ink test and the scabies mite. J Am Acad Dermatol 4:715, 1981

36. Ackerman AB: Histopathology of human scabies. In Orkin M, et al (eds): Scabies and pediculosis. Lippincott, Philadelphia, 1977

37. Orkin M, Maibach HI: Treatment of today's scabies. In Orkin M, Maibach HI (eds): Cutaneous Infestations and Insect Bites. Marcel Dekker, New York, 1984

38. Orkin M, Juranek DD, Maibach HI: Treatment of household and sexual contacts of patients with scabies. In Epstein E Sr (ed): Controversies in Dermatology. Saunders, Philadelphia, 1983

39. Coskey RJ: Scabies-resistance to treatment with crotamiton. Arch Dermatol 115:109, 1979

40. Hernandez-Perez E: Resistance to antiscabietic drugs. J Am Acad Dermatol 8:121, 1983
41. Taplin D: Reply to Reference 40. J Am Acad Dermatol 8:121, 1983
42. Lyle A: Delusions of parasitosis: Michelson lecturer. Br J Dermatol 108:485, 1983
43. Munro A: Monosymptomatic hypochondriacal psychosis. Br J Hosp Med 24:34, 1980
44. Orkin M, Maibach HI: Scabies, a current pandemic. Postgrad Med 66:52, 1979
45. Feldman RH, Maibach HI: Percutaneous penetration of some pesticides and herbicides in man. Toxicol Appl Pharmacol 28:126, 1974
46. Ginsburg CM, Lowry W, Resich JS: Absorption of lindane (gamma benzene hexachloride) in infants and children. J Pediatr 91:995, 1977
47. Davies JE, Dedhia HV, Morgade C, et al: Lindane poisonings. Arch Dermatol 119:142, 1983
48. Cubela V, Yawalkar SJ: Clinical experience with crotamiton cream and lotion in treatment of infants with scabies. Br J Clin Pract 32:229, 1983
49. Scher RK: Subungual scabies. Am J Dermatopathol 5:187, 1983
50. Parish LC: History of pediculosis. In Orkin M, et al (eds): Scabies and Pediculois. Lippincott, Philadelphia, 1977
51. Gratz NG: The current status of louse infestations throughout the world: The control of lice and louse-borne diseases. In Proceedings of the International Symposium on the Control of Lice and Louse-Borne Diseases, Panamerican Health Organization, 1973
52. Orkin M, Maibach HI: Lice Infestation Update; Transmission and Treatment. Marcel Dekker, New York, 1983
53. Felman YM, Nikitas JA: Pediculosis pubis. Cutis 25:482, 1980
54. Chapel TA, Katta T, Kuszmar T, et al: Pediculosis pubis in a clinic for treatment of sexually transmitted diseases. Sex Transm Dis 6:257, 1979
55. Fisher I, Morton RS: Phthirus pubis infestation. Br J Vener Dis 46;326, 1970
56. Epstein E Sr, Orkin M: Pediculosis: clinic aspects. In Orkin M et al (eds): Scabies and Pediculosis. Lippincott, Philadelphia, 1977
57. Orkin M, Epstein E Sr, Maibach HI: Treatment of today's scabies and pediculosis. JAMA 236:1136, 1976
58. Orkin M, Maibach HI: Scabies and pediculosis. In Gellis SS, Kagan BM (eds): Current Pediatric Therapy. Saunders, Philadelphia, 1982
59. Newsom JH, Fiore JL Jr, Hackett E: Treatment of infestation with Phthirus pubis: Comparative efficacies of synergized pyrethrins-benzene hexachloride. Sex Transm Dis 6:203, 1979
60. Feldman RH, Maibach HI: Percutaneous penetration of some pesticides and herbicides in man. Toxicol Appl Pharmacol 28:126, 1974
61. Orkin M, Maibach HI: Current views of scabies and pediculosis pubis. Cutis 33:85, 1984

14

Nonvenereal Diseases of the Genitals

Robert C. Noble

Patients may appear in their physician's office alarmed that they have a skin lesion on their genitals and certain that they have a sexually transmitted disease. This chapter catalogues some of the nonvenereal conditions that may involve the genitals and that may prove puzzling to the general physician who sees patients with sexually transmitted diseases.

LEUKOPLAKIA

DEFINITION.   The term leukoplakia[1] was originally used to describe any white plaque that persisted on a mucous or mucocutaneous surface. At present, there is disagreement as to the exact meaning of the term.

CLINICAL MANIFESTATIONS.   The lesions of leukoplakia are white and hyperkeratotic. They involve the oral mucosa as a response to irritation. In women they are found on the inner aspects of the labia majora, the anterior fourchette, the introitus, the labia minora, and the clitoris. Their appearance is not uniform. The lesions are believed to be potentially malignant. The lesions of leukoplakia may accompany those of lichen sclerosus et atrophicus and also may be present after irradiation.

DIFFERENTIAL DIAGNOSIS.   The differential diagnosis is mostly between leukoplakia and lichen simplex. These two illnesses may be impossible to distinguish based on direct observation.

DIAGNOSIS.   The definitive diagnosis of leukoplakia is made by histologic sections of the involved skin. There is hyperkeratinization with irregular hyperplasia of the malpighian cell layer. The rete ridges are abnormally long and abnormally shaped. These may also show a denticulate process. Atypical cells need not be present.

TREATMENT.   Liquid nitrogen or steroid injections locally may be effective in controlling small areas of leukoplakia. Local excision may be required for areas that do not respond to such measures.

LICHEN SCLEROSUS ET ATROPHICUS

DEFINITION.   Lichen sclerosus et atrophicus (LSA)[1] is a disorder of unknown etiology affecting whites more frequently than

189

other races and women ten times more frequently than men. The lesions are characteristically lichenoid and atrophic in nature. Although LSA can occur in childhood, the incidence is greater in early middle age onward. There is a statistically significant association between LSA and morphea, and LSA and vitiligo.

CLINICAL MANIFESTATIONS. The lesions of LSA are small, atrophic, and pale in color. The hyaline changes in the superficial dermis accompanied by a pigmentary defect are the cause of the white color. Hyperkeratosis may be present at the orifices of the sweat and sebaceous glands. Telangectasia, purpura, and bullae may also occur. Depigmentation may vary in melanized skin. Wrinkled plaques may result from aggregation of the individual lesions. The plaques occur in both sexes on the genitalia with a frequency that is ten times that of other parts of the body. When the vulva is involved, the perianal area is also involved, resulting in an "inverted keyhole" distribution. LSA may also be present on the trunk and limbs, but is not often found on the tongue and buccal mucosa. If present before puberty, LSA may completely resolve. However, lesions appearing after puberty rarely resolve.

LSA may be asymptomatic in women, but itching, soreness, dyspareunia, and dysuria are common complaints. Lesions on the outer aspects of the labia majora may become lichenified, and in anogenital LSA lesions may become macerated and hyperkeratotic. LSA may result in atrophy of the labia minora, and in severe cases there may be contracture of the introitus. In longstanding lesions, there may be transient ulceration and secondary infection. Small adjacent areas of leukoplakia may complicate LSA, and the patient may suffer with itching.

In men, LSA is generally confined to the glans and prepuce. In circumcised men, the

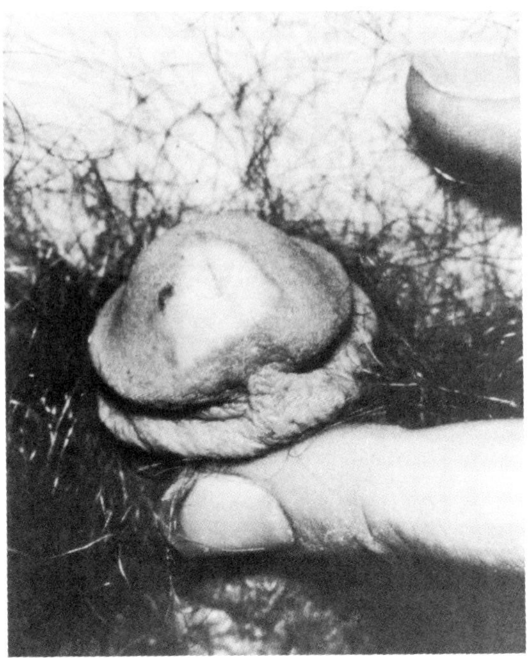

Fig. 14-1 A linear, white, atrophic plaque of lichen sclerosis et atrophicus involving the urethral orifice. (From Fitzpatrick TB, Eisen AZ, Wolf K, et al: Dermatology in General Medicine. 2nd Ed. p 919. McGraw-Hill, New York, 1979, with permission.)

lesions appear anywhere on the glans, including the urinary meatus (Fig. 14-1). This may result in restriction of the urinary flow. Contractures of the foreskin may occur in uncircumcised men, resulting in a need for circumcision. One name given to this disorder is balanitis xerotica obliterans (Fig. 14-2). Leukoplakia and resulting carcinoma may be present in the preputial sac.

DIFFERENTIAL DIAGNOSIS. The differential diagnosis of LSA is difficult in both men and women. In men, it includes any form of balanitis, erythroplasias, and leukoplakia. Severe atrophy and adhesions of the prepuce to the glans may also result from mucosal involvement by pemphigoid. In women, the diagnosis is equally difficult because of the presence of dermatitis, ma-

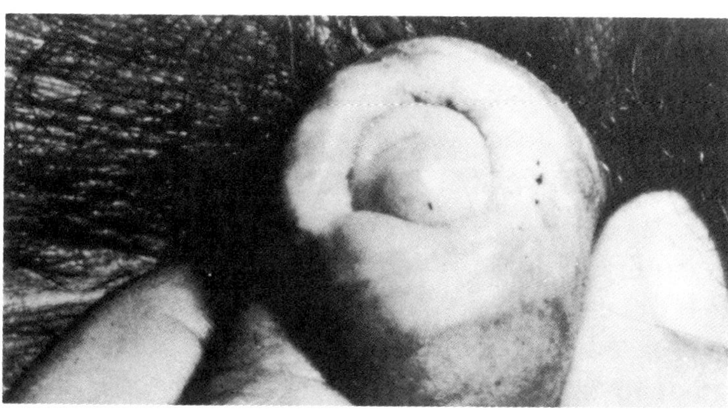

Fig. 14-2 Balanitis xerotica obliterans (lichen sclerosus et atrophicus). (From Fitzpatrick TB, Eisen AZ, Wolf K, et al: Dermatology in General Medicine. 2nd Ed. p 919. McGraw-Hill, New York, 1979, with permission.)

ceration, and the effects of excoriation. Leukoplakia may be confused with LSA and may be present in addition to LSA. Lichen planus may also be confused with LSA. However, lichen planus is usually present at other sites on the body. Macerated and inflamed areas may be confused with *Candida* infections.

DIAGNOSIS. Biopsy is necessary for a definitive diagnosis of LSA. It may be necessary to delay the biopsy in order to clear up any superficial infection and inflammation that would make interpretation difficult.

TREATMENT. Itching is one of the most disturbing symptoms in women. Control of this may require the application of topical steroids. Unfortunately, atrophy is a side effect of this medication, and the weakest preparation that will control the symptoms is the one that should be used. Intralesional steroids or freezing with liquid nitrogen has been effective for particularly persistent lesions. Symptoms may also be lessened by the use of loose cotton underwear and careful genital cleaning. The same type of therapy may also be used for men, except for those unfortunate individuals who require surgery as a result of contractures and phimosis of the prepuce or the presence of a urethral stricture.

BENIGN ERYTHROPLASIAS

DEFINITION. Benign erythroplasias[1] are lesions that must be distinguished from those with malignant potential, such as erythroplasia of Queyrat.

CLINICAL MANIFESTATIONS. Benign erythroplasias are chronic, asymptomatic plaquelike lesions on the vulva in women and in the buccal mucosa. The plaques are velvety, red, and moist. A benign erythroplasia of the penis is called erythroplasia of Zoon.

DIFFERENTIAL DIAGNOSIS. Benign erythroplasias must be distinguished from Bowen's disease, lichen planus, drug eruption, psoriasis, and monilial balanitis. The microscopic picture is similar to that of Bowen's disease.

DIAGNOSIS. Fungal scrapings and culture will rule out *Candida* infection. The history may be helpful in eliminating drug eruptions, and psoriasis and lichen planus lesions will likely be present on other parts of the body. The definitive diagnosis is by biopsy. The epidermis is reduced in thickness with thinning of the subpapillary plates. This results in the red color characteristic of the lesion. A dense infiltrate of plasma cells is present in the upper cutis.

TREATMENT. Erythroplasia may be treated with topical steroids, local excision, cryotherapy, or topical 5-fluorouracil.

ERYTHROPLASIA OF QUEYRAT (BOWEN'S DISEASE; CARCINOMA IN SITU)

DEFINITION. Erythroplasia of Queyrat[2,3] is a genital lesion manifested as a slightly raised plaque on the glans or prepuce in men or on the introitus or labia minora in women. The disease occurs in late life more commonly in men than in women, and it is unusual in men who have been circumcised as an infant. Oral lesions may also occur. This disease is also called Bowen's disease or carcinoma in situ.

CLINICAL MANIFESTATIONS. The lesions take the form of red plaques on the mucosal surface of the prepuce, the glans penis (Plate 14-1), and the corona in men. In women, the lesions are usually present on the labia minora. The lesions may itch or burn, and in women, urination may be painful. Lesions may make intercourse painful. In some patients, the lesions are accompanied by mottled white lesions that give the appearance of leukoplakia. As time passes, the lesions slowly enlarge.

DIAGNOSIS. Some authors see no reason to separate erythroplasia of Queyrat from Bowen's disease, as they are very similar. The crimson color of the lesions is due to the thinning of the suprapapillary plates and the closeness of the papillary vessels to the surface. The granular layer is absent.

DIFFERENTIAL DIAGNOSIS. Bowen's disease is separated from erythroplasia of Queyrat by some clinicians only in that lesions in Bowen's disease are present at other sites on the body. In both diseases, there are persistent red plaques on the genitalia.

TREATMENT. The treatment of choice is excision of the lesion, leaving a wide margin. Radical surgery is not required if cancer has not developed. If the lesion has remained superficial, then another approach is therapy with 5-fluorouracil, as a 1% solution or 5% cream, applied twice daily for 2 to 3 months. Cryotherapy has also been successful.

PAGET'S DISEASE

DEFINITION. Paget's disease[1] is a precancerous lesion generally located on the nipple of the breast in women; however, it can appear in other parts of the body with the same features.

CLINICAL MANIFESTATIONS. Paget's disease most often appears in older individuals. The labia majora is the most frequent site in women, but lesions can be found on the perianal area, the groin, and the perineum (Fig. 14-3 and Plate 14-2). In men, the scrotum is the most commonly involved area, but lesions may also be present on the perianal area and in the groin. Paget's disease presents as a irregularly shaped, erythematous hyperkeratotic plaque, often with areas of erosion. Itching may be the first symptom, but as the lesion becomes more extensive, it becomes infiltrative in character. Early lesions are small and unilateral, but these may increase in size to involve extensive areas.

DIFFERENTIAL DIAGNOSIS. Paget's disease can be confused with erythroplasia if the lesions have erosions. This disease can also mimic Bowen's disease.

DIAGNOSIS. The diagnosis of Paget's disease is made by biopsy. It is suggested by any hyperkeratotic, infiltrative, persist-

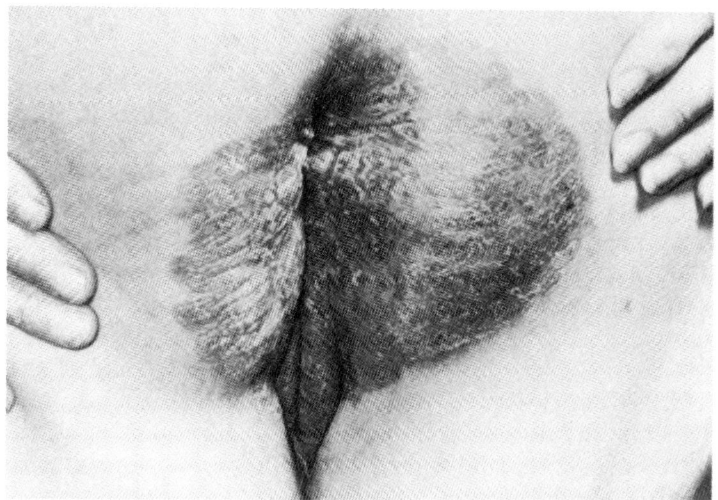

Fig. 14-3 Paget's disease of the anogenital region. (From Hall-Smith P, Cairns RJ: Dermatology, Current Concepts and Practice. 3rd Ed. p 237. Butterworth, Woburn, MA, 1981, with permission.)

ent, erythematous plaque present on the genitals. Erosion or exudation may be present.

THERAPY. In both men and women, wide excision and removal of regional lymph nodes is advised. Often a thorough search of the excised tissue will reveal the presence of an apocrine carcinoma that was unrecognized. Radiotherapy is not recommended. Without therapy, the lesion may remain intraepidermal, but invasion of the dermis is probable with time and untreated disease may be fatal.

SQUAMOUS CELL CARCINOMA OF THE GENITALS

DEFINITION. Squamous cell carcinoma[4] is an epidermal cancer usually arising from a premalignant lesion on the skin.

CLINICAL MANIFESTATIONS. Squamous cell carcinomas usually develop on exposed areas of skin in light-skinned people. These carcinomas do appear, however, in the genital areas of patients. Carcinoma in situ is another name for intraepidermal squamous cell carcinoma. These lesions may be found in lesions already present in the skin, such as Bowen's disease and erythroplasia of Queyrat. At some point in time this cancer crosses the basement membrane and invades the dermis. The tumor then spreads to regional lymphatics and then to more remote sites. The lesions are usually asymptomatic, reddish plaques or nodules that are firm and indurated. Erosions or ulcerations may be present. Cervical carcinoma may have no visual clues to its presence.

DIFFERENTIAL DIAGNOSIS. Any of the causes of genital ulcers could be confused on first visit with carcinoma. The duration of the lesion is one clue. Bowen's disease, erythroplasia of Queyrat, and leukoplakia have been discussed.

DIAGNOSIS. The diagnosis of squamous cell carcinoma is established by biopsy. Early cervical cancers may be diagnosed with a Papanicolaou test.

TREATMENT. The treatment of early lesions is usually by excision or electrocoagulation. Radiation therapy is used for some lesions.

HIDRADENITIS SUPPURATIVA

DEFINITION.   Hidradenitis suppurativa[1] is a chronic disease resulting from obstruction of the apocrine ducts, followed by dilatation and secondary bacterial infection. The apocrine gland areas principally involved are the axillae and anogenital areas (Fig. 14-4). Continued infection and activity of the disease results in scarring and formation of fibrous tissue.

CLINICAL MANIFESTATIONS.   Hidradenitis suppurativa is seen in patients who are between puberty and middle age. Obesity may be a predisposing factor. Axillary involvement is more frequent in women, and perianal involvement is more frequent in men. The initiating event may be local trauma caused by tight-fitting clothes or chemical irritation from deodorants or dipilatories. At first, a small inflammatory swelling unrelated to a hair follicle is seen in the apocrine area. Without therapy, this abscess will open and drain purulent or seropurulent fluid. Over the space of weeks to months, new lesions will develop, which ultimately form sinus tracts and bands of fibrous tissue. Eventually, the patient loses the ability to sweat at the involved site because of the destruction of the apocrine glands. The sinus tracts and draining sites become infected with staphylococci, streptococci, and gram-negative rods, including *Escherichia coli, Proteus mirabilis,* and *Pseudomonas aeruginosa.* Hidradenitis may result in fistula formation in the perianal area.

DIFFERENTIAL DIAGNOSIS.   Early in the course of the illness, hidradenitis suppurativa may be confused with furuncles, carbuncles, infected dermal inclusion cysts, lymphadenitis, or perirectal abscesses. late disease can mimic cutaneous tuberculosis, lymphogranuloma venereum, granuloma inguinale, or actinomycosis. The diagnosis is made by the characteristic distribution and the history of the lesions.

THERAPY.   Initial steps should be directed at removal of any inciting cause of the disease, including chemical irritants, tight clothing, and so on. Draining lesions should be cultured and antimicrobial therapy specifically directed at the offending organism. In early lesions, incision and draining may not be necessary; in addition to

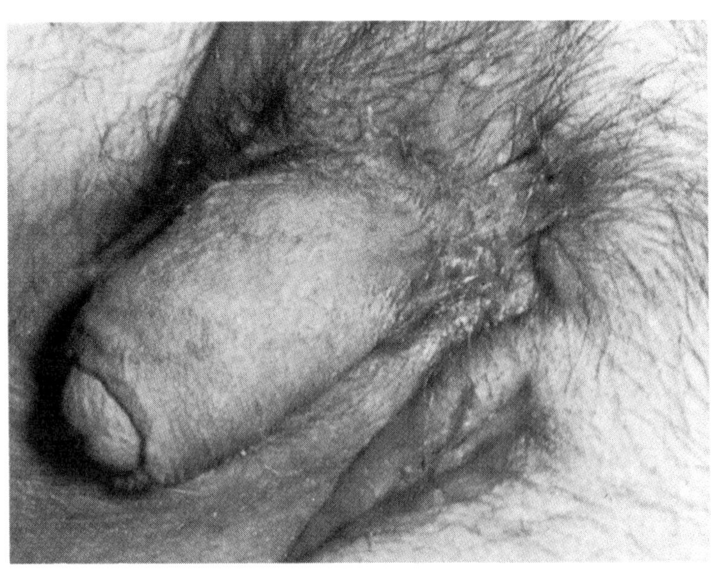

Fig. 14-4 Hidradenitis suppurativa of the genital area. (From Fitzpatrick TB, Eisen AZ, Wolf K, et al: Dermatology in General Medicine. 2nd Ed. p 1827. McGraw-Hill, New York, 1979, with permission.)

antibiotics, the patient should be treated with hot tub baths or soaks for 15 minutes three times daily. In some cases, intralesional steroids may be required. These injections may be administered in the form of triamcinolone, 10 mg/ml. In advanced cases, surgical incision and drainage may be necessary, and the open lesions should be treated with wet to dry saline dressings or a 1:40 dilution of Burow's solution three or four times daily for 30 minutes at a time. In chronic cases resistant to medical therapy, surgical removal is the only effective therapy. Surgery seems to be most effective when the lesions are in a defined area and block removal is feasible. Untreated, chronic lesions can result in fistula formation, fibrosis, and scarring to the point where motion of a limb or extremity may be inhibited.

FOX-FORDYCE DISEASE

DEFINITION. Fox-Fordyce disease[1] is a disorder resulting from plugging and/or rupture of the intraepidermal part of the apocrine gland ducts, resulting in secondary change in the secretory tubule and dermis.

CLINICAL MANIFESTATIONS. Patients complain of itching in the presence of skin-colored or pigmented follicular papules located in follicles of the axilla, pubic area, and mammary areola. The disease is nine times as frequent in women as men, and it is most common between the ages of 13 and 35. Sweating intensifies the itching, and the affected areas may show diminished growth of hair, possibly as the result of excoriation.

DIFFERENTIAL DIAGNOSIS. The differential diagnosis includes syringomas, lichen planus, and neurodermatitis.

DIAGNOSIS. The definitive diagnosis is by biopsy of the affected area. Keratinous plugging of the upper portion of the apo-

crine duct results in intraepidermal apocrine sweat retention and the formation of small vesicles that attract inflammatory cells. This results in the rupture of the intraepidermal part of the apocrine duct. Macroscopically, sweat is absent at the orifice of the duct.

TREATMENT. There is no effective treatment for this chronic condition. Antibiotic therapy may occasionally be required for complicating bacterial folliculitis in some patients.

ECTOPIC SEBACEOUS GLANDS

DEFINITION. Sebaceous glands[1] are not normally found on the mucocutaneous junctions; however, they may on occasion be located high in the cutis, unrelated to hair follicles, and may or may not connect with the surface. These generally do not cause any difficulties.

ANGIOKERATOMAS

DEFINITION. Angiokeratomas[1] are small (2–3 mm) multiple lesions found on the labia and scrotum. There are two types. The angiokeratomas of Fordyce are highly vascular and have little keratin. Although they may rupture and bleed, they are not associated with any internal vascular deformity. The second variety, angiokeratoma corporis diffusum of Fabry, is related to a metabolic disorder of lipids and may be confused with the angiokeratomas of Fordyce on macroscopic examination. These lesions may appear first on the scrotum.

DIAGNOSIS. The diagnosis is made by their characteristic appearance. The two types are distinguished histologically. The lesions of Fabry stain with fat stains and the angiokeratomas of Fardyce do not.

TREATMENT. There is no treatment.

PEARLY PENILE PAPULES (ACRAL ANGIOFIBROMAS)

DEFINITION. Pearly penile papules[5] are located on the corona of the penis and histologically resemble adenoma sebaceum, fibromas of the oral cavity, and fibrous papules of the face.

CLINICAL MANIFESTATIONS. The papules (1–4 mm in size) are present in one to five rows around the coronal sulcus of the penis.

DIFFERENTIAL DIAGNOSIS. There is little to be confused with these lesions except possibly warts and lichen nitidis. The latter lesions appear on the shaft of the penis as well.

DIAGNOSIS. The diagnosis is established by biopsy.

THERAPY. Excision is the common method of therapy of angiofibromas but because of the location this may be difficult.

LICHEN NITIDIS

DEFINITION. Lichen nitidis[1] is a rare, chronic eruption that causes no symptoms and presents as small, normally pigmented papules on the penis, arms, and abdomen. There is no predilection for any sex or race.

CLINICAL MANIFESTATIONS. The papules of lichen nitidis are pinhead in size and polygonal or round in shape. They are slightly raised and this surface has a glistening character. Generally the papules are discrete, but occasionally they may be confluent. They are most often located on the glans and shaft of the penis, the groin, the lower abdomen and the flexor surface of the arms, the palmer surface of the wrists and the breasts.

DIFFERENTIAL DIAGNOSIS. Lichen nitidis must be differentiated from pearly penile papules.

DIAGNOSIS. The characteristic appearance of the lesions and their location suggest the diagnosis, but the definitive diagnosis is by biopsy. Flat warts must be distinguished from lichen nitidis. Warts are generally brown, and their surface is irregular. Lichen planus has a more violaceous color, whereas the lichen nitidis is flesh-colored.

TREATMENT. There is no effective treatment for this disorder.

BENIGN TRANSIENT LYMPHANGIECTASIS (SCLEROSING LYMPHANGITIS OF THE PENIS)

DEFINTION. Benign transient lymphangiectasis of the penis[6–9] is an uncommon condition of unknown etiology believed to be the result of thickening of connective tissue in the wall of lymphatic vessels with partial or total occlusion. Both infection and trauma have been postulated as etiologic agents.

CLINICAL MANIFESTATION. The patient usually notices the sudden appearance of a painless, hard nodular, translucent cord in the penis, most often in the coronal sulcus parallel to the corona of the glans penis. The cord usually appears following sexual intercourse. A number of the reported patients developed their lesions after oral-genital sex.

DIFFERENTIAL DIAGNOSIS. This lesion is uncommon and unlikely to be confused with other conditions.

DIAGNOSIS. The diagnosis is based on the clinical presentation. Stolz and coworkers[9] described a similar lesion in the labium majora and labium minora of two female patients.

TREATMENT. Abstinence from intercourse for a few days is advisable. There is no effective therapy. The condition is self-limiting and patients need only to be reassured.

PENILE VENEREAL EDEMA

DEFINITION. Penile venereal edema[10–12] is a transient, self-limited condition seen in sexually active men. In one venereal disease clinic there was a case rate of 1.7 per 1,000 male visits.[12] The cause is unknown.

CLINICAL MANIFESTATIONS. The patients usually have a painless boggy swelling of the prepuce and shaft of the penis. Although many patients have underlying urethritis and/or infected skin lesions on the penis, other patients associate the appearance of the edema with vigorous sexual activity with a partner who has poor lubrication.

DIFFERENTIAL DIAGNOSIS. Lymphedema of the penis and scrotum can occur in areas of the world where filariosis is endemic. Other causes are severe congestive heart failure, hypoproteinemia, radiation, neoplasms, and prior surgery. Lymphedema may also result from paraffin and silicone injections into the penis and trauma as a result of constrictive rubber bands or devices used to prolong erection.

DIAGNOSIS. The diagnosis is based on the characteristic appearance and the resolution of the lesion with sexual abstinence.

TREATMENT. There is no specific therapy for this disorder, as it resolves without therapy when the patient abstains from sexual intercourse for a few days and has the underlying urethritis or skin infection treated.

FIXED DRUG ERUPTIONS

DEFINTION. Fixed drug eruptions[13,14] of the genitals appear following the ingestion of certain drugs in particular individuals. Some of the drugs incriminated in this reaction are tetracycline, phenolphthalein, antipyrine, quinine, quinidine, barbituates, phenacetin, gold, phenylbutazone, chlordiazipoxide, oxyphenbutazone, penicillin, and sulfonamides.

CLINICAL MANIFESTATIONS. The patient usually notices a burning sensation on the mucous membrane or skin. This is followed by the appearance of a well-demarcated circular or oval erythematous eruption. The lesions become dusky red and vary in diameter from a few millimeters to 3–4 cm in diameter. As the lesions develop, bullae may occur. As they heal, the affected areas become darkly pigmented, and this pigmentation may remain for several weeks to months. Readministration of the drug results in the reappearance of the lesions at the same site.

DIFFERENTIAL DIAGNOSIS. Genital herpes must be in the differential diagnosis because of the recurrent nature of the disease and its presence at the same site. The history of drug ingestion, the pigmented nature of the lesions, and the presence of the large bullae are clues that herpes is not the cause of the eruption.

DIAGNOSIS. The diagnosis is based on the patient's history and the characteristic appearance of the lesions.

TREATMENT. Withdrawal of the offending drug is all that is necessary. The lesions will then resolve in a matter of days.

CONTACT DERMATITIS

DEFINTION. Contact dermatitis[1] is an acute or chronic eruption that results from contact with the skin by a foreign substance.

CLINICAL MANIFESTATIONS. The eruption is usually present in the area of contact and is characterized by a red erythematous, edematous rash with papules and vesicles. In chronic exposures, the skin may be thickened and lichenified. Both hyperpigmentation and hypopigmentation can occur. Papules and vesicles may be present among the areas of chronic changes. Papulovesiculation may be absent on the penis and scrotum, where erythema may be the most prominent feature. The site of appearance, the severity, and the character of the rash may be influenced by perspiration, pressure, and friction. These factors may allow a rash to develop in one area of contact and not in another.

DIFFERENTIAL DIAGNOSIS. The differential diagnosis includes superficial fungal infections, neurodermatitis, and atopic dermatitis.

DIAGNOSIS. The diagnosis of the rash is made generally by the clinical appearance. The definitive diagnosis is made with a patch test of the offending material along with suitable controls. Often this is not necessary, and the disappearance of the rash with the removal of the offending agent is all that is required.

TREATMENT. The principal therapy is removal of the offending substance. There are a number of agents that may be involved. Some things to consider include spermicidal jellies, diaphragms, condoms, colored or scented toilet paper, douches, vaginal deodorants, menstrual pads, dyes in undergarments, and so on. Initial therapy should include the wearing of loose-fitting undergarments and avoidence of binding clothing. The erythematous painful rash may be treated with Burow's solution compresses for 15 minutes three times daily for several days. Topical steroids are generally not required.

VITILIGO

DEFINITION. Vitiligo[15] is a disorder of unknown cause resulting in loss of melanin from the skin. The characteristic lesions are pale white macules that enlarge over a period of time. The disease is most commonly found in individuals between the ages of 10 and 30 years old, and it is more common in women than in men. There is no racial difference in the incidence of the disease. One third of affected individuals have another family member with the disease.

CLINICAL MANIFESTATIONS. Vitiligo lesions are chalky white, a few millimeters to several centimeters in diameter with an oval or round shape. Hair follicles within the depigmented areas may have small areas of pigmentation surrounding the hair, but otherwise pigment within the center of the lesions is lacking. The lesions are located on the extensor bony surfaces and are frequently present over the knees, elbows and digits. They are also found around the eyes, the nose, mouth, rectum, axillae, lower back, the anterior tibal areas, and the flexor areas of the wrists. The genitalia, nipples, lips, and gingiva may also be involved.

DIFFERENTIAL DIAGNOSIS. Vitiligo is not likely to be confused with other diseases.

DIAGNOSIS. The diagnosis is based on the appearance of typical lesions.

TREATMENT. Repigmentation may be attempted with therapy with oral trioxsalen and timed exposure to sunlight or ultraviolet irradiation.

PSORIASIS

DEFINITION. Psoriasis[16] is a chronic skin disease that results in epidermal hyperplasia and an accelerated rate of epidermal turnover. The characteristic lesions are discrete white papules and plaques covered with silvery scales.

CLINICAL MANIFESTATIONS. The typical lesion is an erythematous patch that becomes elevated and then develops a scale. The lesions have irregular borders that are well demarcated. The lesions are most frequently present on the elbows, knees, intertriginous areas, scalp and buttocks. In the groin or the genitals, maceration may develop rather than the typical scaly lesions. Itching is more severe in the eruptive stages. Older lesions may be asymptomatic. One half of patients will have nail abnormalities and 10% will be afflicted with arthritis.

DIFFERENTIAL DIAGNOSIS. The differential diagnosis includes pityriasis rosea, lichen planus, superficial fungal infections, and seborrheic dermatitis.

DIAGNOSIS. A skin biopsy will resolve the question if one cannot make the diagnosis based on the clinical appearance of the lesions.

TREATMENT. Patients with psoriasis are most commonly treated with topical steroids, keratolytic agents, and, in severe cases, tar and possibly long-wave ultraviolet light. The long-term effects of the latter therapy are unknown.

LICHEN PLANUS

DEFINITION. Lichen planus[1] is an eruption of unknown etiology that effects individuals in middle age. Two thirds of the patients are between 30 and 60 years old. There is no sexual or racial predilection. The eruption is a papule with a distinct shape and color. It may be induced by drugs such as antimalarials, thiazide diuretics, gold, phenolphthalein, and barbiturates. The course of the eruption is variable, and patients may have resolution of their lesions within three months or the lesions may continue for up to three years. Usually the lesions resolve within one or two years. Scarring is infrequent, but temporary pigmentation can occur and brown hyperpigmentation can remain for months.

CLINICAL MANIFESTATIONS. Initial lesions frequently appear on the upper extremities often on the flexor surface of the wrist and forearm. The lesion is a small papule that is flat-topped with a glistening surface. Occasionally there is a central umbilication, and the lesion may be covered with a thin scale. The papule may also be covered by a network of white lines called Wickham's striae. Although the genitalia are involved, the lesions are generally distributed symmetrically over the body involving the flexor surface of the arms, forearms and wrists, the sides of the neck, the back, thighs, and shins. Lesions are not commonly found on the soles, palms, and face. If the lesions are hypertrophic, they may be intensely pruritic. Hyperpigmentation is sometimes present. The isomorphic phenomenon or Koebner phenomenon may be induced by trauma.

The genitalia of the male are affected in about one fourth of cases (Fig. 14-5). The glans is involved most often. Lesions are usually papular in nature, but may have an annular configuration. The incidence of lesions in women is unknown, but lesions may be present on the vulva and in the vaginal vault. In this case they are similar in configuration to lesions found in the oral mucosa. Lesions may also be found in the anus.

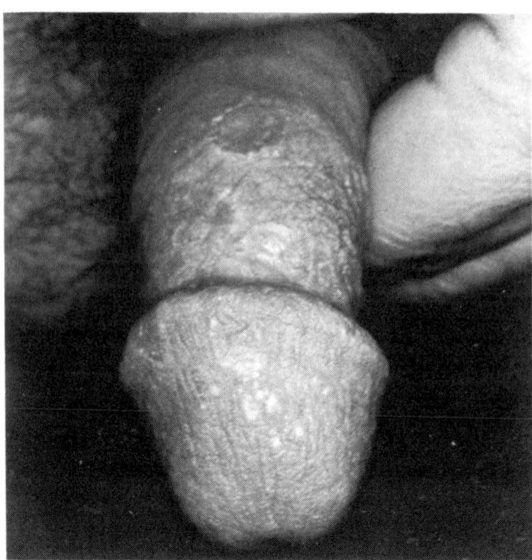

Fig. 14-5 Lichen planus of the penis. (From Bluefarb SM: Scope Monograph on Dermatology. p 10. The Upjohn Company, Kalamazoo, MI, 1972, with permission.)

DIFFERENTIAL DIAGNOSIS. The differential diagnosis includes drug eruptions, psoriasis, leukoplakia, candida infection, mucous patches of secondary syphilis, and seborrheic dermatitis. Severe itching associated with penile lesions may suggest scabies. Papular lesions must be differentiated from secondary syphilis. Hypertrophic lesions must be differentiated from Kaposi's sarcoma, neurodermatitis, and cutaneous amyloid.

DIAGNOSIS. The general appearance of the lesions is suggestive, but the definitive diagnosis is by biopsy.

TREATMENT. There is no definitive treatment for this disorder. It is considered to be benign and self-limited. Regression of the lesions may take place following topical steroids applied under occlusive dressings. Most practitioners recommend avoidance of hot baths, mild soaps, and discontinuance of any offending drugs.

REITER'S SYNDROME

DEFINITION. Reiter's syndrome[17,18] is an illness of unknown etiology originally described by a German physician, Hans Reiter. The syndrome consists of nongonococcal urethritis, arthritis, and conjunctivitis. The original case, a young solider, became ill following an episode of bloody diarrhea without sexual exposure. Mycoplasma and *Chlamydia trachomatis* have been suggested as etiologic agents.

CLINICAL MANIFESTATIONS. Reiter's syndrome is most common in young men and is infrequent in women of any age. Like patients with ankylosing spondylitis, patients with Reiter's syndrome have an increased frequency of HLA-B27 histocompatibility antigen. The illness may be initiated by sexual exposure as well as episodes of bacterial gastroenteritis. Less than 1% of men with nongonococcal urethritis develop Reiter's syndrome. Reiter's syndrome has been described following gastroenteritis caused by *Campylobacter, Shigella, Salmonella,* and *Yersinia.* The frequency of Reiter's syndrome following gastroenteritis of these types is also less than 1%. Around 10% of the postgastroenteritis patients with Reiter's syndrome are women, a group who otherwise have this syndrome rarely. Urethritis in patients with Reiter's syndrome usually starts about one to two weeks after intercourse. Dysuria is not always present, and there is nothing characteristic about the discharge itself. It may be purulent, mucopurulent, or thin and watery. The remainder of the syndrome usually begins within one to five weeks after the onset of the urethritis. The symptom of arthritis usually starts about two weeks after the appearance of the urethritis. The arthritis is asymmetrical and involves the following joints in order of frequency: knees, ankles, metatarsophalangeal joints, sacroiliac joints, and spine. Patients with Reiter's syndrome who are positive for the

HLA-B27 histocompatibility antigen are more likely to develop ankylosing sypondylitis as a complication. Approximately one quarter of patients will develop pain as a result of a calcaneal spur. Those individuals seem to have a poor prognosis. Tendinitis may develop in the plantar fascia and the Achilles tendon. A physical finding in some patients is swelling of the fingers and toes, resulting in a sausage shape. Arthritis may persist for as long as six months and after other features of the syndrome have disappeared. About 80% of patients with Reiter's syndrome develop mucocutaneous lesions. These begin most characteristically over the soles of the feet and palms of the hands as tiny vesicles and enlarge to pustules. The inflammatory reaction at the base of the pustule continues as the material in the pustule dries, and this results in heaped-up keratotic and painless scaling lesions called keratosis blennorrhagia. Similar scaling lesions may appear on the skin, scalp, scrotum, and penis. Erosive and exudative plaques may also be present on the scrotum and penis.

Approximately one fourth of the patients will have a mucosal lesion on the penis called balanitis circinata sicca. This lesion is erythematous, moist, slightly elevated, or eroded and is present on the glans penis. Similar erythematous patches and erosions may develop in the oropharynx or buccal mucosa. Painless erosions may also be present on the tongue. The nails are also affected in Reiter's syndrome. Yellow pustules may develop under the nail and enlarge to erode through the nail plate. This process may result in loss or deformity of the nail. Among the components of the Reiter's syndrome, the eye findings occur least frequently, and often for the shortest duration. Although inflammation of the iris and cornea may occur, bilateral conjunctivitis is more common, sometimes lasting for only a few days.

Reiter's syndrome may develop over a few days with arthritis as the most promi-

nent manifestation, and the first attack may last for several months. The skin lesions heal without scarring. Approximately 80% of patients will have some continuing manifestation with arthritis as the most disabling symptom. Half of the individuals with recurrent disease will have permanent joint damage. There is an increased prevalence of sacroilitis and chronic uveitis in patients who are HLA-B27-positive.

Some of the more unusual manifestations of Reiter's syndrome include pericarditis, myocarditis with atrioventricular heart block, aortitis, which may lead to aortic insufficiency, acute meningoencephalitis, seizures, and polyneuritis.

DIFFERENTIAL DIAGNOSIS. Diseases to be included in the differential diagnosis of Reiter's syndrome include gonococcal arthritis or the gonococcal arthritis-dermatitis syndrome, ankylosing spondylitis, or spondylitis associated with regional enteritis or ulcerative colitis. The spondylitis associated with psoriasis may be confused with the arthritis of Reiter's disease in that they both have skin-associated findings.

DIAGNOSIS. The diagnosis of Reiter's syndrome is made difficult in that it depends upon the recognition of a constellation of clinical features. The principal features include urethritis, arthritis, conjunctivitis, circinate balanitis, shallow ulcerations of the buccal mucosa, and keratoderma blenorrhagicum. At least three of these findings should be present before the diagnosis is established. Not all of the findings need to be present at the same time. Unfortunately there is not a definitive diagnositic test nor is there a diagnostic pathologic finding. About 80% of whites and 50% of blacks with Reiter's syndrome are HLA-B27-possitive. The absence of the HLA-B27 histocompatibility antigen does not exclude the diagnosis. Certain laboratory tests may be helpful. The erythrocyte sedimentation rate is usually elevated. The joint fluid examination reveals an inflammatory response, yellow to opalescent, with a low viscosity. The joint fluid leukocyte counts are in the range of 2,000–100,000/mm^3, and of these cells, 50% or more are polymorphonuclear leukocytes. The mucin clot is friable and the joint fluid glucose is generally greater than 25 mg/100 ml but lower than that in the blood glucose. Roentgenograms may show severe demineralization of the bone next to involved joints and, less commonly, destructive changes in the joints themselves. Sacroiliac involvement may be present on x-ray film, and periosteal formation may be seen at the insertion of the Achilles tendon. Also calcification of the paraspinus ligaments may take place.

TREATMENT. No specific therapy is available for Reiter's syndrome. Although almost universally used, antiinflammatory agents are not always effective. If aspirin is used, blood levels of 20 mg/100 ml should be attained. Prednisone may be administered in initial dosage of 60 mg daily, followed by tapering to a maintenance level. Indomethacin may also be administered in daily dosages from 75 to 150 mg orally. There is no evidence that this is effective in shortening the course of disease. Nonsteroidal antiinflammatory agents are also worthy of trial.

BEHÇET'S DISEASE

DEFINTION. Behçet's disease[19,20] is a disease of unknown etiology. The name is derived from a Turkish dermatologist who, in 1937, described a number of patients with recurrent oral and genital ulceration and relapsing iridocyclitis. Behçet's disease is twice as common in men than in women, and the illness occurs most often in patients between the ages of 19 and 40 years old. Behçet's disease is more frequent in certain areas of the world. These include the Middle East, Israel, Turkey, Greece, Cyprus, and Japan. The disease is also found in northern European countries, especially England and France. Perhaps because of its lack of recognition, Behçet's disease is infrequently reported in the United States. There may be a genetic predisposition to Behçet's disease, and some investigators believe that the manifestations are secondary to vascular immune complex deposition. If this is so, the nature of the antigen is unknown.

CLINICAL MANIFESTATION. As with many rheumatic diseases, Behçet's disease exists as it is defined. One diagnostic schema suggests the following as major manifestations of the disease: apthous stomatitis, genital ulceration, and iridocyclitis. Minor manifestations include cutaneous lesions, recurrent thrombophlebitis, thrombosis of the venae cava, arteritis, and meningoencephalomyelitis. The diagnosis of Behçet's disease is established when two major and one minor manifestation are present. Another diagnostic schema includes the following suggestive criteria: aphthous stomatitis, aphthous genital ulceration, uveitis, cutaneous vasculitis, synovitis, and meningoencephalitis. In this schema, the diagnosis is established when three of the suggested criteria are present, one being recurrent aphthous ulceration. An incomplete form of Behçet's disease is diagnosed if there are two criteria present, one being recurrent aphthous ulceration. The major features of the disease often do not occur at all the same time and their appearance may be transient in character.

In most patients aphthous stomatitis presents as painful recurrent oral ulcers that persist for one to two weeks, heal spontaneously, then reappear at irregular intervals from several weeks to several months. They may be present on the lips, buccal mucosa, tongue, gums, larynx, or tonsils. The ulcers may present as a single lesion or they may appear in clusters. The ulcers vary in diameter (2–10 mm) and in depth. The deep ulcers may have a central necrotic base.

The genital ulcers are also painful and have a similar appearance and course as the oral ulcers. The ulcers may be present on the vulva or vagina in women and on the penis and scrotum in men. Other skin lesions include a nonspecific inflammatory response to infections and superficial scratches as well as a variety of other skin lesions. The latter include erythema nodosum-like lesions, vesicles, papules, pustules, acnelike lesions, pyodermas, abscesses, and folliculitis. These nonspecific lesions also disappear in one to two weeks and recur irregularly.

The eye findings in patients with Behçet's disease may vary in character. Patients may have anterior segment involvement (in order of frequency): relapsing iridocyclitis, conjunctivitis, and corneal ulceration. Posterior segment involvement includes choroiditis. Patients may complain of photophobia, blurred vision, and pain. They may have retinal vessel involvement (phlebitis and/or arteritis), optic papillitis, and inflammatory or hemorrhagic involvement of the vitreous humor. The retinal veins may be engorged and permeable to fluorescein dye. Unfortunately, some patients may be blinded by this disease, approximately one third of those with uveitis. Other patients may have cataracts and glaucoma as a result of Behçet's disease.

Neurologic involvement is present in 10 to 25% of patients with Behçet's disease and usually occurs at the same time as the ulcerative lesions. Neurologic manifestations may not develop until several months after the appearance of the disease. Patients with neurologic involvement generally have fever, headache, and abnormal spinal fluid findings. The latter consist of mildly elevated protein concentrations and pleocytosis (5–500 cells/mm^3) with predominant lymphocytosis. The neurologic manifestations may be varied and include transient ocular palsies, corticospinal tract disease,

pseudobulbar palsy, cerebellar ataxia, and meningoencephalitis. Papilledema may be present. The illness in some patients may resemble an organic confusional state. The mortality rate in patients with neurologic disease is approximately 40%.

Arthritis is one of the most common features of Behçet's disease. Patients have arthralgias initially that later develop into arthritis. The most frequently involved joints are the knees, followed by the ankles, fingers, wrists, elbows, and feet. The arthritis usually resolves without permanent damage to the joint, and only a minority of cases show radiologic evidence of cartilage destruction and bone erosion. The arthritis is generally accompanied by fever, mouth, and genital ulcers, and other skin lesions, including the erythema nodosum-like lesions.

Other manifestations of the disease include thrombophlebitis, colon arterial thrombosis, colitis, aneurysm of the systemic and pulmonary circulations, orchitis, epididymitis, glomerulonephritis, recurrent pneumonitis, pericarditis, and amyloidosis.

DIFFERENTIAL DIAGNOSIS. The differential diagnosis of Behçet's disease includes systemic lupus erythematous, inflammatory bowel disease, Reiter's syndrome, herpetic infections, Mollaret's meningitis, sarcoidosis, Vogt-Kayanagi's syndrome, herpes-virus meningoencephalitis, confusional states, and small strokes.

DIAGNOSIS. The diagnosis of Behçet's disease depends on the recognition of the clinical manifestations of the disease previously described. These may not appear all at the same time. Laboratory tests are not helpful: complete blood counts and blood chemical analysis are within normal limits. The erythrocyte sedimentation rate and the plasma globulins are both generally elevated. The common histopathologic lesion of all of the clinical manifestations is a vasculitis characterized by perivascular infiltrates with mononuclear cells, resembling the lesion seen in a delayed hypersensitivity reaction to an intradermal antigen.

TREATMENT. The therapy of Behçet's disease is unsatisfactory and difficult to evaluate, in part because of the unpredictability of the natural course of the illness. Some investigators begin therapy with oral prednisone, 50 mg daily. This drug is then tapered over several days to a maintenance dose between 5 and 20 mg. Other investigators would add cytotoxic agents such as azathioprine to the prednisone. No controlled studies are available that identify the ideal medical therapy.

REFERENCES

1. Fitzpatrick TB, Eisen AZ, Wolff K, et al: (eds): Dermatology in General Medicine. 2nd Ed. McGraw-Hill, New York, 1979
2. Burket JM: Dark plaques in nether regions. A sign of carcinoma in situ. JAMA 230:439, 1974
3. Lupulescu A, Mehregan AH, Rahhari H, et al: Venereal warts vs Bowen disease. A histologic and ultrastructural study of five cases. JAMA 237;2520, 1977
4. Chapel TC, Rahbari H: Genital bowenoid papulosis-squamous cell carcinoma in situ. Sex Transm Dis 7:139, 1980
5. Akerman AB, Kornberg R: Pearly penile papules. Acral angiofibromas. Arch Dermatol 108:673, 1973
6. Fiumara NJ: Nonvenereal sclerosing lymphangitis of the penis. Arch Dermatol 111:902, 1975
7. Hutchens P, Dunlop EMC, Rodin P: Benign transient lymphangiectasis (sclerosing lymphangitis) of the penis. Br J Vener Dis 53:379, 1977
8. McMillan A: Lymphocoele and localized lymphoedema of the penis. Br J Vener Dis 52:409, 1976
9. Stolz E, van Kampen WJ, Vuzevski V: Sklerosierende Lymphangitis des Penis, der Oberlippe und des Labium minus. Hautarzt 25:231, 1974
10. Malloy TR, Wein AJ, Gross P: Scrotal and penile lymphoedema: Surgical consideration and management. J Urol 130:263, 1983
11. Wilde H, Canby JP: Penile venereal edema. Arch Dermatol 108:263, 1973
12. Wright RA, Judson FN: Penile venereal edema. JAMA 241:157, 1979
13. Fiumara NJ, Yaqub M: Pigmented penile lesions (fixed drug eruptions) associated with tetracycline therapy for sexually transmitted diseases. Sex Transm Dis 8:23, 1981
14. Pasricha JS: Drugs causing fixed eruptions. Br J Dermatol 100:183, 1979
15. Moss TR, Stevenson CJ: Incidence of genital vitiligo. Report of a screening programme. Br J Vener Dis 57:145, 1981
16. Fiumara NJ: Psoriasis of the penis: Koebner reaction following oral genital exposure. J Am Vener Dis Assoc 3:59, 1976
17. Calin A: HLA-B27: To type or not to type? Ann Intern Med 92:208, 1980
18. Paronen I: Reiter's disease: A study of 344 cases observed in Finland. Acta Med Scand [Suppl] 212:1, 1948
19. Chajek T, Fainaru M: Behçet's disease: A report of forty-one cases and a review of the literature. Medicine 54:179, 1975
20. Lehner R, Barnes CG (eds): Behçet's syndrome: Clinical and immunological features. Academic Press, London, 1979

15

Homosexuality and Sexually Transmitted Diseases

David G. Ostrow

HOMOSEXUALITIES AND HOMOSEXUAL BEHAVIOR

The inclusion of a chapter on homosexuality in a book on sexually transmitted diseases (STDs) reflects the growing awareness that specific sexual behaviors contribute to the incidence of sexually transmitted diseases. Further, there is a growing body of information implicating specific sexual practices common among homosexual males in the emergence of "new" STDs. Along with information regarding the enteric infections such as hepatitis B, shigellosis, and *Entamoeba histolytica,* this chapter will review those aspects of homosexual behavior that are relevant to the general practice of medicine and STD diagnosis and treatment. In addition, we will include information useful to the primary care provider in his or her work with homosexual patients. Throughout this chapter, the emphasis is on the gay male patient, since it is with this patient that specific sexual practices are most clearly related to the incidence and treatment of STDs. There is little if any evidence linking lesbian sexual practices to specific aspects of STDs.[1]

The prevalence of homosexuality in modern Western civilizations has been variously estimated to be anywhere from 2 to 10% of the adult male population. However, we must be careful to differentiate between the prevalence of homosexuality as a pattern of exclusive or near-exclusive choice of same-gender partners for sexual activities and the practice of specific homosexual acts. In their landmark study, Kinsey, Pomeroy, and Martin[2] defined a spectrum of adult sexual gender preference ranging from exclusive heterosexuality to exclusive homosexuality. Those same studies revealed that the occurrence of same-sex activities at some time in an individual's lifetime were the rule rather than the exception, and that a significant portion of the adult heterosexual male population continued to have occasional homosexual activities.

These findings are of major importance to any discussion of homosexual behavior and its relationship to infectious or traumatic illness. It is not sufficient for the physician to determine the predominant gender preference, homosexual or heterosexual, of a patient. Rather, the physician must be aware of the full range of specific sexual practices and their relative frequencies for that patient. Many physicians may find it difficult to inquire about some specific sexual practices, and thus are content with a patient's verbal or nonverbal acquiescence to a statement such as "you don't do any of *that* stuff!" Such an approach to sexual practice history-taking will result in incomplete and potentially dangerous omissions in the examination and workup of a significant number of patients. If we assume that at least 5 to 10% of patients are either primarily homosexual in orientation or occasionally participate in same-gender sexual relations, then we are dealing with a relatively important segment of the patient population. In many large urban centers and clinics specializing in the treatment of sexually transmitted diseases the percentage may be considerably higher. Therefore, it is important that all physicians and allied primary health care professionals be aware of the specific sexual practices and their risks to the homosexual male patient. If the practitioner cannot bring himself or herself to inquire adequately into these aspects of a patient's history, then that practitioner should not hesitate to refer any patient with real or suspected STD problems to a colleague or service organization competent to handle such patients in a nonjudgmental fashion.

Several recent population-based surveys have attempted to define patterns of male homosexual behavior in ways that are more valid than the stereotyped versions of homosexual behavior used so visibly in our culture. In a recently published study entitled *Homosexualities: A Study of Diversity Among Men and Women,* Kinsey Institute researchers Alan P. Bell and Martin S. Weinberg[3] attempt to update the Kinsey scales in a manner which takes into account the various aspects of behavior, both sexual and nonsexual, that define an individual's lifestyle in relation to gender preference.

Acknowledging that no single behavioral parameter can adequately be used to describe groups or typologies, the authors describe the "homosexualities" according to a number of criteria, including the level of sexual activity, the stability and types of coupling, the degree of functional and physical problems encountered in sexual activities, and the individual's acceptance of his or her homosexuality. Applying cluster analysis to the large number of respondents interviewed in the San Francisco area, Bell and Weinberg arrived at five general clusters of male homosexual behavior:

I. *Close-coupled.* Men living in a stable monogamous relationship with a sexual partner. Their standard scores on number of sexual problems, number of sexual partners, and amount of cruising were low. We would expect close-coupled individuals to have few, if any, sexually transmitted infections.

II. *Open-coupled.* Men involved in a "marital" relationship with another man but still having a variety of sexual contacts. Such individuals would be expected to be exposed to a variety of sexually transmitted infections depending on their frequency and type of sexual contacts.

III. *Functional.* Men who are "single" and have high numbers of sexual partners and level of sexual activity. Members of this group would be expected to have the highest rate and extent of sexually transmitted disease problems.

IV. *Dysfunctional.* Men who are "single" and sexually active, but have high scores on number of sexual problems and regret over their homosexuality (12% of respondents). Depending on their actual level and types of sexual activity, such individuals may range widely in their actual STD exposure.

V. *Asexual.* Men who are neither coupled nor reporting multiple numbers of partners or amount of cruising. While at very low risk for sexually transmitted diseases, such individuals may actually be frequent seekers of consultation for real or imagined STD problems.

Whatever the limitations of descriptive clusters based on a selected population of respondents, the classification of homosexual males based on general characteristics of sexual and psychologic functioning can be utilized in delineating general levels of risk for sexually transmitted diseases and in designing education and control measures aimed at reducing the incidence of STDs in the gay male population.

One of the most important areas of physician activity in controlling the epidemic of STDs and AIDS in the homosexual population is, in fact, education and counseling of patients. It is the physician's responsibility to counsel patients at risk for the STDs on ways in which they can reduce that risk. Such educational information can be given to patients in a positive, nonjudgmental, and noncoercive manner. At the very least, sexually active patients with multiple partners need to be counseled on the importance of periodic STD checkups, the value of self-examinations for lesions and discharges, and the importance of sexual abstinence during the symptomatic or treatment period in order to prevent spread or reinfection. Again, the recognition that AIDS is a sexually transmitted disease, with the risk of acquiring it strongly associated with the number of different sexual partners, makes counseling patients regarding the risks involved in multiple sexual contacts extremely important.

While the 1960s and 1970s saw the repeal of many state laws against "sodomy" and the passage of "gay rights bills" in several states and communities, there continue to be both real and imagined risks to admitting openly to a homosexual preference. The existence of legal and cultural biases against homosexual persons results in a distortion of the doctor-patient relationship from one of open communication to one of subtle denial. While this chapter makes the point that a complete sexual practices history is an essential and necessary part of the workup of any patient presenting with a real or potential STD, some patients will inevitably view such questioning as unnecessarily intrusive or even insulting. In large part, this will depend on both the patient's and practitioner's own comfort in dealing with sexuality and, in particular, homosexuality. Most medical texts either omit discussion of homosexuality and homosexual behavior altogether or refer to the subject under the category of "sexual dysfunction," "deviancy," or "perversions." Likewise, medical professionals are no more comfortable with the subject of sexuality than are members of the general population, and homosexual patients will often assume that the physician or health care worker is negatively biased against homosexuality. This distortion of the doctor-patient relationship results in the withholding of important information regarding sexual practices and experiences which are necessary to a complete and accurate diagnostic workup or treatment plan. More serious is the fact that medical problems are sometimes not brought to the attention of the health care system for fear that the nature of the problem will reveal the individual's sexual orientation and/or adversely affect future medical treatment.

These impediments to treatment are magnified for the young individual who has not yet "come out," especially if he is a minor or still in the care of a pediatrician or family physician. Individuals may assume that revealing their sexual orientation to their physician will result in their parents' discovering their homosexuality. Such patients frequently present at Board of Health STD clinics, gay community clinics, or hospital emergency rooms, precisely because of the relative anonymity such services provide. However, at least in the case of emergency room visits, this is an inappropriate use of a service and can lead to inadequate follow-up. In addition, minors will often assume that any medical service will automatically report the visit to their parents, and thus will delay seeking diagnosis and treatment of STD problems. Many patients split their medical care between a private physician and gay community clinics, oftentimes arbitrarily deciding which problems are sexually related and thus require witholding from their private physician.

There are no simple solutions to the above problems, just as there are no simple solutions to the attitudes and myths about homosexuality that underlie homophobia. Some states and communities have passed ordinances and regulations allowing health care providers to treat minors for STDs without having to report to the patient's parents or obtain their consent. However, the existence of such laws and ordinances does not automatically ensure sufficient trust in the doctor-patient relationship and the health care institutions to produce an open and truthful relationship with the health care provider. Ironically, in order to protect their patient's anonymity, many private physicians customarily do not report a patient's STD results to the local board of health. This has resulted in a massive underreporting of STD information and has hindered the development of adequate diagnostic and treatment regimens.[4] In order to provide confidential and dignified STD diagnostic and treatment services to the gay community, community-sponsored STD clinics have been formed. Such clinics have developed systems of reporting STD incidence statistics to the local Department of Health, and from there to the Centers for Disease Control, that ensure confidentiality, utilizing clinic visit numbers rather than names. These systems have enabled gay community clinics to establish a level of trust and truthfulness with their patients that optimizes STD services for gay patients.

THE SEXUAL PRACTICES HISTORY

The preceding discussion has emphasized the need for a complete sexual practices history for all patients presenting with a real or potential STD. In fact, until it has been established that an individual is either celibate or obtaining STD services elsewhere, all patients require sexual practice history information as part of their overall evaluation process.

The most difficult part of taking a sexual practice history is introducing the subject in the course of a general medical history in a way which will produce the most open and truthful response from the patient. Obviously, the attitude of the health care provider will affect the ability to establish such a setting. By leaving the sexual practices history to the very end of the history-taking process in the hope that the patient will bring up the subject or that it can be totally avoided, the physician will signal to the patient the practitioner's own discomfort with the subject and thus limit the results of any subsequent questioning. Likewise, close-ended questions or comments such as "You don't do any of *that* stuff?!" or "I assume that you are only having sex with your wife?" will severely limit the accuracy of sexual practice information. From personal experience, it appears much better to approach the sexual practice history in the context of the overall social history. Thus, you can begin with a statement to the effect that "in order to provide you with optimal care, there are a number of areas of your personal habits and practices which I need to understand and be aware of. These include the use of any nonprescription drugs, alcohol use, special diets, sexual practices, and foreign travel." Such an introductory statement alerts your patient to your interest in their sexual practices, but places that concern within the overall context of an open and honest doctor-patient relationship.

Table 15-1. Specific Sexual Practices and Possible Associated Disease Problems

Sexual Practice (Street terms)	Disease Problem (Listed in approximate order of frequency)
Close body contact	Pediculosis pubis Scabies Fungal infections
Masturbation (jacking off, beating off)	Physical abrasions Conjunctivitis
Douches, lubricants	Allergic reactions Rectal fatty tumors
Amyl nitrite, butyl nitrite ("poppers")	Amyl and butyl nitrite burns Contact dermatitis AIDS
Fellatio active (Do you suck your partner's penis?)	Physical abrasions Oral gonorrhea Oral herpes simplex virus (especially type 2) Nongonococcal pharyngitis (chlamydia and others) Oral condyloma acuminatum Syphilis Hepatitis B Enteric infections Lymphogranuloma venereum (LGV) Oral donovanosis (granuloma inguinale) Oral chancroid
Fellatio passive (Does your partner suck your penis?)	Physical abrasions Bites Genital herpes simples (especially type 1) Nongonococcal urethritis (?) Gonococcal urethritis Meningococcal urethritis
Anal intercourse active (Do you put your penis into your partner's rectum?)	Nongonococcal urethritis Gonococcal urethritis Genital herpes Molluscum contagiosum Condyloma acuminata Syphilis Trichomoniasis Epididymitis/prostatitis Fungal infections Lymphogranuloma venereum Donovanosis (granuloma inguinale)

Table 15-1. (*continued*)

Sexual Practice (Street terms)	Disease Problem (Listed in approximate order of frequency)
Anal intercourse active (Do you put your penis into your partner's rectum?)	Chancroid Cytomegalovirus (?) Hepatitis B
Anal intercourse passive (Does your partner put his penis into your rectum?)	Traumatic proctitis Rectal gonorrhea Anal condyloma acuminata Molluscum contagiousium (rare) Nonspecific proctitis (chlamydia and others) Anorectal herpes Anorectal syphilis Hepatitis B Rectal trichomoniasis (?) Lymphogranuloma venereum Anorectal granuloma inguinale Anorectal chancroid Cytomegalovirus infection Anorectal candidiasis AIDS
Anilinction active	Enteric infections shigellosis *Campylobacter fetus* Enterotoxigenic *Escherichia coli* AIDS
Scat (Do you rim or do scat?)	Hepatitis A, B(?), non-A/non-B Amebiasis Giardiasis Salmonellosis *Enterobius vermicularis* *Strongyloides stercoralis* Oral infections Oral warts Oral gonorrhea Syphilis Lymphogranuloma venereum Oral donovanosis Oral chancroid Oral herpes simplex AIDS
Anilinction passive (Do you get rimmed?)	Rectal herpes simplex (especially type 1) Syphilis Anorectal meningococcal infection (?)

(*Continues.*)

Table 15-1. (*continued*)

Sexual Practice (Street terms)	Disease Problem (Listed in approximate order of frequency)
Fist/finger fornication passive (Have you been fist-fucked?)	Internal scrapes Anal sphincter tears Perforations of the colon Acute abdomen AIDS
Fist/finger fornication active (Do you fist-fuck?)	Enteric infections
Toys/apparatus (cock rings, dildoes, leather, tit clamps, etc.)	Allergic reactions—metal plastic, rubber, leather Friction dermatitis Physical torsions Varicocoeles Peyronie's disease Fungal infections Lost rectal foreign bodies Testicular strangulation
S & M, piercing, bondage (Are you into S & M, piercing, or bondage?)	Lacerations Cutaneous infections Trauma
Group sex	See Anilinction, active and passive

Modified from Ostrow DG, Sandholzer TA, Felman Y (eds.): Sexually Transmitted Diseases in Homosexual Men: Diagnosis, Treatment, and Research. Plenum, New York, 1983, with permission.

The reader is referred to several sources for complete listings of the various sexual practices which need to be covered in a sexual practices questionnaire.[5–7] As stressed above, it is usually necessary to inquire about specific practices as well as the broad categories of homosexual/heterosexual orientation because of the large overlap in specific sexual practices in persons admitting to one or the other orientations. Asking "Do you have sex only with men, only with women, or with both?" will establish the presence or absence of same-sex activity. Questions regarding specific sexual practices with same and/or opposite sex partners should follow. Table 15-1 lists each of the specific male homosexual practices and specific infections or traumatic problems which may be associated with each prac-

tice. The list is not exhaustive, nor has a specific causal relationship between each practice and the pathologic conditions listed been firmly established in all cases. Because patients will frequently use the vernacular terms and be unfamiliar with medical terminology, the lay term(s) for each practice is included in parentheses.

INTERRELATIONSHIP BETWEEN SEXUAL BEHAVIOR AND SEXUALLY TRANSMITTED DISEASE TRANSMISSION/PRESENTATION IN HOMOSEXUAL MALES

It should be obvious from the information in Table 15-1 that certain sexual practices have greater associated STD risks than others. For each specific sexual practice listed, the number and type of partners (i.e., anonymous or known) and the setting in which the practice occurred, will significantly affect the actual risk associated with that practice. For example, the risk of acquiring amebiasis from fecal-oral contact, as in anilingus, depends on whether the sexual partner is infected, and, if so, on the frequency and extent of contact, stage of infection, personal hygiene, and so on. Perhaps the most complete analysis of these interrelated risk factors for STDs in homosexual men is the information obtained in the Centers for Disease Control-sponsored study of risk factors for hepatitis B transmission performed at five locations during the period of 1978–1980.[8] That study established the number of years of homosexual activity and the number of different nonsteady sexual partners during the last four months as the two most important risk factors for retrospective prevalence of seropositivity for hepatitis B. When viewed from a prospective incidence perspective, specific sexual practices were found to add independently to the overall risk of acquiring hepatitis B. These were, in order of relative importance:

1. Receptive ("passive") anal-genital intercourse.

2. "Active" oral-anal intercourse (anilingus).

3. Insertive ("active") anal-genital intercourse.

4. Rectal douching in association with receptive anal-genital intercourse.

5. Receptive manual-anal intercourse ("passive" partner in anal insertion of finger or fist).

These observations were extended to the other STDs frequently seen in homosexual men (syphilis, hepatitis B, and gonorrhea) in a study recently performed at three screening sites in Chicago's gay male community.[9] These sites were the Howard Brown Memorial Clinic, a mobile testing van that visited gay bars, and a gay bathhouse STD testing station. The populations sampled at the three sites were quite similar in terms of age, race, and education. The mean number of nonsteady homosexual partners in the last 4 months was quite different among the three groups, with the bathhouse group being higher than the clinic group, and the van group being lowest. This same relative ordering (baths, highest; van, lowest) was observed for *prevalence* rates for the three STDs, as measured by the patient's report of past history and serology results for syphilis and hepatitis B. Differences between gonorrhea *prevalence* rates at the three testing stations were not statistically significant because of the low number of positive cultures. Table 15-2 shows the relationship between two sex practice variables: number of nonsteady partners and number of years homosexually active and each STD. Combining patients from all three screening sites showed that those with a positive serology or those reporting a past history of one of the STDs had significantly higher mean number of partners than those with nonreactive serologic tests or no history of an STD. As expected, past history of one STD (particularly hepatitis B) was correlated with past history or positive serology for the other two STDs.

Several conclusions can be drawn from these studies. First, it appears that number of nonsteady sexual partners is the most important risk factor for any of the major STDs seen in gay men. As bathhouse patrons have the greatest opportunity for mul-

Table 15-2. Number of Partners and Years of Homosexual Activity as Predictors of Sexually Transmitted Disease History and Serology

| | Survey Item | | | | | |
| | Mean No. Partners[a] | | | Mean No. Years Activity[b] | | |
Presence of	No	Yes	t	No	Yes	t
Past hepatitis	17.4	22.7	3.1[c]	10.8	12.6	2.4[c]
Past syphilis	17.2	24.6	3.7[d]	10.4	14.9	5.3[d]
Past oral gonorrhea	18.3	24.4	2.2[e]	7.5	10.3	NS
Past urethral gonorrhea	17.5	20.7	NS	10.5	12.8	5.9[d]
Past rectal gonorrhea	16.5	26.4	5.0[d]	8.6	10.5	NS
Hepatitis B seropositive[f]	14.6	22.5	4.7[d]	8.7	12.8	5.9[d]
VDRL reactive	18.6	26.8	1.8[e]	10.8	16.0	3.0[d]

[a] Defined as number of nonsteady same sex partners patient has had contact with during prior four-month period.

[b] Defined as number of years patient had been homosexually active on a regular basis (at least one contact per month).

[c] $p < .01$.

[d] $p < .001$.

[e] $p < .05$.

[f] Defined as HB_sAg and/or anti-HB_s and/or anti-HB_c.

tiple anonymous partners and did, in fact, have significantly higher numbers of partners than respondents questioned at either the clinic or van,[9] it follows that bathhouse patrons are an especially high-risk group for STD infection. Accordingly, screening and education programs should be targeted to this group as well as to patients discovered to currently have one or more STDs. Second, it appears that specific sexual practices such as anal-genital intercourse and anilingus can provide introduction into the STD catalogue of a large number of enteric pathogens, including hepatitis B, *Giardia lamblia, Entamoeba histolytica,* and shigellosis.

UNIQUE ASPECTS OF SEXUALLY TRANSMITTED DISEASES IN HOMOSEXUAL MALES

Aspects of STDs that are unique or particularly relevant to the gay patient have been the subject of several recent excellent review articles[9–11] and an entire monograph.[7] In order to illustrate some of the special considerations necessary during the workup of a homosexual patient, some of the more important or interesting examples of STDs in gay men are listed below.

Syphilis

Because primary chancres are often painless, syphilis of the rectum can easily be overlooked. It is perhaps fortunate for homosexual men that rectal chancres are frequently painful or cause symptoms such as bloody diarrhea, constipation, dyschezia, tenesmus, or bleeding. The more developed primary lesions or condylomata may often be confused with nonspecific fissures, polyps, herpetic lesions, or anal warts. The tendency of some homosexual men to have anonymous sexual partners severely limits the usefulness of traditional syphilis epi-

demiology work with this subpopulation. We have found that aggressive outreach into such areas as bathhouse STD testing and mobile "VD vans" can lead to the identification of a significant number of cases of syphilis while, at the same time, helping to educate persons at high risk of STDs and AIDS to the need for regular STD testing.

Gonorrhea

Special aspects of gonococcal infection in gay men relate to the practice of orogenital and anogenital intercourse and the resulting high rates of oral and anal infection, in addition to urethral gonorrhea. Both the overall high incidence of gonococcal infection in the homosexual male population and the possibility for multiple sites of infection make the risk of infection substantially greater than in the heterosexual patient. The problem is compounded by the fact that both anal and pharyngeal gonococcal infections are frequently asymptomatic.[12] The diagnosis of gonococcal infection in these two sites is further complicated by the high rate of colonization with meningococci, which are difficult to differentiate from the gonococcus with routine laboratory procedures.[13] Thus, diagnostic laboratories receiving specimens from oral or anal sites should use sugar utilization or immunologic tests to identify *Neisseria* recovered from these sites on selective medium. The value of Gram stain of material obtained from anoscopic examination of symptomatic patients is somewhat controversial. This technique, when restricted to symptomatic patients and material obtained directly under anoscopic visualization, yields correct diagnosis in a significant number of cases of rectal gonorrhea and allows for immediate treatment without having to wait for the culture result.[9,14,15]

The high prevalence of asymptomatic pharyngeal infection in homosexual men[13,14] suggests that there could be significant risk of disseminated gonococcal infection (DGI) in this population. However, there have been very few reports of DGI in homosexual patients. This may reflect differences in the virulence of strains of *Neisseria gonorrhoeae* isolated from gay men when compared to isolates from heterosexuals, in whom DGI is more common.[16]

Nongonococcal Urethritis

Several studies have confirmed the relatively low rate of nongonococcal urethritis (NGU) in homosexual men as compared to heterosexual men.[17,18] Bowie and colleagues[19] have further shown that, while approximately 40% of heterosexual men with NGU have *Chlamydia trachomatis* infection, only 10 to 20% of homosexual men with NGU have *C. trachomatis* infection.[19] *C. trachomatis* is also a major cause of postgonococcal urethritis in heterosexual men but not in homosexual men. The etiology of NGU and postgonococcal infection in gay men is unknown at the present time.[18]

Intestinal Parasites

During the past several years, a number of studies have confirmed an extremely high rate of enteric protozoal infection in gay men living in New York City,[20–22] San Francisco,[23] and Cleveland.[24] Particularly the New York studies of William and collaborators[20,21] have linked amebiasis and giardiasis in homosexual men to the practice of anilingus, consistent with the well-known fecal-oral route of transmission of these infections. What is most important in the context of this review is that an infectious etiology of acute or chronic gastrointestinal symptoms must be considered in all patients practicing anilingus or other sexual practices in which fecal-oral contact is possible. The situation is further complicated in that a large proportion of protozoal carriers will be asymptomatic or only intermittently ill. A recent report has implicated fecal-contaminated objects, such as enema apparatuses and examination instruments, in the direct anal-anal transmission of giardiasis.[25] This suggests that fomite-transmitted protozoal infection could take place in bathhouse and other group-sex situations. The workup of homosexually active male patients with bowel symptoms is outlined in Figure 15-1.[7] This rather elaborate scheme is made necessary by the relatively low sensitivity of existing diagnostic tests. While more sensitive serologic and stool antigen tests for *Entamoeba histolytica* are being developed, their relatively low specificity limits their current usefulness. In addition, some investigators have argued that even asymptomatic gay men may harbor parasitic infections and that these chronic infections may contribute to the reduced immunocompetency leading to the development of AIDS. This would argue for empiric treatment for amoebic infection in persons with negative stool examinations but suffering from chronic lymphadenopathy, reduced cellular immune function, or other prodromal symptoms. These same workers are also questioning the distinction between "pathogenic" and "nonpathogenic" parasites, again arguing for aggressive amoebicidal therapy in any gay male with parasites present on examination. The treatment schedules for *E. histolytica* and *Giardia lamblia* are given in Table 15-3.

Shigellosis and Salmonellosis

According to a recent review by William,[7] shigellosis is the most common cause of bacterial dysentery in homosexually active men. The prevalence of sexually transmitted salmonellosis in this population is unknown. Since *Shigella*, unlike salmonella, have no intermediate host outside of man, transmission is usually person-to-person via the fecal-oral route. *Shigella* are

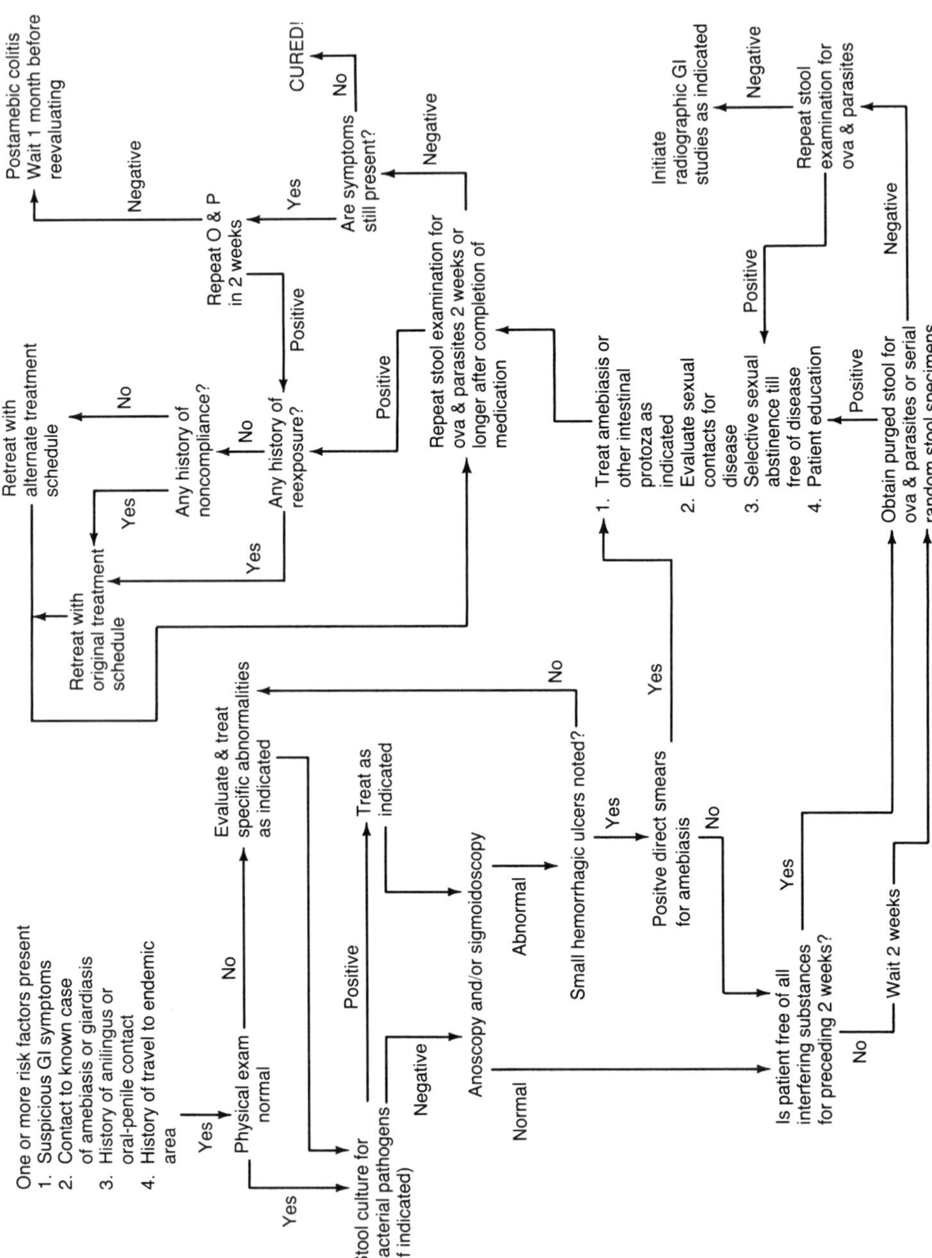

Fig. 15-1 Flowchart for the diagnosis and treatment of suspected amebiasis. (From Williams DC: Amebiasis. In Ostrow DG, Sandkolzer TAS, Felman, YM (eds): Sexually Transmitted Diseases in Homosexual Men: Diagnosis, Treatment, and Research. Plenum, New York, 1983)

Table 15-3.   Treatment Schedules for Enteric Infections

Amebiasis
  For asymptomatic cyst carrier.
    Diiodohydroxyquin, 650 mg PO tid for 20 days   *or*
    Metronidazole (Flagyl), 750 mg PO tid for 5 to 10 days   *or*
    Diloxanide furoate (Furamide), 400 mg PO tid for 10 days
  For patients with mild to moderate intestinal disease
    Diiodohydroxyquin, 650 mg PO tid for 20 days *plus* paromomycin sulfate (Humatin), 25 to 30 mg/kg in three doses per day for 5 to 10 days   *or*
    Diiodohydroxyquin, 650 mg PO tid for 20 days *plus* metronidazole (Flagyl), 750 mg PO tid for 5 to 10 days
  For patients with recurrent or resistent disease, a third drug may be added to the above regimen
    Erythromycin   *or*
    Tetracycline   *or*
    Carbazone   *or*
    Chloroquine

Giardiasis
    Quinacrine hydrochloride (Atabrine), 100 mg PO tid for 5 to 10 days   *or*
    Metronidazole (Flagyl), 250 mg PO tid for 10 days *or*
    Furazolidone (Furoxone), 100 mg PO qid for 7 days

Shigellosis
    Sulfamethoxazole-trimethoprim (Bactrim or Septra), 800 mg: 160 mg PO bid for 5 days   *or*
    Ampicillin, 500 mg PO every 6 hours for 5 days

highly infectious, requiring an inoculum of less than 200 bacteria to cause clinical disease. The treatment of shigellosis is given in Table 15-3. It is not recommended to treat salmonellosis, as this disease is usually self-limited and antibiotic or antidiarrhial therapy may prolong the carrier state.

Hepatitis

There has been a virtual explosion of information regarding sexually transmitted hepatitis since the recognition of high rates of both hepatitis A[26] and B in gay men. Detailed discussion of hepatitis infections in gay men is the subject of Chapter 8 of Ostrow, Sandholzer, and Felman's textbook on STDs in gay men.[7] One of the positive aspects of this discovery has been the abil-

ity to rapidly test the recently developed hepatitis B vaccine for safety and efficacy in gay men.[27,28] Despite this enormous breakthrough in disease prevention, the vaccine's application to prevent the venereal spread of hepatitis B has been very limited. This is the result of several factors, including the relative high cost of the vaccine (approximately $100 per series of three injections) and the time required (six months) for complete vaccination. However, one additional factor that has limited the use of the vaccine has been the irrational fear among physicians and some sectors of the public that the Heptavax B[r] is contaminated with an AIDS-producing agent. Recent review of safety data involving both early developmental lots of the vaccine and the currently available commercial lots has unequivocally demonstrated the safety of the vaccine.[29] Not one single case of AIDS has occurred in vaccine recipients who are not members of one of the groups at high risk for development of AIDS. And the actual number of AIDS cases among gay vaccine recipients in New York City was lower than that of matched control groups who did not receive the vaccine.

Given the slow rate of acceptance of the hepatitis B vaccine by the medical profession and the public, we can expect both acute and chronic hepatitis B infections to continue to be quite common as sexually transmitted diseases. Figure 15-2 outlines the diagnostic procedures useful in the workup of a patient with acute hepatitis infection. Since treatment is only supportive, the main purpose of determining the etiology of acute hepatitis is for counseling of the patient and his sexual contacts. With the increasing availability of rapid and inexpensive tests to determine preexisting immunity to both hepatitis A and B, it is usually possible to test sexual contacts of acute cases before prescribing prophylactic immune globulin injections.

We have been especially interested in determining the long-term sequelae of hepa-

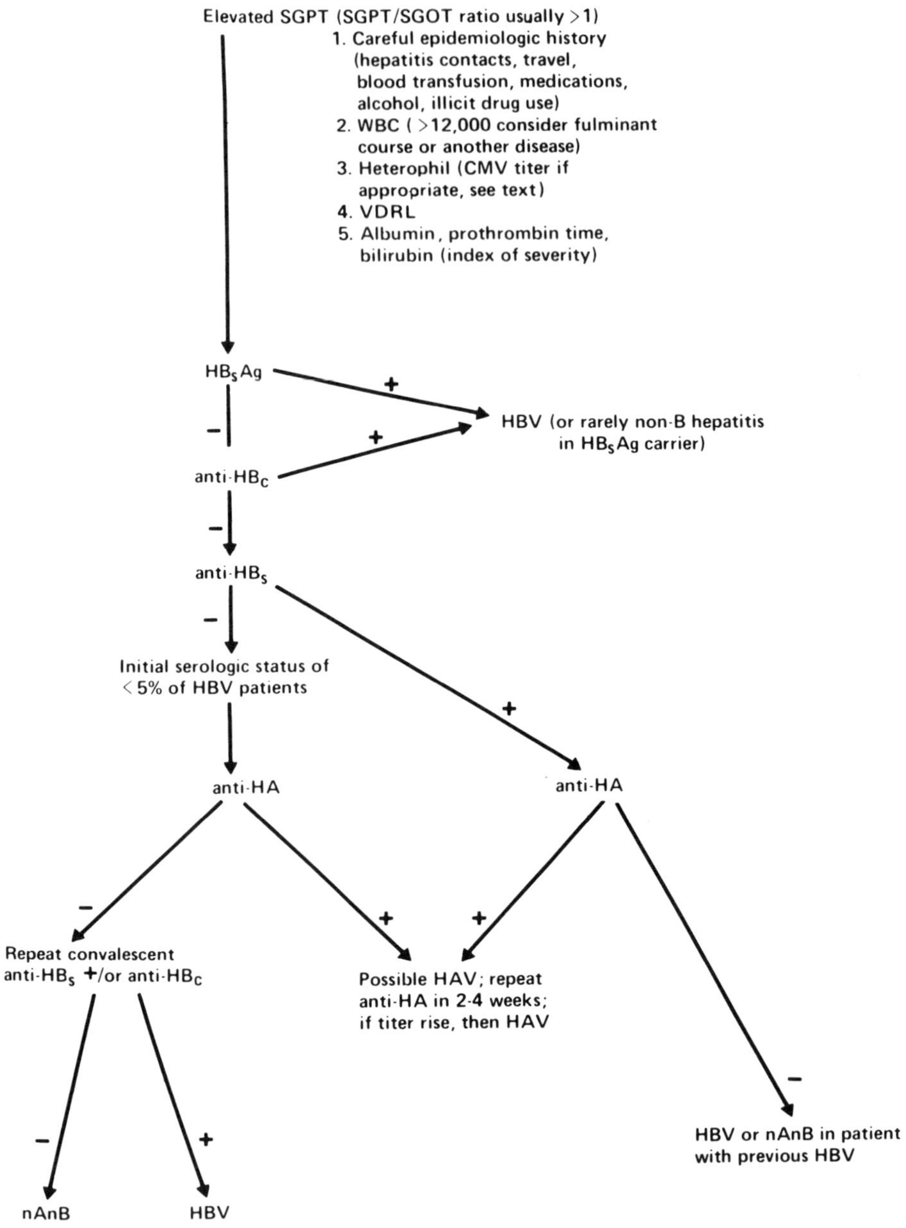

Fig. 15-2 Laboratory evaluation of acute hepatitis. (From Ostrow DG, Gayle TC: Viral hepatitis. In Ostrow DG, Sandholzer TAS, Felman YM (eds): Sexually Transmitted Diseases in Homosexual Men: Diagnosis, Treatment, and Research, Plenum, New York, 1983)

titis B infection. Approximately 10% of acute infections were observed to go on to chronic hepatitis infections in our series of 866 cases.[30] The chronic infections appear to be evenly divided between asymptomatic "carriers" and persons with clinical or laboratory evidence of chronic viral replication. The overall outcomes of acute hepatitis B infections in gay men are illustrated in Figure 15-3.

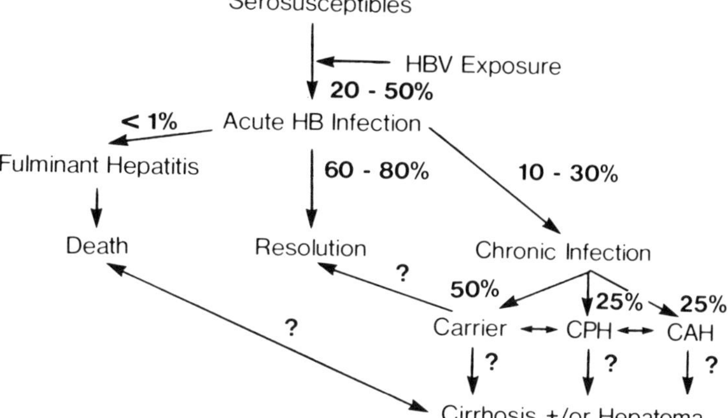

Fig. 15-3 Sequelae of hepatitis B exposure in homosexual men. CPH = chronic persistent hepatitis B; CAH = chronic active hepatitis B.

Obviously, prophylactic immunization of all sexually active gay men is the only currently available effective means for decreasing the significant acute and chronic sequelae of this major STD problem. Approximately 90% of gay men vaccinated with three 20-µg doses of the Heptavax B (Merck) will develop protective surface antibody levels.[27,28] Of the remaining group of initial vaccine "nonresponders," approximately half will respond to a second set of immunizations.[31] The immunologic findings in the remaining group of gay men, comprising between 2 and 5% of the total population studied by us, are suggestive of a mild form of acquired immune deficiency state.[31] This finding suggests that there is a preexisting state of immune deficiency that predates the appearance of opportunistic infection or Kaposi's sarcoma in gay men.

ACQUIRED IMMUNODEFICIENCY SYNDROME, KAPOSI'S SARCOMA, AND PNEUMOCYSTIS PNEUMONIA

In July of 1981, the Centers for Disease Control published reports[32] concerning an outbreak of Kaposi's sarcoma in gay men. These reports were quickly followed by reports of outbreaks of *Pneumocystis carinii* pneumonia among gay men in Los Angeles, New York City, and San Francisco. It has since been established that a profound state of cellular immune suppression underlies both these unusual conditions appearing in homosexual male populations, giving rise to the term "acquired immune deficiency syndrome" or "AIDS."

In the few years since the initial recognition of AIDS, approximately 20,000 cases of this usually fatal disease have been identified throughout the United States. In addition to homosexual men, who comprise approximately two thirds of total AIDS cases, intravenous drug users, Haitian entrants, and hemophiliacs receiving pooled plasma clotting factor concentrates have been identified as being at increased risk for AIDS. This syndrome is described in detail in Chapter 8 of this monograph.

The discovery of the AIDS virus and its widespread appearance as a sexually transmitted or related disease condition denote an event of immense significance in the history of venereal disease. Large-scale prospective epidemiologic investigations are now underway in a number of United States cities in order to define the natural history and mode(s) of transmission of AIDS. In addition, extensive investigations into the immunosuppressive properties of a variety of sexually transmitted disease pathogens, such as cytomegalovirus, herpes simplex, and hepatitis B, and retroviruses such as

Table 15-4. Guidelines for the Prevention of AIDS and Other Sexually Transmitted Diseases in Gay Men

1. Reduce the number of different sexual partners.
2. Know the health status of your partners and exchange information so that you can contact each other in case of a subsequent health problem.
3. Refrain from any sexual contact if you are suffering from a viral infection or have unexplained symptoms of an infection, such as swollen lymph nodes, diarrhea, or respiratory symptoms.
4. Modification of sexual practices to avoid the exchange of any bodily materials, such as semen, saliva, urine, feces, or blood, will reduce the chances of transmission of viruses during intercourse. The use of condoms during rectal intercourse has been advocated, but their effectiveness in preventing the transmission of AIDS has not been established.
5. Seek medical attention for any symptoms which indicate the possibility of infection or decreased immune competency.

human T-cell lymphotropic virus, type III (HTLV-III) promise to greatly increase our understanding of the immune consequences of exposure to the wide spectrum of STDs seen in the homosexual population. Until a vaccine against HTLV-III is developed, preventive measures remain our only defense against even wider spread of AIDS. The current recommendations for AIDS prevention of the American Association of Physicians for Human Rights and the National Coalition of Gay STD Services are summarized in Table 15-4.

EFFECTIVE PREVENTIVE MEASURES FOR SEXUALLY TRANSMITTED DISEASES IN THE GAY MALE COMMUNITY

It should be obvious from the above discussion that the current epidemic of STDs in the gay population is the result of multiple interacting factors and circumstances operating not only at the level of the individual and the infectious agents themselves, but also the social milieu, the health care system and the society at large. For any control measures to be effective, they must address these interacting factors rather than isolated single aspects of the problem. As with any population with endemic illness, control measures embodying education and motivation of those persons at highest risk for the disease to seek preventive action have the greatest chance for major impact. Unfortunately, there is little emphasis on preventive medicine or patient education in most STD control programs, or generally in modern medicine.

Gay community-sponsored STD clinics were organized as a direct result of the growing awareness of STDs as a major health hazard among sexually active gay men. As a result, they have been notably successful in motivating patients to seek routine diagnostic and treatment services. Despite this success, STDs continue to be epidemic in the community and "new" etiologic agents or disease presentations continue to be discovered. Even more innovative programs must be designed if we are ever to motivate a large enough proportion of the homosexual community to preventive health measures.

Programs that simultaneously increase awareness of STD problems and make testing/treatment services more accessible and attractive to the young gay person may be successful, but require a coordinated effort involving the community, public and private sectors of the health care system, and educational media. An example of such a program has been the multicenter hepatitis B research program described above, which, through the vaccination of high-risk individuals, may ultimately have a significant impact on the venereal spread of hepatitis B. The retrenchment of public funding of such programs will obviously limit their immediate effects. However, a significant portion of the gay community is now motivated and involved in STD programs and there is a growing appreciation by the population-at-large of the importance of preventive health care. Ultimately, it is the motivation of the persons at risk for STDs that will have the greatest impact on controlling the significant health problems discussed in this chapter.

REFERENCES

1. Robertson P, Schacter J: Failure to identify venereal disease in a lesbian population. Sex Transm Dis 8;75, 1981
2. Kinsey AC, Pomeroy WB, Martin CE: Sexual Behavior in the Human Male. Saunders, Philadelphia, 1948
3. Bell AP, Weinberg MS: Homosexualities: A Study of Diversity Among Men and Women. Simon & Schuster, New York, 1978
4. Darrow WW: Social and psychologic aspects of the sexually transmitted diseases: A different view. Cutis 27:307, 1981
5. Group for the Advancement of Psychiatry: Assessment of Sexual Function: A guide to Interviewing. Aronson, New York, 1974
6. Owen WF Jr: The clinical approach to the homosexual patient. Ann Intern Med 93:90, 1980
7. Ostrow DG, Sandholzer TAS, Felman, YM (eds): Sexually Transmitted Diseases in Homosexual Men: Diagnosis, Treatment, and Research. Plenum, New York, 1983
8. Schreeder MT, Thompson SE, Hadler SC, et al: Epidemiology of hepatitis B in gay men. J Homosex 5:307, 1980
9. Ostrow DG, Altman NL: Sexually transmitted diseases and homosexuality. Sex Transm Dis 10:208, 1983
10. Felman YM: Homosexual hazards. Practitioner 224:1151, 1980
11. Owen WF Jr: Sexually transmitted diseases and traumatic problems in homosexual men. Ann Intern Med 92:805, 1980
12. Wiesner PJ, Tronca E, Bonin P, et al: Clinical spectrum of pharyngeal gonococcal infection. N Engl J Med 288;181, 1972
13. Janda WM, Bohnhoff M, Morello JA, et al: Prevalence and site-pathogen studies of Neisseria meningitidis and N. gonorrhoeae in homosexual men. JAMA 244:2060, 1980
14. Ostrow DG, Shaskey D, Steffen G, et al: Epidemiology of gonorrhea infections in gay men. J Homosex 5:285, 1980
15. William DC, Felman YM, Riccardi NB: The utility of anoscopy in the rapid diagnosis of symptomatic anorectal gonorrhea in men. Sex Transm Dis 8:16, 1981
16. Handsfield HH, Knapp JS, Diehr PK, et al: Correlation of auxotype and penicillin sensitivity of Neisseria gonorrhoeae with sexual preference and clinical manifestations of gonorrhea. Sex Transm Dis 7:1, 1980
17. Judson FN, Penley KA, Robinson ME, et al: Comparative prevalence rates of sexually transmitted diseases in heterosexual and homosexual men. Am J Epidemiol 112:836, 1980
18. Holmes KK: Nongonococcal urethritis: General considerations and specific considerations for homosexual men. J Homosex 5:295, 1980
19. Bowie WR, Alexander ER, Holmes KK: Etiologies of postgonococcal urethritis in homosexual and heterosexual men: Roles of Chlamydia trachomatis and Ureaplasma urealyticum. Sex Transm Dis 5:151, 1978
20. William DC, Shookhoff HB, Felman YM, et al: High rates of protozoal infections in selected homosexual men attending a VD clinic. Sex Transm Dis 5:155, 1980
21. William DC, Felman YM, Marr JS, et al: Sexually transmitted enteric pathogens in male homosexual populations. NY State J Med 77:2050, 1977
22. Schmerin MJ, Gelston A, Jones TC: Amebiasis, an increasing problem among homosexuals in New York City, JAMA 238:1386, 1977
23. Dritz SK, Ainsworth TE, Back A, et al: Patterns of sexually transmitted enteric diseases in a city. Lancet 2:3, 1977
24. Kazal HL, Sohn N, Corrasco JI, et al: The gay bowel syndrome: Clinicopathologic correlation in 260 cases. Ann Clin Lab Sci 6:184, 1976
25. Simmons R, Klein MG, Canfield T, et al: Amebiasis associated with colonic irrigation-Colorado. MMWR 30(13):101, 1981
26. Corey L, Holmes KK: Sexual transmission of hepatitis A in homosexual men. N Engl J Med 302:435, 1980
27. Szmuness W, Stevens CE, Harley EJ, et al: Hepatitis B vaccine: Demonstration of efficacy in a controlled clinical trial in a high-risk population in the United States. N Engl J Med 303:833, 1980

28. Francis DP, Hadler SC, Thompson SE, et al: The prevention of hepatitis B with vaccine: Report the CDC multi-center efficacy trial among homosexual men. Ann Intern Med 97:362, 1982

29. Stevens C: Hepatitis B and AIDS. Paper presented at the Central Society for Clinical Research Meeting, Chicago, IL, November 5, 1983

30. Shah N, Ostrow DG, Altman N, Baker AL: Evolution of acute hepatitis B in homosexual men to chronic hepatitis B. Arch Intern Med 145:881, 1985

31. Ostrow DG, Kalish SB, Phair JP, et al: Nonresponse to hepatitis B vaccine in homosexually active males. p. 33 Proceedings of the Fifth International STD Research Meeting, Seattle, WA, August, 1983

32. Centers for Disease Control: Kaposi's sarcoma and pneumocystis pneumonia among homosexual men—New York City and California. MMWR 30(25), July 3, 1981

16

Kaposi's Sarcoma— Acquired Immune Deficiency Syndrome in the Spectrum of Sexually Transmitted Diseases

Bijan Safai
Nancy Wolfin

Until recently, Kaposi's sarcoma (KS) was believed to be an uncommon multifocal cancer which occurred in endemic areas with a cluster distribution. There has been a current revival of interest in Kaposi's sarcoma with the epidemic of this cancer in association with acquired immune deficiency syndrome (AIDS). Many investigators have recently been involved in research upon various aspects of the disease, that is, clinical manifestations of the disease as well as its course and associated immunologic aspects. The following is a general review of the information that presently is known about KS.

HISTORICAL PERSPECTIVE

Moritz Kaposi, a Hungarian physician in the mid-1800s, is first credited with describing a condition in 1872 which consisted of an "idiopathic multiple pigmented sarcoma of the skin."[1] In 1891 Koebner suggested that this symptom complex be designated "Kaposi's sarcoma." Dr. Kaposi, however, preferred to refer to this disease as "sarcoma idiopathicum multiplex hemorrhagicum." He felt this terminology better described the actual tumor and the source of the pigment contained in the lesions.

Over the ensuing years, multiple reports of the entity were made throughout the world. In 1882 a five-year-old child was described with the disease. The first disseminated form of the disease was then reported by Dr. Kaposi in 1887. Smith and Elmes[2] studied a series of 500 neoplasms from Africa, of which 10 cases (2% of the series) were found to be KS. This report appeared some 20 years after the initial reported African case by Hallenberger[3] in 1914. Multiple other large series of cases were reported from Africa, prompting the meeting of the International Union Against Cancer in Uganda in 1961. A monograph of the proceedings of the conference were published by Ackerman and Murray[4] in 1962.

Over the next two decades, KS was recognized with increasing frequency among renal transplant recipients and patients requiring immunosuppressive therapy.[5–7] In 1981 multiple reports of young homosexual men with KS came from New York and California.[8] Since that time, the association of KS in the population with acquired immune deficiency syndrome has been well established.[9–12]

GEOGRAPHICAL DISTRIBUTION

KS has been noted to occur in a cluster distribution with a predilection for certain endemic areas. In Africa, the highest occurrence rates are reported from the hill and open savannah bush country at an altitude of 1200 to 1500 meters. This endemic belt primarily includes the countries of Zaire, Kenya, and Tanzania. In these areas, however, it has been noted that native blacks are affected at a far greater frequency than nonblacks. In Europe, several series have been reported from a vast diversity of locations. However, the greatest concentration of cases is found in eastern Europe, Italy, and among individuals of Jewish extraction. In North America, the ancestry of the majority of affected patients can be traced back to these same endemic areas.[13] These findings have been used by Rothman[14] to postulate a racial predisposition to the development of Kaposi's sarcoma.

Multiple cases of KS have been reported from other regions around the world, including western Europe, Armenia, India, China, and Japan. They occur, however, at a markedly lower frequency than those reported from endemic areas.

In the new epidemic form of KS/AIDS, KS is more often present in homosexual men than among intravenous drug abusers, hemophiliacs, or Haitians who have also presented with the AIDS syndrome. Other recent observations include a greater frequency of KS in New York AIDS cases, as compared to those reported from Florida, as well as a higher incidence among Caucasian patients than among black individuals.[15,16]

OCCURRENCE RATES

KS is a relatively rare tumor, except in the previously stated endemic areas. In Uganda, it has been found to account for approximately 9% of all neoplasms.[17] Its occurrence has been estimated to be 200 times greater in Africa than in the United States, where its incidence is estimated to be far less than 1%.[18] In a review of the tumors diagnosed over a 38-year period at the Mayo Clinic, Reynolds and coworkers[19] reported only 70 cases of KS, which represented merely 0.06% of all neoplasms diagnosed at that center. An even lower incidence of 0.02 per 100,000 has been put forth by Templeton,[20] and Dorn and Cutler.[21]

AGE AND SEX

In Africa, the peak incidence of the lymphadenopathic cases occur in the first decade, with rare cases reported in the second decade. There is, however, an increasing frequency of other forms of KS throughout adult life on that continent.[2,2] In the classical form of the disease occurring in non-African patients, 80% of all cases are found in the fifth to eighth decades of life. DeGiovanna and Safai[23] reported a mean age of 63 years upon analysis of 90 such cases.

A male predominance, 10–15:1, has been cited from several centers.[19,20,24,25] In a study done at Memorial Sloan-Kettering Hospital a male:female ratio of 3:1 was elucidated.[26] Of note is the reversal of this sex ratio, which has been found in cases reported among the white population in South Africa and Algeria.[27,28]

In the new epidemic form of the disease, the average age of affected patients has been found to be 39 years. The vast majority of these individuals are male, with very few cases being reported in women.[15,16]

CLINICAL PRESENTATION AND COURSE OF THE DISEASE

KS most often presents as a multifocal disease with red-purple nodules, plaques, or macules found most frequently on the lower extremities, although they might appear anywhere on the skin, mucous membranes, or gastrointestinal tract. There is also rare involvement of the lymph nodes and various internal organs. In 75% of cases, the site of initial involvement is the lower extremity, primarily the foot or the ankle.[25] In 15% of cases, the hand or forearm is the initial site of involvement. The trunk or the head and neck areas are the next most frequent primary sites of presentation, comprising 10% of cases. Other sites of initial manifestation that have been reported include the penis,[25] ear,[29] mouth,[30] eyelid,[30] conjunctiva,[31] and nose.[32] Symptoms often associated with the cutaneous disease include pruritis, pain in the lower extremities, as well as nonpitting edema.

In the new epidemic form of the disease, KS generally presents on the trunk, the head and neck area, or the upper extremities. The cutaneous lesions have been noted by many observers to be elongated and ovoid in shape. They have also been noted to follow lines of cleavage, as do the lesions of pityriasis rosea.[33,34] Characteristically, there is frequent involvement of the mucous membranes, lymph nodes, and the gastrointestinal tract. Several individuals have been reported with sole involvement of these internal areas without cutaneous manifesta-

tions of the disease.[35] Other investigators have reported lesions in the lungs, pancreas, liver, adrenal glands, spleen, testes, and larynx.[9] The systemic complaints of these patients generally consist of fatigue, weight loss, malaise, and anorexia.

KS is felt to progress from a macular and patch stage to a plaque and nodular stage. Appearance of new lesions may be noted on the trunk and upper extremities, as well as, although less frequently, on the head, neck, and internal organs.[19] The disease is felt to be multifocal in origin, therefore the occurrence of new lesions is not believed to represent metastatic disease. The occurrence of involvement of internal organs is most likely higher than clinically appreciated, with estimates ranging from 10 to 70%.[36,37] Internal sites of involvement that have been observed are the gastrointestinal tract, adrenal glands, pericardium, and liver. Brain involvement has been reported in only 4 cases.[38]

A wide diversity has been noted in the course of the disease, ranging from a slow, indolent course to a rapid and fulminant decline with metastatic dissemination. In the American series, the mean survival time has been reported to be 8 to 13 years. Of note are cases of spontaneous tumor regression, as well as survivals up to 50 years.[19,20,25,28,39–41] In the American and European cases, the ultimate cause of death in most patients with KS is usually not as a direct result of the disease. It is, rather, more often due to second primary malignancies or other diseases found with great frequency in the elderly population.[9]

In the new epidemic form of KS, a mean survival of 18 months has been postulated. This disease appears to be far more aggressive than the classical form, with rapid dissemination and a high incidence of intercurrent opportunistic infections. It is these infections which are most frequently responsible for the cause of death, rather than the fulminant spread of the KS tumor.[9,35]

A moderately aggressive form of KS has

been found in renal transplant patients. In some patients, regression of KS has been noted after discontinuation or tapering of immunosuppressive therapy.[5–7]

HISTOPATHOLOGY

The pathologic process is felt to begin in the dermis and progress upward toward the epidermis. Histopathologically, KS consists of interweaving bands of spindle cells and vascular structures which are embedded in a network of reticular and collagen fibers. The vascular component appears as delicate capillaries of cleftlike spaces between the spindle cells. A wide range of nuclear pleomorphism may be noted in the spindle cells. Other histologic characteristics of KS lesions include extravasated erythrocytes, hemosiderin-laden macrophages, as well as lymphocytic infiltration. In African KS, three different histologic patterns of KS lesions have been described based on the varying quantities of the vascular component, spindle cells, fibrosis, and nuclear pleomorphism found in individual tumors. These are (1) a mixed cellular pattern, which consists of equal proportions of spindle cells, vascular slits, and well-formed vascular channels; (2) a mononuclear pattern, which is characterized by an abundance of spindle cells, and (3) an anaplastic pattern, which demonstrates cellular pleomorphism with frequent mitoses.[42]

Little significant difference has been noted in the histologic features of KS in the classical form of the disease as compared to the new epidemic form.[34]

THE CELL OF ORIGIN

The exact origin and nature of the cell responsible for KS has not as yet been elucidated. Several theories have been postulated, with controversial results from various studies.[44–50] A reticuloendothelial cell of origin[49,50] has been supported by the increased association of KS with various lymphoreticular malignancies.[26] The theory of an endothelial cell of origin[48] is more widely accepted, secondary to the recent work of Guarda and coworkers[51] who have demonstrated that KS cells can react with antifactor VIII antibodies. It has been found that platelets and endothelial cells are responsible for the secretion of factor VIII.

It is widely believed that KS is a malignant neoplasm. This view is supported by the aggressive course of the disease as seen in African children and homosexual men with KS. However, the rare recurrence of metastases and the inability to grow KS in tissue culture of laboratory animals favors the more benign nature of the disease. It has therefore been speculated that KS is a proliferative process of endothelial cells to certain, as yet uncharacterized, stimuli.

IMMUNE STATUS

The development of KS appears to be extremely sensitive to the normal function of the immune system of the host. KS lesions have developed in patients with systemic lupus erythematosus during treatment with immunosuppressive medications,[52] as well as in patients with immune deficiencies, plasma cell dyscrasias, thymoma, polymyositis, and temporal arteritis.[7,53–57] Occasionly these lesions regress when immunosuppressive therapy is decreased or discontinued. Given these observations, in addition to the high incidence of second primary malignancies in patients with KS,[26,28] a possible association between the malfunctioning immune system and the development of KS has been suggested.

In African KS, immunologic studies have shown an improvement in the delayed hypersensitivity reaction to dinitrochlorobenzene (DNCB), as well as a decrease in autologous tumor cell killing.[59–63] The recent association of the epidemic form of KS with acquired immune dysfunction may account for the development of an aggressive, disseminated form of KS with concurrent severe, and often fatal, opportunistic infections. This observation possibly suggests a link between immune dysfunction and suppression with the pathogenesis of KS.[26]

GENETIC ASPECTS

A possible genetic predisposition to the development of KS may be inferred from the cluster distribution of the disease. However, the absence of consanguinity and infrequent occurrence of familial KS argues against simple Mendelian dominant or recessive inheritance.

The study of major histocompatibility antigens in patients with both forms of KS[35,64] have shown an increased frequency of HLA-DR5, found in approximately 60% of patients with the disease. It has also been found that HLA-BW35 antigen occurs with a greater prevalence in KS patients. In patients with AIDS who have had solely opportunistic infections, no specific increase or decrease in the frequency of HLA antigens have been demonstrated as compared to the general population. Other conditions in which HLA-DR5 has been found to be increased include scleroderma,[65] rheumatoid arthritis,[66] renal cell carcinoma,[67] and mycosis fungoides.[68]

ASSOCIATED CONDITIONS

Many reviews have been published in which KS has been associated with a variety of disease conditions. Moertel[69] reviewed 565 cases of lymphoreticular neoplasms in which KS developed in 51 patients as a second primary cancer. In contrast, of 4,475 cases of lymphoreticular tumors at the Mayo Clinic, only 2 cases of KS were subsequently observed.[70] Conversely,

the development of lymphoreticular malignancies have been observed in patients with KS.[26,71] In one review, 9 out of 63 cases of KS eventually developed lymphoreticular diseases.[72]

A study at Memorial Sloan-Kettering Cancer Center reported 34 of 92 patients with KS have had one other primary malignancy, 58% of whom developed a second primary cancer which involved the lymphoreticular system.[26] This contrasts with a general 8% incidence of all patients with one primary cancer who develop a subsequent lymphoreticular disorder. Other malignancies found in association with KS were of the gastrointestinal tract (two cases), skin (four cases), breast (two cases), and urinary tract (one case).

The association between dysfunctions of the immune system and the development of Kaposi's sarcoma has been addressed in this article. An increased occurrence of diabetes mellitus in patients with KS has been suggested. Hurlburt and Lincoln[43] analyzed 13 KS cases and found diabetes mellitus in 6 of these patients. DeGiovanna and Safai found 16 cases of diabetes mellitus in a survey of 90 cases of KS.[23] Another condition reported to be coincident with KS is anemia.[23,73–75]

CAUSAL FACTORS

The etiology of KS remains unclear. The aspect of cluster distribution of cases of KS has suggested a possible role of geographical influences, genetic factors, and an infectious etiology. Simple Mendelian dominance or recessive inheritance has been felt to be unlikely, given the rarity of familial occurrences of the disease. These genetic patterns could only be invoked if one postulated an unusually great number of cases with incomplete penetrance.

Environmental factors do not appear to play an important role in the etiology of KS. This is suggested by studies such as that of

Oettle,[17] who found a 10 times greater incidence of KS in South African Bantus as compared to Caucasians inhabiting the same geographical zone. A case of two brothers with KS was reported from Memorial Sloan-Kettering Cancer Center: one brother was born in Russia, whereas the other was born in the United States. This observation was felt to be indicative of a greater contribution of hereditary factors in the development of KS as compared to geographical influences. This observation is also supported by the increased incidence of HLA-DR5 in cases of both the classical and the epidemic forms of KS.[35,64]

An infectious basis of the disease has frequently been discussed. Giraldo and coworkers[76–79] postulated a possible role of cytomegalovirus (CMV) in the pathogenesis of KS. They demonstrated the presence of herpesviruslike particles in the tissue culture lines of patients with KS. A close serologic association between CMV and KS has also been demonstrated in European and American cases. In addition, the DNA sequences occurring in CMV have been shown to be the same as those found in tissue from classical KS tumors. These observations have been substantiated in the epidemic form of the disease as well. Renal transplant recipients, who have been found to be at high risk for KS, have also been found to have a higher incidence of CMV infections. It is also of note that CMV antibodies are found in approximately 94% of homosexual men as compared with 54% of heterosexual men.[80] These observations point toward a possible link between CMV infection and KS and suggest a role for CMV in the epidemic form of KS.

THERAPEUTIC MODALITIES

It has been repeatedly demonstrated that the KS tumor is very sensitive to both radiation and chemotherapy. Radiation therapy has become an established treatment for localized disease. Chemotherapy has become a mainstay of therapy where x-ray facilities are not available, as well as in cases where the disease is aggressive and disseminated.

Solitary lesions are often treated with radiation therapy. In general, early stages of the disease, that is, early nodules and macules, are more radiosensitive than older infiltrative plaques. Due to the multifocal nature of the disease, dosimetric problems are often encountered at junction points of multiple ports of radiation. Therefore, hemibody radiation or total and subtotal skin electron beam therapy has been used in cases of KS involving significant areas of the body surface. Radiation necrosis has been found to be a problem in doses of greater than 2500 rads or when portal size exceeds 20 cm.[81] Complete responses were found in 9 of 11 patients studied by Holecek and Harwood[82] who were treated with extended field radiation of 800 rads in a single dose.[82] Five of these patients experienced a recurrence of their disease. Total or subtotal skin electron beam therapy was used on 20 patients by Nisce and colleagues,[83] with complete responses reported in 17 of these patients. In 36 and 43 months of follow-up, only 2 of these 17 patients relapsed with recurrent disease.[83] Successful results have been reported by Goldman[84] with the use of laser irradiation.

Chemotherapy has been used extensively in Africa, where x-ray facilities are limited. Cook[85] treated 75 KS patients in Uganda with intralesional nitrogen mustard; 60% of these patients demonstrated partial responses, which were, unfortunately, short-lived remissions. Kyalwazi[86] used a different alkylating agent, trenimon (2,3,5,-tres-(1-azuredinye)-*P*-benzoquinone), and reported complete regression in 11 patients with partial response in 9 patients. Only two of the patients, however, maintained a complete response for two years.[86] In more aggressive forms of KS, combination drug regimens have been discussed. A three-drug combination of actinomycin D, DTIC, and vincristine has so far been found to be the most effective.[87] The combination was found to be more advantageous than either drug alone or in dual combination.[88,89] Odom and Goette[90] have attempted the local use of vincristine with excellent results reported with the intralesional use of the drug in the case of nodular KS of the lower extremities. Another drug combination that has shown some promise is bleomycin and BCNU.[91] The standard chemotherapeutic agent used in the United States since the mid-1960s has been vinblastine.[92–94] Cyclophosphamide has been ineffective in the treatment of this disease. In fact, the observation has been made that renal transplant recipients have developed KS while receiving immunosuppressive therapy consisting of cyclophosphamide, azathiooprine, and prednisone. Other treatments that have been used for patients with KS include razoxane,[95] peptochemio,[96] methotrexate, topical application of dinitrochlorobenzene (DNCB), and intralesional injections of purified protein derivative (PPD) or *Candida* extract.

In the new epidemic form of KS, combination and single-agent chemotherapy has resulted in variable responses in the patients treated. However, a potentially fatal outcome resulted in most patients secondary to intercurrent opportunistic infections. In addition to the previously mentioned chemotherapeutic modalities, VP-16 (4'-demethylepipodophyllotoxin-3-D-ethylidene glucoside) has been used with several complete responses.

An attempt to use immune-modulating therapy in the treatment of the epidemic form of KS has been made, thereby directing therapy primarily toward the host rather than the disease. The immunodeficiency syndrome, which is such an integral part of the KS/AIDS syndrome, is possibly the result of a transmissible agent of AIDS, perhaps a viral agent. Although at the present time this causative agent remains unknown, immune-modulating agents directed at improving the host's immune status may be beneficial. Recombinant alpha-interferon has been used in treatment trials with an observed 20% complete response rate.[97]

SUMMARY

Far more investigation is necessary to better elucidate the origin and nature of the cells responsible for the development of KS. It would thereby clarify whether this disease is truly a malignant process or a proliferative disorder in light of an overriding immune dysfunction. The possible roles of hereditary and genetic factors, such as the increased incidence of HLA-DR5, require further investigation.

While the cutaneous Kaposi's sarcoma tumor appears to be sensitive to both radiation and chemotherapeutic agents, patients with internal involvement seem to respond poorly to these modalities, with death ensuing within a relatively short period of time. The coincidence of KS with lymphomas, in renal transplant recipients, and in patients with acquired immune deficiency syndrome, suggests a significant association between immune dysfunction and the development of the KS tumor. Therefore, immune-modulating therapies may show promise in the treatment of KS in the future. In conclusion, the epidemic of KS/AIDS may serve as a model to study the interrelation between infections, immunity, and malignant disease.

ACKNOWLEDGMENT

This work was supported in part by U.S. Public Health Service Grants CA-31643, CA-23766, CA-16599, CA-34995, and CA-34822 from the National Institute of Health, and the Ancell Fund.

REFERENCES

1. Kaposi M: Idiopathisches multiples Pigmensarkom der Haut. Arch Dermatol Syphilol 4:265, 1872
2. Smith EC, Elmes BGT: Malignant disease in the natives of Nigeria. An analysis of 500 tumors. Ann Trop Med Parasitol 28:461, 1934
3. Hallenberger O: Multiple Angiosarkome der Haut bei einem Kammerunneger. Arch Schiffs Trop Hyg 18:647, 1914
4. Ackerman LV, Murray JF: Symposium on Kaposi's sarcoma. S. Karger, Basel, 1963
5. Harwood A, et al: Kaposi's sarcoma in recipients of renal transplants. Am J Med 67:759, 1979
6. Myers B, et al: Kaposi's sarcoma in kidney transplant recipients. Arch Intern Med 133:307, 1974
7. Ettinger D, Humphrey R, Skinner M: Kaposi's sarcoma associated with multiple myeloma. Johns Hopkins Med J 137:88, 1975
8. Centers for Disease Control: Kaposi's sarcoma and Pneumocystis penumonia among homosexual men—New York City and California. MMWR 30:305, 1981
9. Urmacher C, et al: Outbreak of Kaposi's sarcoma in young homosexual men. Am J Med 72:569, 1982
10. Siegal F, et al: Severe acquired immunodeficiency in male homosexuals manifested by chronic perianal ulcerative herpes simples lesions. N Engl J Med 305:1439, 1981
11. Masur H, et al: An outbreak of community-acquired Pneumoncystis carinii pneumonia. N Engl J Med 305:1431, 1981
12. Gottlieb M, et al: Pneumocystis carinii pneumonia and mucosal candidiasis in previously healthy homosexual men. N Engl J Med 305:1425, 1981
13. Bluefarb SM: Kaposi's sarcoma. Charles C Thomas, Springfield, IL, 1957
14. Rothman S: Some clinical aspects of Kaposi's sarcoma in the European and North American populations. Acta Unio Internationales Contra Cancrum 18:364, 1962
15. Centers for Disease Control: Epidemiologic aspects of the current outbreak of Kaposi's sarcoma and opportunistic infections. N Engl J Med 306:248, 1982
16. Haverkos HW, Curran JW: The current outbreak of Kaposi's sarcoma and opportunistic infections. CA 32:330, 1982
17. Oettle AG: Geographical and racial differences in the frequency of KS as evidence of environmental or genetic causes. Acta Unio Internationales Contra Cancum 18:330, 1962
18. Rothman S: Medical research in Africa. Arch Dermatol 85:311, 1962
19. Reynolds WA, Winkelmann RK, Soule EH: Kaposi's sarcoma. Medicine (Baltimore) 44:419, 1965
20. Templeton AC: Kaposi's sarcoma. In Andrade R, et al (eds): Kaposi's Sarcoma in Cancer of the Skin. Vol. 2. p 1183. Saunders, Philadelphia, 1976
21. Dorn HF, Cutler SJ: Morbidity from cancer in the United States. Part I. Variation in incidence by age, sex, marital status, and geographic region. Public Health Monogr 29:121, 1955
22. Davies JNP, Lothe F: Kaposi's sarcoma in African children. In Ackerman LV, Murray JF (eds); Symposium on Kaposi's Sarcoma. S Karger, Basel, 1963
23. DiGiovanna J, Safai B: Kaposi's sarcoma: Retrospective study of 90 cases with particular emphasis on the familial occurrence, ethnic background, and prevalance of other diseases. Am J Med 71:779, 1981
24. Rothman S: Remarks on sex, age, and racial distribution of Kaposi's sarcoma and on possible pathogenetic factors. Acta Unio Internationales Contra Cancrum 18:322, 1962
25. Lothe F: Kaposi's sarcoma in Ugandan Africans. Acta Pathol Microbiol Scand [Suppl] 161:1, 1963
26. Safai B, et al: Association of Kaposi's sarcoma with second primary malignancies. CA 45:1472, 1980
27. Oettle AG: Geographic and racial differences in frequency of Kaposi's sarcoma as evidence of environmental or genetic causes. p 330. In Ackerman LV, Murray JF (eds): Symposium on Kaposi's Sarcoma. S Karger, Basel, 1963
28. Palmer PES: Haemangiosarcoma of Kaposi. Acta Radiol Rev 12:640, 1972
29. Symmers D: Kaposi's sarcoma. Arch Pathol 32:764, 1941
30. McLaren DS: Kaposi's sarcoma of the eyelids of an African child. Arch Opthalmol 63:859, 1960

31. Mortada A: Conjunctival regressing Kaposi's sarcoma. Br J Opthalmol 51:275, 1967
32. Hansson CJ: Kaposi's sarcoma. Clinical and radiotherapeutic studies on 23 patients. Acta Radiol (Stockh) 21:457, 1940
33. Myskowski PL, Romano JF, Safai B: Kaposi's sarcoma in young homosexual men. Cutis 29:31, 1982
34. Gottlieb GJ, Ackerman AB; Kaposi's sarcoma: An extensively dissseminated form in young homosexual men. Hum Pathol 13:882, 1982
35. Friedman-Kien AE: Disseminated Kaposi's sarcoma syndrome in young homosexual men. J Am Acad Dermatol 5:468, 1981
36. Ecklund RE, Valaitis J: Kaposi's sarcoma of lymph nodes. Arch Pathol 74:224, 1962
37. Cox FX, Helwig EB: Kaposi's sarcoma. Cancer 12:289, 1959
38. Rivomushana RJW, Bailey IC, Kyalwazi SK: Kaposi's sarcoma of the brain. Cancer 36:1127, 1975
39. Taylor JF, et al: Kaposi's sarcoma in Uganda: A clinicopathological study. Int J Cancer 8:122, 1971
40. Rothman S: Some clinical aspects of Kaposi's sarcoma in the European and North American populations. Acta Unio Internationalis Contra Cancrum 18:364, 1962
41. Keen P: The clinical features of Kaposi's sarcoma in the South African Bantu. Acta Unio Internationalis Contra Cancrum 18:380, 1962
42. Slavin G, Cameron HM, Singh H: Kaposi's sarcoma in mainland Tanzania: A report of 117 cases. Br J Cancer 23:249, 1969
43. Lothe F: Kaposi's sarcoma in Ugandian Africans. Acta Pathol Microbiol Scand 1962 [supl]:1–71
44. Safai B, Good RA: Kaposi's sarcoma. A review and recent developments. Clin Bull 10:62, 1980
45. Becker BJP: The histogenesis of Kaposi's sarcoma. Acta Unio Internationalis Contra Cancrum 18:477, 1962
46. Hashimoto K, Lever WF: Kaposi's sarcoma: Histochemical and electron microscope studies. J Invest Dermatol 43:539, 1964
47. Mustakallio KK, Leponen E, Ralkallio J: Histochemistry of Kaposi's sarcoma. I. Hydrolases and phophorylase. Exp Mol Pathol 2:303, 1963
48. Loring WE, Wolman S: Idiopathic multiple hemorrhagic sarcoma of lung (Kaposi's sarcoma). NY State J Med 65:668, 1965
49. Dorffel J: Histogenesis of multiple idiopathic hemorrhagic sarcoma of Kaposi. Arch Dermatol Syphilol 26:608, 1932
50. Dayan AD, Lewis PD: Origin of Kaposi's sarcoma from the reticuloendothelial system. Nature 213:889, 1967
51. Guarda LG, et al: Factor VIII in Kaposi's sarcoma. Am J Clin Pathol 76:197, 1981
52. Klein M, Pereira F, Kantor I: Kaposi's sarcoma complicating systemic lupus erythematosus treated with immunosuppression. Arch Dermatol 110:602, 1974
53. Leung F, Fam A, Osoba D: Kaposi's sarcoma complicating corticosteroid therapy for temporal arteritis. Am J Med 71:320, 1981
54. Kapadia S, Krause J: Kaposi's sarcoma after long-term alkylating agent therapy for multiple myeloma. South Med J 70:1011, 1977
55. Mazzaferre E, Penn G: Kaposi's sarcoma associated with multiple myeloma. Arch Intern Med 122:521, 1968
56. Dantzig P: Kaposi's sarcoma and polymyositis. Arch Dermatol 110:605, 1974
57. Law I: Kaposi's sarcoma and plasma cell dyscrasia. JAMA 229:1329, 1974
58. Moertel C: Multiple primary malignant neoplasms, their incidence and significance. Recent Results in Cancer Res 7:34, 1966
59. Master S, et al: Immunological studies in Kaposi's sarcoma in Uganda. Br Med J 1:600, 1970
60. Safai B, et al: Cell-mediated immune reaction in KS. Clin Res 28:9, 1980
61. Taylor J, et al: Lymphocyte transformation in Kaposi's sarcoma. Int J Cancer 8:468, 1971
62. Taylor J: Lymphocyte transformation in Kaposi's sarcoma. Lancet 1:883, 1973
63. Taylor J, Ziegler J: Delayed cutaneous hypersensitivity reactions in patients with Kaposi's sarcoma. Br J Cancer 30:312, 1974
64. Pollack MS, et al: Frequency of HLA and GM Immunogenetic markers in Kaposi's sarcoma. Tissue Antigens 21:1, 1983
65. Gladman DD, et al: Increased frequency of HLA-DR5 in scleroderma. Arthritis Rheum 24:854, 1981

66. Tosato G, Steinberg A, Blaese M: Defective EBV-specific suppressor T-cell function in rheumatoid arthritis. N Engl J Med 305:1238, 1981

67. DeWolf WC, et al: Association of HLA and renal cell carcinoma. Hum Immunol 1:41, 1981

68. Safai B, et al: Association of HLA-DR5 with mycosis fungoides. J Invest Dermatol 80:395, 1983

69. Moertel CG: Multiple primary malignant neoplasms. Recent Results Cancer Res. 7:1, 1966

70. Moertel CG, Hagedorn AB: Leukaemia or lymphoma and coexistent primary malignant lesion. A review of the literature and a study of 120 cases. Blood 12:788, 1957

71. O'Brien PH, Brasfield R: Kaposi's sarcoma. Cancer 19:1497, 1966

72. Klein MB, Pereira FA, Kantor I: Kaposi's sarcoma complicating systemic lupus erythematosus treated with immunosuppression. Arch Dermatol 110:602, 1974

73. Hogeman D: Hyperhemolysis of nonsplenic origin. Acta Med Scand 144:247, 1953

74. Martensson J, Henrikson H: Immunohemolytic anemia in Kaposi's sarcoma with visceral involvement only. Acta Med Scand 150:175, 1954

75. Cook J: The clinical features of Kaposi's sarcoma in the East African Bantu. Acta Unio Internationales Contra Cancrum 18:388, 1962

76. Giraldo G, Beth E, Hanguenau F: Herpestype virus particles in tissue culture of Kaposi's sarcoma from different geographic regions. J Natl Cancer Inst 49:1509, 1972

77. Giraldo G, et al: Antibody patterns to herpes virus in Kaposi's sarcoma. Serological association of European Kaposi's sarcoma with cytomegalovirus. Int J Cancer 15:839, 1975

78. Giraldo G, et al: Antibody patterns to herpes viruses in Kaposi's sarcoma. II. Serological associations of American Kaposi's sarcoma with cytomegalovirus. Int J Cancer 22:126, 1978

79. Giraldo G, Beth E, Huang E: Kaposi's sarcoma and its relationship to cytomegalovirus. III. CMV, DNA, and CMV-early antigens in Kaposi's sarcoma. Int J Cancer 26:23, 1980

80. Drew W, et al: Prevalence of cytomegalovirus infection in homosexual men. J Infect Dis 143:188, 1981

81. Cohen L: Dose time and volume parameters in irradiation therapy of Kaposi's sarcoma. Br J Radiol 35:485, 1962

82. Holecek MJ, Harwood AR: Radiotherapy of Kaposi's sarcoma. Cancer 41:1733, 1978

83. Nisce L, Safai B, Poussin-Rosello H: Once weekly total and subtotal skin electron beam therapy for Kaposi's sarcoma. Cancer 47:640, 1981

84. Goldman L: Laser radiation of malignancy in man. Cancer 18:533, 1965

85. Cook J: The treatment of Kaposi's sarcoma with nitrogen mustard. Acta Unio Internationales Contra Cancrum. 18:494, 501, 1962

86. Kyalwazi SK: Chemotherapy of Kaposi's sarcoma: Experience with trenimon. East Afr Med J 45:17, 1968

87. Oliveny CLM, et al: Treatment of Kaposi's sarcoma by a combination of actinomycin-D, vincristine, and imidazole carboxamide. Results of a randomized clinical trial. Int J Cancer 14:649, 1974

88. Vogel CL, et al: Treatment of Kaposi's sarcoma with actinomycin-D: Results of a randomized clinical trial. Int J Cancer 8:136, 1971

89. Vogel CL, et al: Treatment of Kaposi's sarcoma with a combination of actinomycin-D and vincristine: Results of a randomized clinical trial. Cancer 31:1382, 1973

90. Odom RB, Goette DK: Treatment of cutaneous Kaposi's sarcoma with intralesional vincristine. Arch Dermatol 114:1693, 1978

91. Vogel CL, et al: Phase II clincal trails of 1,3-bis-(2-chlorolthyl-1-nitrosurea),(BCNU, NSC 4099621) and bleomycin (NSC 125066) in Kaposi's sarcoma. Cancer Chemother Rep (part I) 57:325, 1973

92. Scott WP, Voight JA: Kaposi's sarcoma management with vincaleukoblastine. Cancer 19:557, 1966

93. Tucker SB, Windelmann RK: Treatment of Kaposi's sarcoma with vinblastine. Arch Dermatol 112:958, 1976

94. Klein E, et al: Treatment of Kaposi's sarcoma with vinblastine. Cancer 45:427, 1980

95. Oliveny CLM, et al: Treatment of Kaposi's

sarcoma with ICRF-159 (NSC 129943). Cancer Chemother Rep 60:111, 1976

96. Cottafava F, et al: Kaposi's sarcoma. Report on a case treated with peptochemio. Minerva Pediatr 29:247, 1977

97. Krown SE, et al: Preliminary observations on the effect of recombinant leukocyte A interferon in homosexual men with Kaposi's sarcoma. N Engl J Med 308:1071, 1983

17

Amebiasis and Giardiasis

John D. Frame

An association between intestinal protozoal infections and the homosexual lifestyle was mentioned by Most[1] in 1967. Statistical evidence of a relationship of amebic infections and homosexuality was presented by Dritz and associates[2] and by William and associates[3] in 1977. Numerous case reports of giardiasis as well as of infection with *Entamoeba histolytica* and nonpathogenic amebae have shown that an array of intestinal protozoa may be found in homosexual males.[4]

Presumably the intestinal parasites are spread among them by their sexual practices. Anilingus and other practices permit direct oral infection with fecal material. Attendance at "baths" where frequent sexual contacts occur with numerous partners, often anonymous, allows for widespread distribution of infections. It is also possible that contamination of food prepared by a carrier of protozoal cysts may also serve as a source of infection, though in view of the anally oriented sexual practices already mentioned this route of infection is likely to be of relatively low importance.

Anilingus and anal intercourse are practiced by heterosexuals as well, and sexually transmitted intestinal protozoal infection is not confined to homosexual men. Knowledge of this possibility may elucidate the source of otherwise inexplicable amebiasis and giardiasis in heterosexual patients.

AMEBIASIS

Etiology

Amebiasis generally refers to infection with *Entamoeba histolytica* Schaudinn 1903. Other intestinal amebae which have been reported in homosexual patients include *E. hartmanni* von Prowazek 1912, *E. coli* (Grassi 1879) Casagrandi; Barbagallo 1895, and *Endolimax nana* (Wenyon and O'Connor 1917) Brug 1981, and *Iodamoeba butschlii* (von Prowazek 1911) Dobell 1919. These nonpathogenic organisms are indicative of human fecal contamination by the oral route, and encourage further examination of stool specimens of patients in whom *E. histolytica* was not found on initial testing. *Dientamoeba fragilis* Jepps and Dobell 1918, now considered a flagellate, may cause relatively mild intestinal symptoms.

The diagnosis of *E. histolytica* infection has been complicated in recent years by the recognition that not all organisms morphologically similar to *E. histolytica* are pathogenic. *E. hartmanni* differs by its size, with cysts smaller than 10 μm in diameter. Even among amebae, which by present criteria must be considered *E. histolytica* on structural grounds, there are differences in pathogenicity.

Among the nonpathogenic amebae are the *E. histolytica*-like organisms, which cannot be distinguished from *E. histolytica* by morphologic criteria including their size, but which differ in a number of characteristics. The first known ameba of this group was the strain which was used in the classical transmission experiments of amebiasis.[5] During early investigations it was found that subjects infected with this Laredo strain had diarrhea no more frequently than did controls. Subsequently, the Laredo strain was found capable of culture at room temperature,[6] and in hypotonic media,[7] qualities not shared by known pathogenic strains of *E. histolytica*. In vitro tolerance to emetine was ten times that of pathogenic strains.[8] *E. histolytica*-like organisms include other strains that share these characteristics. Biochemical differences of this

group from *E. histolytica* have been demonstrated by serologic tests[9] and isoenzyme electrophoresis.[10]

The most sensitive tests distinguishing the intestinal amebae have been developed by Sargeaunt and Williams and their colleagues[11] who have investigated them by means of thin-layer starch-gel electrophoresis. They have been able to divide the many strains of *E. histolytica* they have cultured into 18 zymodemes, or groups of amebic strains that share common electrophoretic enzyme patterns. Only seven of these zymodemes have been obtained from patients with clear-cut clinical disease[12] (Fig. 17-1).

It has long been held that *E. histolytica* is often a commensal. It was never certain under what conditions the organism might become pathogenic. It was assumed that this occurred because of poorly understood changes in the host. The recent reports of Sargeaunt and his colleagues[10–12] suggest

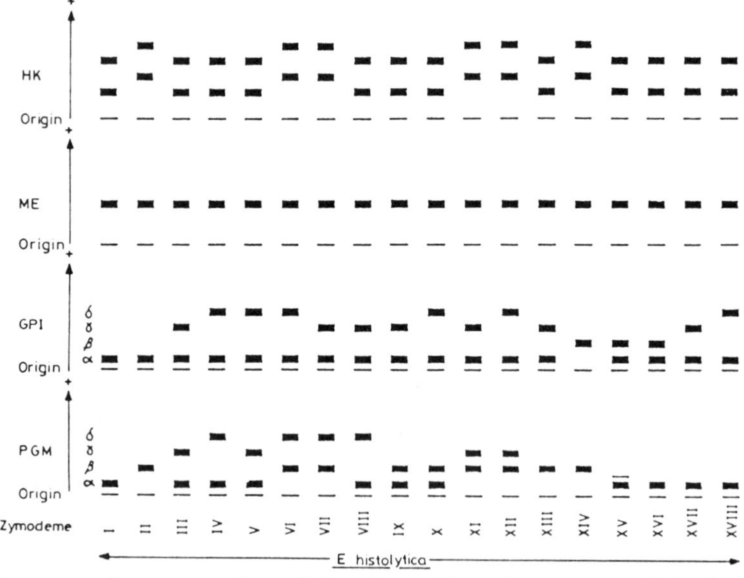

Fig. 17-1 Diagrammatic presentation of the electrophoretic patterns of the isoenzymes of *Entamoeba histolytica*. Enzymes used: EC 5319 glucose phosphate isomerase (GPI); EC 11140 L-maleate: NADP⁺ oxidoreductase (oxaloacetate decarboxylating) (ME); EC 2751 phosphoglucomutase (PGM); and FC 2711 hexokinase (HK). Zymodemes II, VI, VII, XI, XII, XIII, and XIV are from patients; other zymodemes from carriers. (Sargeaunt PG, Oates JK, Maclennan I, et al: Entamoeba histolytica in male homosexuals. Br J Vener Dis 59:193, 1983, with permission.)

that morphologically similar organisms are either nonpathogenic commensals or essentially pathogenic invaders. It is still not clear whether host factors may in some way influence the isoenzymes of the amebae so that a nonpathogenic form may become pathogenic.

In the intestinal tract *E. histolytica* is found as the trophozoite and cyst. The trophozoite is the stage in the life cycle capable of causing symptomatic disease. When stained it measures from 15 to 25 μm in diameter, and contains a single nucleus characterized by a rim of rather evenly distributed chromatin on a delicate nuclear membrane and a central nucleolus or karyosome. The pathogenic form may also contain remnants of ingested erythrocytes. The living trophozoite moves by progressive extension of pseudopods into which the cytoplasmic material flows (Fig. 17-2).

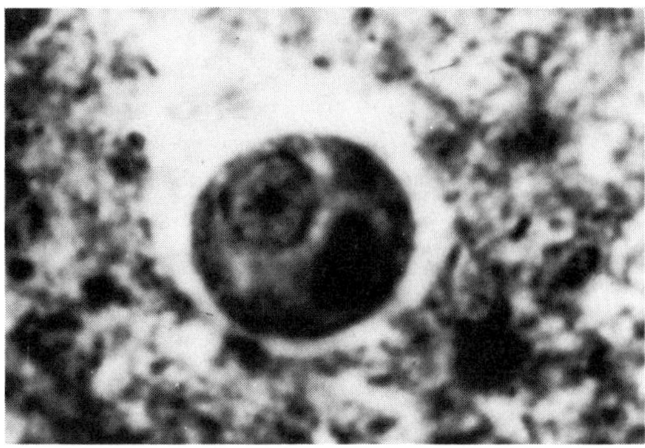

Fig. 17-3 *Entamoeba histolytica* cyst, showing a single nucleus with cenplaced karyosome, and chromatoidal bar with rounded ends.

The cyst, 10 to 20 μm in diameter, is spherical. It contains from one to four nuclei, again with finely distributed chromatin margins and centrally placed karyosomes. At times chromatoidal bodies with blunt ends are seen in the cytoplasm. Cysts form under adverse environmental conditions and are able to survive outside the host; they are therefore the forms involved in transmission and infection of a new host (Fig. 17-3).

Epidemiology

Infection with *E. histolytica* is generally acquired by the ingestion of its cyst. Although direct infection through the anus may be possible, this is probably not the usual mode of acquisition of the parasite. Traditionally amebic infections have been considered the result of ingestion of contaminated food or water. However, the oral-anal sexual practices already described are also efficient means of transmission of amebae.

The prevalence of sexually acquired amebiasis is not known. In a Canadian study 27% were found to be infected with amebae in a group of 200 homosexuals who voluntarily submitted specimens for examination.[13] This may represent a higher than av-

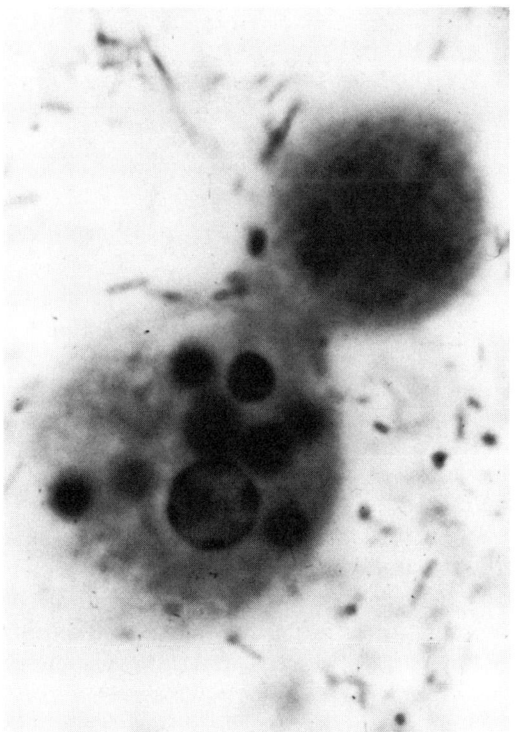

Fig. 17-2 Trophozoite of *Entamoeba histolytica*, with large pseudopod and ingested erythrocytes. Nucleus poorly visible.

erage prevalence; it is likely that many volunteers in the sample submitted specimens because they were symptomatic. A group of 100 male controls, presumably not homosexual, included one person with a specimen positive for *E. histolytica*. In a British investigation in which the stools of 470 homosexual patients were cultured, 52 were positive for *E. histolytica*, a prevalence of 11%,[12] compared to 0.5% in the general population of the communities where they lived. A prospective investigation of homosexual males attending a venereal disease clinic in New York City revealed 20% positive for *E. histolytica*.[14]

It is generally impossible to determine the ultimate source of the chain of infection resulting in a given case of amebiasis. In one patient I observed, it appeared likely that an infection incurred in Singapore was successfully treated, and was followed by another acquired in a commune in the American southwest. The frequency of sexual contacts in the group suggests that an imported infection will likely spread widely through the community within a relatively short period of time. It is probable that there is a wide variety of strains with varying pathogenicity and responses to treatment in people who have acquired *E. histolytica* infections sexually.

Pathology

The essential pathology in amebiasis appears to result from the production by the trophozoite of lysosomal proteolytic enzymes with destruction of host tissues. There is no neutrophilic response, probably because of the production of cytotoxins that destroy leukocytes.

The earliest specific lesions of intestinal amebiasis are very small ulcerations of the colonic mucosa, described typically as flask-shaped; the deeper parts are wider than the more superficial. They are most commonly found in the cecum, ascending

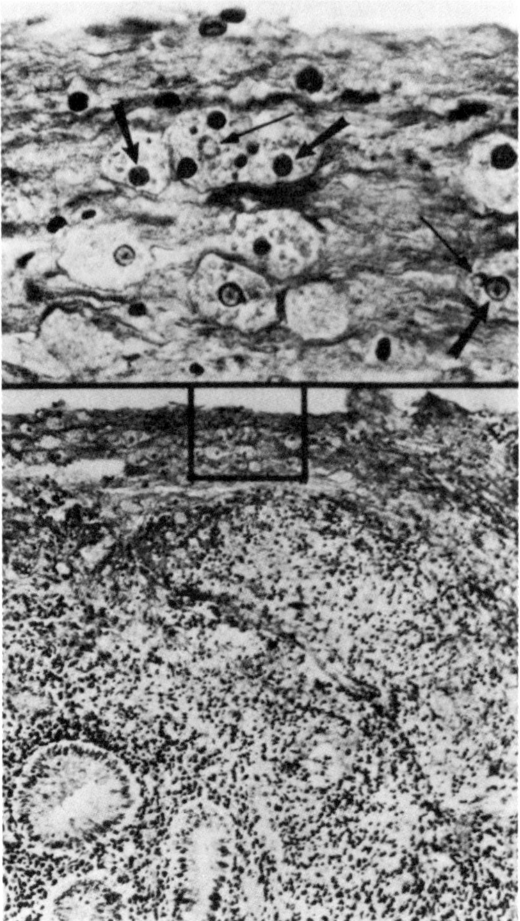

Fig. 17-4 Rectal pathology. *Above*: A high-power view showing trophozoites of *Entamoeba histolytica*; large arrows point to typical nuclei with central karysomes and small arrows to ingested erythrocytes. *Below*: A low-power view showing crypt destruction, inflammation, and overlying exudate.

colon, sigmoid, and rectum (Fig. 17-4). As the ulcers progress they extend into the submucosa and even into the muscularis layer; they may penetrate through the wall of the intestine into the peritoneal cavity, leading to localized abscess formation or to peritonitis. Occasionally fistulae may form through the abdominal wall or into the vagina in females.

Another intestinal lesion is the formation of an ameboma, a mass of granulation tissue with lymphocytes, plasma cells, and eosinophils present as well. Often occurring in the cecum, the tumor may be confused with colonic carcinoma.

Trophozoites of *E. histolytica* are found in the base of ulcers; they are present in scanty numbers in amebomas.

Amebic abscesses of the liver are characterized by the development of necrotic cavities containing chocolate-colored thick pus, often described as resembling achovy sauce. The abscesses grow and coalesce, and can become very large. Amebic trophozoites are not likely to be found in the midst of the thick pus, but are present in large numbers in the margins of the abscess.

The liver abscess may perforate Glisson's capsule; if the perforation is superior a subphrenic abscess may develop, or penetration into the pleural cavity will result in a pleural effusion or empyema.

Mestastatic spread to the lungs, brain, and other structures may occur; these complications are relatively uncommon.

Clinical Findings

E. histolytica may be found on stool examination in patients with no symptoms of intestinal origin, or in those with a wide variety of syndromes. The classification of the World Health Organization[15] permits an orderly presentation of what is in practice often a very confusing matter.

Asymptomatic patients do not have symptoms referable to their infection. Patients who are symptomatic may have intestinal amebiasis or extraintestinal amebiasis.

Intestinal amebiasis includes dysentery, nondysenteric colitis, ameboma, and amebic appendicitis. A large tender liver may be found in some dysenteric cases; this probably does not reflect actual invasion of the liver by *E. histolytica*, but rather a reaction to toxins associated with the dysentery. Intestinal amebiasis may be complicated by perforation with peritonitis, hemorrhage, intussusception, postdysenteric colitis, and stricture.

Extraintestinal amebiasis includes liver abscess, which may rupture or extend into adjacent spaces such as the pleural cavity. The skin, lungs, brain, spleen, and other organs are at times infected with *E. histolytica*.

It appears that about 50% of patients infected with *E. histolytica* are asymptomatic[16]; these people are generally found in routine surveys. This group also includes persons who know of amebiasis, have heard of its potential risks, and wish to be assured that they do not have amebic infection.

Patients may also present with flatulence, irregularity of bowel habit, and mild abdominal cramping. They are the most difficult group to evaluate if they are found to be infected with intestinal parasites. It is not always clear that their symptoms are in fact due to the presence of the protozoa discovered in their feces. The question is applicable to all patients, but has been investigated specifically among male homosexuals. In the Canadian survey[13] gastrointestinal complaints occurred in 59% of those in whom pathogenic protozoa were found on stool examination, and in 52% of those in whom none were present. The difference between the two groups was not clinically significant.

Serologic investigation of homosexual males infected with *E. histolytica* also casts doubt on the clinical significance of the amebae found on stool examination. Positive indirect fluorescent antibody tests have indeed been reported in two patients, one asymptomatic and the other with amebic proctitis.[17] On the other hand, I observed that none were found positive for indirect hemagglutination antibodies (IHA) in a series of 20 homosexual males actively infected at the time of serologic testing in whom the parasitologic diagnosis had been made by stool examination in expert laboratories. General experience with this test suggests that up to 80% of patients with mild intestinal amebiasis may be expected to be IHA-positive.[18]

Tests for isoenzymes of *E. histolytica* performed on strains isolated from homosexuals raise further questions about the pathogenicity of many amebae found in this population. In the British investigation of Sargeaunt and his coworkers,[12] none of the 52 strains cultured from stools were classified in any of the seven zymodemes associated with amebic disease. This was also true of 18 strains obtained from a group of homosexual patients in New York City tested at the Centers for Disease Control.[19]

It is likely that in many patients their mild gastrointestinal symptoms are not due to the *E. histolytica* harbored in their intestinal tracts.

More severe cases of amebic diarrhea are characterized by the passing of several loose or liquid stools daily. The patient complains of abdominal cramps, and the abdomen is generally tender on examination. Small flecks of blood-tinged mucus will often be found on careful examination of the stools. Sigmoidoscopic examination will generally reveal rather nonspecific inflammation or shallow ulceration of the colonic mucosa.

In acute amebic dysentery, numerous liquid stools are passed daily. In about one half of instances the onset is sudden, with headache, nausea, chills and fever; abdominal cramps are severe, and there is likely to be tenesmus. Stools may be grossly bloody. Sigmoidoscopic examination will often reveal ulceration of the rectosigmoid; ulcers typically have overhanging margins. The liver is enlarged and tender in about a quarter of cases, most likely because of toxins released from the bowel and not because of amebic invasion. The white blood count may range from normal values to a leukocytosis of 15,000/μl with a marked predominance of neutrophilic polymorphonuclears.

Amebic liver abscess is often considered a late complication of amebiasis, but may occur relatively early even after apparently mild amebic intestinal disease. Cases of amebic abscess have been reported in male homosexual patients[20] (Fig. 17-5). The onset of symptoms may be acute or gradual. Fever and a sense of fullness and then pain in the upper abdomen are found in most patients. Pain is likely to be accentuated by respiration, and is at times referred to the shoulder. Amebic abscesses are more common in the right lobe than in the left; the area of pain depends upon the lobe that is involved. Upon examination the liver is generally tender, except in early abscess located deep in the liver. The fever tends to be spiking in nature, and is often followed by profuse sweating. In some instances with necrosis of large portions of the liver slight jaundice may be found; this occurred in one third of instances in a large series.[21] Leukocytosis in the range of 15,000 to 35,000/μl is common. Though a single abscess is found in most patients, multiple abscesses do occur; the single lesion may be due to relatively late diagnosis after several abscesses have coalesced.

Amebiasis of the penis presents as a painful ulcerating lesion, rapidly progressing and with a purulent exudate.[22,23] Amebiasis of the uterine cervix is characterized by the presence of a profuse dark vaginal discharge, with ulcers found on examination.[24] Carcinoma of the cervix has been the initial diagnosis in some instances. Amebiasis of the cervix has generally been found as a complication of intestinal amebiasis and is probably not common as a sexually transmitted infection, but may lead to penile amebiasis in the sexual partner.[25]

Laboratory Diagnosis

The definitive diagnosis of amebiasis is made by the identification of *E. histolytica* in an appropriate specimen by a competent laboratory.

In the case of intestinal amebiasis a single

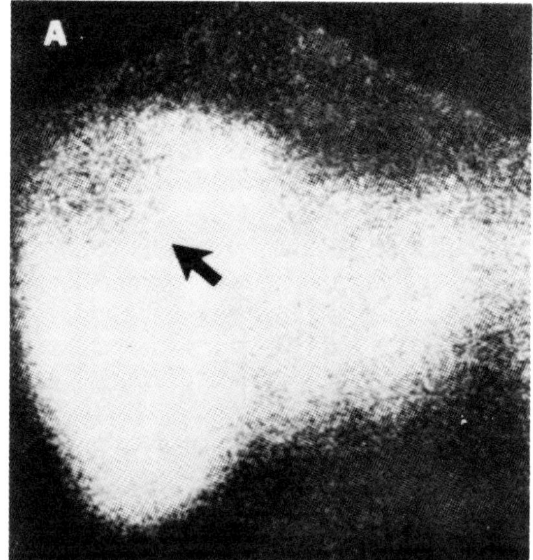

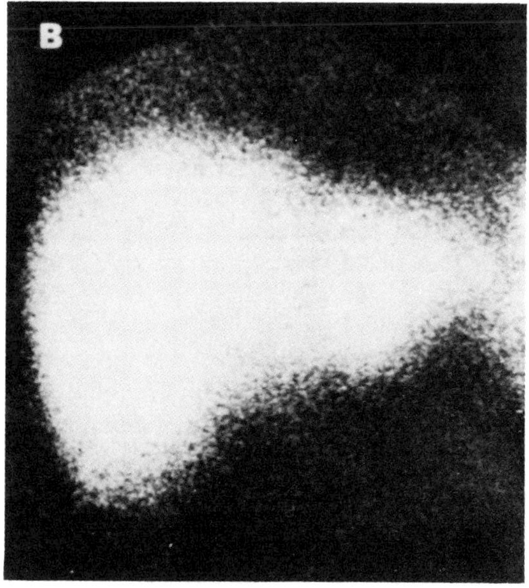

Fig. 17-5 Technetium liver scans. *A:* During the patient's acute illness, showing a solitary 5 cm defect in the right lobe (arrow). *B:* Five months later, showing a normal liver. (From Ylvisaker JT, McDonald GB: Sexually acquired amebic colitis and liver abscess. West J Med 132:153, 1980, with permission.)

stool examination by the most capable of technicians will be positive in about 70% of patients ultimately proved to have amebic infection. If the clinical suspicion of amebiasis is strong, up to three examinations of properly collected fecal samples should be performed if the first is negative. Even then a few infections may be missed.

A good specimen is one that is freshly passed and examined microscopically or fixed for later study immediately after passage. Desiccation of the stool in the rectum will destroy trophozoites; it is best to obtain material from higher regions in the colon. The administration of a saline purge to the patient and the collection of a soft or liquid stool in the laboratory will provide a specimen suitable for diagnosis. The second movement after the purge will generally be the most appropriate for the demonstration of motile trophozoites.

In some laboratories the "two-vial" technique is used. The patient is given two specimen bottles or tubes, one containing formalin and the other polyvinyl alcohol (PVA) as fixatives. The specimen is collected at home; a convenient receptable is a plastic refrigerator food storage bag with one side torn open to form a conical trough. This is attached to the toilet seat by adhesive cellulose tape. The patient is instructed not to urinate into the bag. Samples are collected from the last part of the bowel movement to ensure that they include contents of the proximal colon, and are placed in the vials immediately following defecation.

Examination of fresh warm specimens mounted in saline may reveal trophozoites with the progressive locomotion characteristic of *E. histolytica*. The addition of a drop of iodine solution such as Lugol's will cause rounding up of the trophozoites, but will clearly demonstrate cysts and will facilitate the characterization and counting of nuclei. Specimens fixed in PVA are stained by Wheatley-Gomori trichrome stain in order to delineate the organism's structure. Concentration of formalin-fixed stools may permit the discovery of cysts present in small numbers.

The presence of erythrocytes within the trophozoite cytoplasm indicates that the organism is a pathogenic strain. The presence of amebic cysts or of trophozoites without included erythrocytic fragments leaves the question of pathogenicity unresolved.

False-positive stool examinations are due to the confusion of leukocytes, nonpathogenic amebae, or other elements with *E. histolytica*. False negative results may arise from mishandling of specimens, or from testing too soon after the administration of antibiotics or amebicides that depress the number of organisms to a point too low to be found by the technician. The use of antidiarrheal kaolin or bismuth preparations will obscure whatever protozoa are present in a "sandstorm" of particulate matter.

Culture of the stools for amebae will increase the recovery rate to almost 100%; the technique, however, is not practiced in most diagnostic laboratories. Culture of amebae and subsequent isoenzyme electrophoresis would be a highly specific means of diagnosis of infection with pathogenic amebae, but the procedure has not yet been adopted in this country; in Great Britain Sargeaunt and his group perform the test on a referral basis.

Material obtained by curette, glass aspirator, or punch biopsy from amebic ulcers discovered on proctosigmoidoscopic examination is examined fresh for the discovery of motile trophozoites, or after fixation in PVA. The cotton swab is not as successful a means to this end, since the trophozoites tend to adhere to the fibers.[26]

A technique for the testing of stools for *E. histolytica* antigen by enzyme-linked immunosorbent assay (ELISA) was promising, but was withdrawn from the commercial market because of problems in quality control.

Serologic tests will help determine whether the patient is infected with pathogenic amebae; positive results likely indicate the presence of an invasive strain, though actual invasion may not be demonstrable in all instances. Over 95% of patients with severe intestinal amebiasis will have positive serologic results. Antibodies to *E. histolytica* persist for some time after infection has been cured, a factor to be considered in the evaluation of the results of serologic testing. Counterimmunoelectrophoresis, indirect hemagglutination, and complement fixation are the usual tests available in various laboratories.

In amebic liver abscess stool examinations are positive for *E. histolytica* in only 12 to 15% of patients at the time the abscess is diagnosed. Serologic tests are usually, but not universally, positive.[27] Routine radiologic examination of the abdomen may show an enlarged liver, elevation of the right hemidiaphragm, pleural effusion or infiltrates, or atelectatic changes in the lung. Special techniques such as radionuclide scans, computerized tomography, and ultrasound will generally demonstrate the presence of amebic abscess. Diagnostic aspiration of the abscess is rarely indicated now that these techniques are available. If aspiration is carried out, trophozoites of *E. histolytica* will be found in only about one half of instances; cysts will not be present.

Examination of the exudate of genital amebic infection will usually demonstrate the presence of trophozoites; the diagnoses in most reported cases have been made in biopsy material obtained because of the suspected diagnosis of carcinoma.

Differential Diagnosis

The differential diagnosis of sexually transmitted amebiasis includes not only general gastroenterologic disorders but also other specific infections acquired through sexual activity. The term "gay bowel syndrome",[28] has been coined to summarize the host of lower bowel ailments that lead the male homosexual to seek proctologic attention. The range in the symptomatology of amebic infection is reflected in the number of conditions from which it is to be distinguished. The clinician must exercise judgment whether to seek these confounding disorders at the onset of the management of the patient.

Irritable bowel syndrome is at times difficult to differentiate from mild to moderate amebiasis. The history of fragmented or pencillike stools, a tendency to several bowel movements early in the day and the presence of mucus without blood in the absence of amebae on repeated stool examinations are characteristic of this functional disorder. It may be a sequel to amebiasis.

Other noninfectious conditions that simulate more severe amebic infection include trauma and the presence of a foreign object in the rectum or sigmoid.[28,29] Sigmoidoscopic examination will establish the diagnosis.

Idiopathic ulcerative colitis, granulomatous colitis, and pseudomembranous proctitis may well simulate amebic dysentery and are to be distinguished by appropriate clinical and radiologic investigations; carcinoma of the colon must also be excluded in some patients. Acquired immunodeficiency syndrome (AIDS) may be heralded by symptoms of persistent diarrhea; several patients under my observation were treated repeatedly for amebiasis by various physicians, and have now proved to be afflicted with AIDS.

A number of intestinal infections may be confused with amebiasis, or occur concomitantly. *Shigella,*[30] *Salmonella,*[31] *Yersinia,* and *Chlamydia* are among the agents that can be identified by appropriate bacteriologic culture. Gonorrheal proctitis may be asymptomatic, but at times is associated with anal discharge and abdominal cramping; special cultures will identify this infection. Syphilitic chancre is likely to give symptoms more localized to the anus than does amebic infection.

In patients who have had repeated courses of metronidazole or the tetracyclines for amebiasis candidiasis may occur as a suprainfection. The presence of *Candida* sp. in the stool is generally not reported by the parasitologic laboratory. *Blastocystis hominis* appears to be found increasingly among homosexuals in recent years.[32] In some instances, at least, this organism has apparently been associated with the development of gastroenterologic symptoms.

Giardiasis is the most common sexually transmitted parasitic infection to be distinguished from amebiasis; diagnosis may at times be difficult to discover. *Cryptosporidium* sp. has been increasingly reported,[33,34] especially in the immunocompromised host such as the patient with AIDS.

Pyogenic liver abscess must be distinguished from amebic abscess. Serologic tests for amebiasis are usually positive in the latter; at times the distinction can only be made by aspiration of the abscess and microscopic examination and bacteriologic culture of its contents.

Treatment

The dictum that the patient and not the disease must be treated is pertinent to the management of sexually acquired amebiasis. The patient has in most instances received dire warnings of the dangers of "ameba," may have been treated previously with repeated courses of toxic amebicides, and is often convinced that the infection is incurable and fears development of amebic liver abscess. The physician is aware that the *E. histolytica* strain harbored by the patient may not be pathogenic. Until tests for pathogenicity are readily available, the decision whether to treat will be based on clinical grounds.

Acknowledgment of the patient's lifestyle by both physician and patient will encourage improved compliance with whatever therapeutic measures are needed.[35] Interference with a person's erotic life leads to anxiety and anger. An objective discussion of the relationship of sexual practices and infection may encourage him to avoid reinfection. Realistic assessment of the status of infection and the likelihood of cure will promote a response of trust very important in the management of an illness so closely related to a way of life.

Among the most difficult patients are those who have been treated elsewhere and now present themselves with persistent clinical symptoms. Review of the medical history may reveal that the original diagnosis was not based on firm laboratory findings, and that the "clinical failure" was due to inappropriate treatment of a nonamebic disorder.

Persistent infection following appropriate treatment is most often due to reinfection.[4] In some cases, however, drug resistance may play a part.[36] It is known that *E. histolytica*-like organisms are resistant to concentrations of some amebicides that are lethal to the strains that have been used in the testing of the drugs.[8] It has been suggested that most drug trials have been performed with strains representing a single zymodeme of *E. histolytica*[37]; some of the strains circulating in the homosexual population may be unusually resistant to the available amebicides.

The asymptomatic cyst passer is treated with diiodohydroxyquin, 650 mg three times daily for 20 days. If cysts (but not trophozoites) are still present upon examination and the patient is still asymptomatic, diloxanide furoate may be administered, 0.5 g three times daily for 10 days. The latter is an investigational drug in the United States and may be obtained only from the Drug Service, Centers for Disease Control in Atlanta.* The physician will be requested to complete forms needed for the use of an investigational drug, including a report of the patient's response to the treatment. If

the subsequent stool examinations are still positive, the patient should ordinarily not be treated further, but should be advised to return for further evaluation in the event symptoms develop in the future.

Mildly symptomatic patients in whom only amebic cysts are found should receive the same treatment. If the patient is moderately ill or trophozoites are present in the stool, metronidazole may be administered concurrently with the diiodohydroxyquin at a dose of 750 mg three times daily for 5 to 10 days. The patient should be advised to avoid all alcohol intake during the treatment with metronidazole and for at least five days thereafter, for the drug has an disulfiramlike effect. He should be warned of the common side effects of the drug—metallic taste, nausea and occasional vomiting, dizziness, and a sense of weakness. An alternative drug is paramomycin, 25 to 30 mg/kg/day divided into three doses and given for 5 to 10 days.

The combination of diiodohydroxyquin and metronidazole is appropriate also for the patient with dysentery. An alternative treatment is the substitution of dehydroemetine for the metronidazole; it is administered in a daily deep subcutaneous or intramuscular dose of 1 to 1.5 mg/kg/day for five days. Dehydroemetine must be obtained from the Drug Service of the Centers for Disease Control. Yet another drug is emetine given similarly at a dose of 1 mg/kg/day to a maximum of 60 mg daily. Emetine and, to a lesser extent, dehydroemetine are cardiotoxic, and electrocardiagrams should be obtained before treatment and daily during its course, stopping treatment if major conduction irregularities develop.

Tetracycline is administered by some physicians with all the above regimens except that of paramomycin; tetracyclines depress the bacterial flora that form a major source of nutrition for amebae.

Amebic liver abscess is treated with any of the courses used for amebic dysentery. Intravenous metronidazole is available if oral drugs cannot be tolerated.[38] If emetine

---

* The telephone number is 404-329-3670.

or dehydroemetine is used, chloroquine phosphate is added to the regimen at a dose of 1.0 g daily for the first two days, then 0.5 mg daily for another 2 to 3 weeks. Aspiration of the abscess with a trocar is no longer generally needed, unless exquisite tenderness over the abscess suggests that it is likely to rupture. In most cases a single course of treatment will lead to rapid improvement of the patient's clinical status; the abscess will slowly decrease in size over a period of months.

Genital amebiasis reponds to the prescribed course of diiodohydroxyquin and metronidazole.

The use of carbarsone should be avoided, though it may clear up an amebic infection not responding to the other drugs. Carbarsone may cause a hemorrhagic encephalapathy, a complication certainly more dreadful than the relatively mild cases of amebiasis for which it is frequently being used.

If symptoms persist, but no amebae are found on stool examination, the physician may repeat the search for amebae from time to time. However, the most likely cause for continued illness is the presence of one of the conditions mentioned in the section on differential diagnosis, particularly suprainfection with *Candida* sp., not uncommon after the use of metronidazole, tetracycline, and paramomycin. The presence of postamebic irritable bowel syndrome should also be considered as a possible diagnosis.

In the face of what appears to be persistent infection repeated use of amebicides should be undertaken with caution because of their toxicities and side effects. Diiodohydroxyquin in prolonged courses has been implicated in the development of subacute myelooptic neuropathy; less severe complications of its use include generalized furunculosis, drug fever, dermatitis, pruritus, abdominal discomfort, and headache. Diloxanide furoate is generally well tolerated. Metranidazole has been found mutagenic in bacteria and, in large doses, carcinogenic in

rodents. Relatively common side effects are the development of a metallic taste, glossitis and stomatitis, nausea, anorexia, diarrhea and abdominal pain, headache, and vomiting. Metronidazole causes a disulfiram-like effect if alcohol is taken during the course of treatment. Suprainfection with *Candida* sp. may follow its use. Neutropenia has been observed in some patients; the white-cell count returns to normal after completion of the course of therapy.

Treatment with paramomycin may be accompanied by diarrhea and followed by an overgrowth of *Candida*. Tetracycline at times causes gastrointestinal symptoms and may result in suprainfection with *Candida* sp. and various bacteria.

Emetine is cardiotoxic and nephrotoxic; its use should be avoided in patients with heart or kidney disease, except for those with amebic abscess in whom metronidazole is ineffective or contraindicated. Gastrointestinal symptoms are apparently the result of individual hypersensitivity to the drug. Weakness and muscular aching and tenderness may presage more severe reactions. These symptoms are usually not significant in patients receiving the short courses of treatment advised above. Dehydroemetine is less toxic than emetine. Patients receiving either of these drugs should be treated with strict bed rest.

Chloroquine may cause mild and transient headaches, visual disturbances, gastrointestinal symptoms, and pruritus. The macular retinopathy complicating prolonged courses of large doses will not occur in the relatively short duration of treatment prescribed for amebiasis.

In addition to the hemorrhagic encephalopathy mentioned earlier, adverse reactions from the use of carbarsone include gastrointestinal symptoms, sore throat, hepatitis, pruritus, dermatoses, neuritis, visual disorders, and swelling of ankles, knees, and wrists. Exfoliative dermatitis and hepatic necrosis have been reported as well.

Prevention of sexually acquired amebiasis requires avoidance of oroanal or genitoanal contact with patients who have the disease.

GIARDIASIS

Etiology

Giardiasis is the state of infection with *Giardia lamblia* Stiles 1915, a flagellate protozoan. *Giardia* parasites are found in a wide range of vertebrate species, and it was long thought that the organisms were host-specific. However, it has been found that in many instances infection can be transmitted from one animal host to another of a different species. It is likely that two species infect mammals, *G. muris* in rodents, and *G. lamblia,* at times called *G. duodenalis,* in other warm-blooded vertebrates. *G. intestinalis* and *Lamblia intestinalis* are synonyms used in Western and Eastern Europe, respectively.[39]

The possibility has been raised that there are variations in strains associated with the variability of symptoms found in giardial infection. Recent work, in which *Giardia* from asymptomatic, mildly symptomatic, and more severely ill subjects were used to infect mice, suggested that there were intrinsic differences in virulence among the parasites.[40] It has been my observation, however, that it is not uncommon to find both asymptomatic and moderately symptomatic infections in members of the same family. Evidence for differences among the strains of *G. lamblia* is not as strong as in the case of *E. histolytica.*

The pear-shaped motile trophozoite lives in the upper two thirds of the small intestine, in the duodenum and jejunum. It is 10–20 μm long and 7–10 μm in diameter. Two prominent nuclei and a ventral disklike depression in its anterior portion are characteristic features, as well as four pairs of flagellae by which it moves in a fluttering fashion. The trophozoite is normally at-

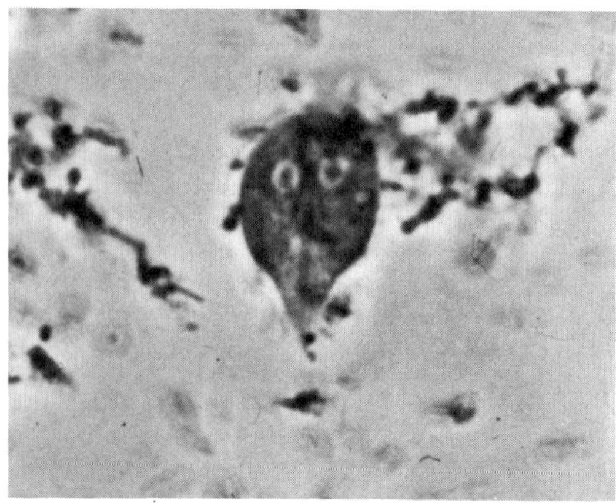

Fig. 17-6 *Giardia lamblia* trophozoite.

tached to the small bowel epithelial surface by means of its disk; in diarrheal cases it may be found in the feces (Figs. 17-6, 17-7).

The cyst of *G. lamblia* is oval, and measures 8–12 by 6–10 μm in size. There are four, occasionally two, nuclei, with a longitudinal division formed by two axostyles and groups of fibrils representing the flagellae (Fig. 17-8). The cyst is the infective stage; it is able to withstand environmental conditions outside the host destructive to the trophozoite. Upon ingestion by a new host, each cyst divides into two motile forms, which leave the cyst and are capable of further binary division as trophozoites.

Epidemiology

Giardiasis is a sporadic infection among people living in countries where sanitary practices are deficient, and it is often found in family clusters with parents and children infected. It is also common among children living in institutions and among adults and children in communal settings.[41] It is believed that in family and institutional environments the parasite is transmitted by fecal contamination from hand to mouth. In larger outbreaks waterborne infection has been implicated. Citywide epidemics and outbreaks in resorts have been traced to in-

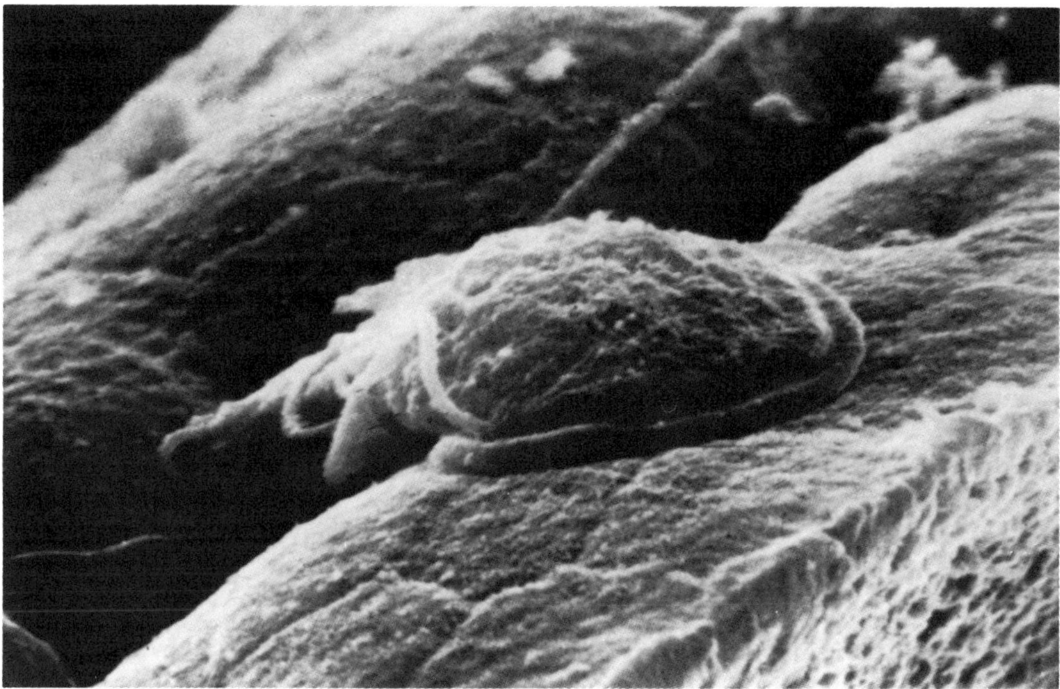

Fig. 17-7 Scanning electron micrograph of a biopsy specimen of the duodenum with a trophozoites of *Giardia lamblia* attached to the surface of the columnar epithelium. (Courtesy of Dr. R. L. Owen. From Katz M, Despommier DD, Gwadz R: Parasitic Diseases. Springer-Verlag, New York, 1982, with permission.)

adequate purification of the water supply. Giardiasis has also affected people undergoing wilderness hardship training, presumably from the ingestion of water infected by wild animal reservoirs.[42]

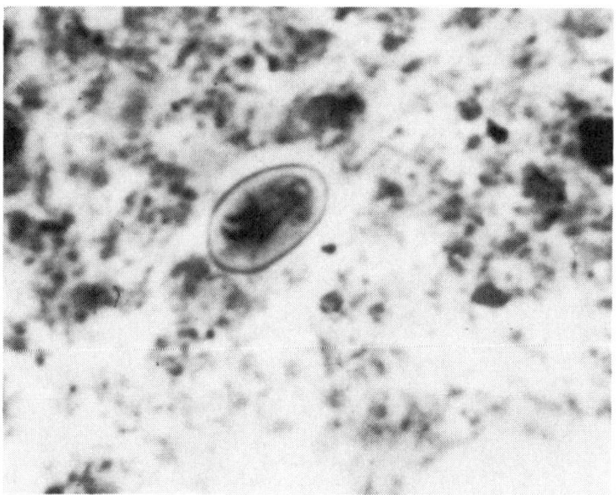

Fig. 17-8 Cyst of *Giardia lamblia*; only two of the nuclei are visible, as the others are out of the focal plane.

Sexual transmission of giardiasis was suggested by Shookhoff[43] and Lynch.[44] The study of the progression of infection within a group of male homosexuals strongly supported this hypothesis.[45] A prospective investigation of intestinal protozoa among homosexuals in New York City demonstrated that 17% harbored *G. lamblia*,[14] and 13% were found infected in a Canadian investigation, whereas there were three infections among 100 presumably heterosexual male controls.[13]

Infection of the human may not require the ingestion of more than 10 cysts.[46] Host factors also play a part in infection. Susceptibility to giardiasis is increased in persons with gastric achlorhydria. Secretory IgA appears to interfere with the adherence of giardial trophozoites to the intestinal mucosa; deficiency of IgA in the intestinal lumen is associated with increased severity of symptoms.

Pathology

In the small intestine trophozoites of *G. lamblia* wander over the mucosal surface and may adhere to the brush border or microvilli of the upper two thirds, the duodenum and jejunum. They have been found between epithelial cells; it is not known what relationship this has to the pathologic change in giardiasis. At times the imprints of the ventrally placed disks are seen in scanning electron micrographs of the mucosa.[42] Villous shortening and even atrophy have been described in giardiasis associated with malabsorption; these findings are often accompanied by lymphocytic infiltration of the lamina propria and epithelium.

Functional changes associated with giardial infection include decreases in disaccharidase activities. They are generally temporary, but occasional patients do have persistent lactase deficiency and lactose intolerance after parasitologic cure of their infection.[47] Diminished fat and vitamin B_{12} absorption indicate that ileal function is impaired even though pathologic changes have not been described in this portion of the small intestine.

The characteristic functional result in giardiasis is the malabsorption syndrome.[42] The reasons for malabsorption are not clearly understood. Direct damage to the microvilli has been described as the cause of the functional changes, but malabsorption may occur even in patients in whom large areas of the mucosa appear to be intact. Physical interference with absorption due to the covering of the surface by trophozoites, and competition between parasite and host for nutritive elements are not likely to be significant reasons for absorptive problems; the number of parasites is probably not enough to cover the absorptive surface nor their mass to preempt nutrition of the host.

The inflammatory response in the submucosa has also been implicated as a possible cause of malabsorption. The production of a soluble toxin has been suggested as an explanation for the functional changes, but evidence for its presence is not conclusive.

Bacterial overgrowth with the presence of fecal organisms in the upper small intestine is common in giardiasis associated with malabsorption; it is not yet clear what part these changes in the microbial flora play in the severity of giardial infection.[48,49]

Clinical Findings

Giardiasis often occurs as an asymptomatic infection. When symptoms are present they range from the mildest epigastric distress and flatulence through diarrheas of increasing severity to malabsorption syndrome with significant weight loss.

Persistent diarrhea is the most common single symptom. A history of diarrhea with abdominal cramping, flatulence, and the passage of foul-smelling stools should arouse strong suspicions of the presence of giardial infection in a person whose travel history or sexual lifestyle indicates a high risk of acquisition of the parasite. Stools tend to be pale and bulky, and tend to float on the surface of the water in the toilet bowl. These signs are also true of the bowel movements of patients with acute viral and bacterial infections, but symptoms tend to be prolonged in giardiasis.

Inasmuch as *G. lamblia* is the most common protozoal disease in the United States it should be sought in all cases of chronic small bowel illness. Instances of giardial proctitis have been described,[50] but cases are rare enough that the diagnosis will in most instances likely be made only after the review of pathologic material from rectal biopsy.

Diagnosis

The diagnosis of *G. lamblia* infection is made by the discovery of trophozoites or cysts in appropriately collected specimens.

The likelihood of finding the parasite on examination of the stool is related to the patterns of excretion that have been demonstrated in series of patients in whom the diagnosis has been established by means of various tests.

In some patients numerous parasites may be found in most specimens examined, and in others the cysts may be so scant that they are missed on routine examination. In still other patients periods of low parasite concentration will alternate with times when organisms are abundant. There is no correlation between the concentration of parasites and the severity of symptoms. *G. lamblia* will be found on initial examination in about one half of infected persons.

Because of the periodicity which has been described, patients in whom giardiasis is strongly suspected should be tested with several stool examinations performed at weekly intervals. The use of a laxative will not increase the likelihood of diagnosis, and may actually diminish the probability of finding organisms.

In addition to the examination of fecal material a number of other techniques are used in the diagnosis of giardiasis. A braided nylon cord in a weighted gelatin capsule, which is swallowed (Enterotest, Hedeco, Palo Alto, California), is withdrawn after a period of four hours, and trophozoites sought in the duodenal contents attached to it.[51] Duodenal aspiration and jejunal biopsy are also used to effect diagnosis. No one technique has been found successful in all instances.

It has been suggested that with the difficulty in making certain that a person does not have giardiasis treatment may be given on the basis of presumptive findings, even though the etiologic agent has not been found. This "therapeutic test" may be disappointing for sexually transmitted giardiasis. There are so many possible alternative diagnoses that the probability of some other cause for the patient's symptoms is relatively high.

Serologic tests for giardiasis may be helpful in reaching a diagnosis,[39] unfortunately such tests are not easily available.

Differential Diagnosis

Many of the conditions listed under the differential diagnosis of amebiasis must be considered when one is attempting to establish the diagnosis of giardiasis. The viral, bacterial, and protozoan infections are frequent causes of confusion. *Candida* suprainfection and irritable bowel syndrome are often difficult to differentiate.

Other causes of malabsorption must also be considered. Gluten enteropathy (celiac sprue) will ordinarily present with a history of childhood disease. Tropical sprue should be considered if the patient has traveled to regions of poor sanitation. It has been noted that malabsorption caused by *Giardia* responds to anti-*Giardia* treatment, while that due to tropical sprue is improved with tetracycline alone.[47]

Treatment

The treatment of sexually transmitted giardiasis is subject to the same general comments made for the management of amebiasis. Gaining the confidence of the patient will help to prevent reinfection, and will make easier the handling of instances in which apparent resistance to treatment leads to the patient's anxiety.

All patients with giardiasis should be treated, even those who are asymptomatic, since they may become sources of infection for others.

Metronidazole is particularly useful in treatment of cases with severe malabsorption as it not only destroys *G. lamblia*, but affects as well the small bowel infection with fecal bacteria that is frequently present. It is administered at a dose of 250 mg three times daily for seven days. It has been reported to clear up to 90% of infections in a single course; treatment may be repeated if necessary. The untoward effects of metronidazole have been described in the section on the treatment of amebiasis.

Quinacrine hydrochloride administered at a dose of 100 mg three times daily for seven days will cure about 80% of patients in a single course; it, too, may be repeated if needed.

The common side effects of the use of quinacrine include dizziness, headaches, nervous symptoms, bad dreams, nausea, and vomiting. The skin (but not the sclerae) may develop a faint yellow tint by the end of treatment. Quinacrine must be avoided in patients with psoriasis in whom it may precipitate exfoliative dermatitis. It is also contraindicated in patients with a history of psychosis.

Furazolidine has also been effective in the treatment of giardiasis at a dose of 100 mg four times daily. Complications of treatment include a disulfiram-type reaction after the ingestion of alcohol. A metabolite is a monoamine-oxidase inhibitor, and hypertension may result if furazolidine is taken with adrenergic agents, certain antidepressants, and foods rich in tyramine. Common symptoms with the use of furazolidine include nausea and vomiting; pruritic rashes have been reported as well.

Prevention of giardiasis requires avoidance of oroanal contacts with infected persons. The patient should also be informed of the widespread distribution of the parasite, and the need to avoid the ingestion of contaminated water in countries of poor sanitation, as well the risks of drinking from what appear to be uncontaminated streams in the wilderness.

REFERENCES

1. Most H: Manhattan: "A tropical isle?" Am J Trop Med Hyg 17:333, 1968
2. Dritz SK, Ainsworth TE, Garrard WF, et al: Patterns of sexually transmitted enteric diseases in a city. Lancet 2:3, 1977
3. William DC, Felman YM, Marr JS, Shookhoff HB: Sexually transmitted enteric pathogens in male homosexual population. NY State J Med 77:2050, 1977
4. Hurwitz AL, Owen RL: Venereal transmission of intestinal parasites. West J Med 128:89, 1978
5. Beaver PC, Jung RC, Sherman HJ, et al: Experimental Entamoeba histolytica infections in man. Am J Trop Med Hyg 5:1000, 1956
6. Dreyer KA: Growth of a strain of Entamoeba histolytica at room temperature. Texas Rep Biol Med 19:393, 1961
7. Richards CS, Goldman M, Cannon LT: Cultivation of Entamoeba histolytica and Entamoeba histolytica-like strains at reduced temperature and behavior of the amebae in diluted media. Am J Trop Med Hyg 15:648, 1966
8. Entner N, Evans LA, Gonzalez C: Genetics of Entamoeba histolytica: Differences in drug sensitivity between Laredo and other strains of Entamoeba histolytica. J Protozool 9:466, 1962
9. Goldman M: Entamoeba histolytica-like amoebae occurring in man. Bull WHO 40:355, 1969
10. Sargeaunt PG, Williams JE, Neal RA: A comparative study of Entamoeba histolytica (NIH:200, HK9, etc), "E. histolytica-like" and other morphologically identical amoeba using isoenzyme electrophoresis. Trans R Soc Trop Med Hyg 74:469, 1980
11. Sargeaunt PG, Williams JE: Electrophoretic enzyme patterns of Entamoeba histolytica and Entamoeba coli. Trans R Soc Trop Med Hyg 72:164, 1978
12. Sargeaunt PG, Oates JK, Maclennan I, et al: Entamoeba histolytica in male homosexuals. Br J Vener Dis 59:193, 1983
13. Keystone JS, Keystone DL, Proctor EM: Intestinal parasitic infections in homosexual men: Prevalence, symptoms and factors in transmission. Can Med Assoc J 123:512, 1980
14. William DC, Shookhoff HB, Felman YM, DeRamos SW: High rates of enteric protozoal infections in selected homosexual men attending a venereal disease clinic. Sex Transm Dis 5:155, 1978

15. World Health Organization: Amoebiasis. WHO Tech Rep Ser 421, 1969
16. William DC: Enteric diseases. Cutis 27:278, 1981
17. Finch R, Burnham WR, Reeve RS: Letter. Br Med J 283:1545, 1981
18. Milgram EA, Healy GR, Kagan IG: Studies on the use of the indirect hemagglutination test in the diagnosis of amebiasis. Gastroenterology 50:645, 1966
19. Matthews HM, Moss DM, Mildvan D, Healy GR: Isoenzyme patterns of Entamoeba species isolated from male homosexuals. The American Society of Parasitologists Annual Meeting, San Antonio, Texas, Dec 4–8, 1983. (Abstract No. 177)
20. Ylvisaker JT, McDonald GB: Sexually acquired amebic colitis and liver abscess. West J Med 132:153, 1980
21. Manson-Bahr PEC, Apted FIC: Amoebiasis, giardiasis and balantidiasis. p 119. In Manson's Tropical Diseases. 18th Ed. Baillière Tindall, London, 1982
22. Purpon I, Jimenez D, Engelking RL: Amebiasis of the penis. J Urol 98:372, 1967
23. Thomas JA, Antony AJ: Amoebiasis of the penis. Br J Urol 48:269, 1976
24. Cohen C: Three cases of amoebiasis of the cervix uteri. Br J Obstet Gynecol 80:476, 1973
25. Mylius RE, ten Seldam REJ: Venereal infection by Entamoeba histolytica in a New Guinea native couple. Trop Geog Med 14:20, 1962
26. Krogstad DJ, Spencer HC, Healy GR, et al: Amebiasis: Epidemiologic studies in the United States 1971–1974. Ann Intern Med 88:89, 1978
27. Stevens DL, Taylor RG, Everett ED, et al: Amebic liver abscess: Report of a case presenting with nonreactive serologic tests for Entamoeba histolytica. Am J Gastroenterol 72:234, 1979
28. Kazal HL, Sohn N, Carrasco JL, et al: The gay bowel syndrome: Clinicopathological correlation in 260 cases. Ann Clin Lab Sci 6:184, 1976
29. Quinn TC, Corey L, Chaffee RG, et al: The etiology of anorectal infections in homosexual men. Am J Med 71:395, 1981
30. Mildvan G, Gelb AM, William D: Venereal transmission of enteric pathogens in male homosexuals; two case reports. JAMA 238:1387, 1977
31. Dritz SK, Braff EH: Letter. N Engl J Med 23:1359, 1977
32. May RG, MacLeod CL, Whiteside ME: Intestinal colonization of Blastocystis hominis in a homosexual male community. The American Society of Tropical Medicine and Hygiene Annual Meeting, San Antonio, Texas, Dec 4–8, 1983, Program No. 148 (Abstract)
33. Centers for Disease Control: Cryptosporidiosis: Assessment of chemotherapy of males with acquired immune deficiency syndrome. MMWR 31:589, 1982
34. Ma P, Soave R: Three-step stool examination for cryptosporidiosis in 10 homosexual men with protracted watery diarrhea. J Infect Dis 14:824, 1983
35. Felman YM, Morrison J: Examining the homosexual male for sexually transmitted diseases. JAMA 238:2046, 1977
36. Kean BH: Venereal amebiasis. NY State J Med 76:930, 1976
37. Sargeaunt PG: Letter. J R Soc Med 75:920, 1982
38. Kovaleski T, Malangoni MA, Wheat LJ: Treatment of an amebic liver abscess with intravenous metronidazole. Arch Intern Med 141:132, 1981
39. Meyer EA, Jarroll EL: Giardiasis. Am J Epidemiol 111:1, 1980
40. Aggarwal A, Bhatia A, Naik SR, Vinayak VK: Variable virulence of isolates of Giardia lamblia in mice. Ann Trop Med Parasitol 77:163, 1983
41. Millet VE, Spencer MJ, Chapin MR, et al: Intestinal protozoan infection in a semicommunal group. Am J Trop Med Hyg 32:54, 1983
42. Stevens DP: Giardiasis: Host-pathogen biology. Rev Infect Dis 4:851, 1982
43. Shookhoff HB: Letter. JAMA 222:1310, 1972
44. Lynch VD: Letter. JAMA 222:1309, 1972
45. Meyers JD, Kuharic HA, Holmes KK: Giardia lamblia infection in homosexual men. Br J Vener Dis 53:54, 1977
46. Rendtorff RC: The experimental transmission of human intestinal protozoan para-

sites. II. Giardia lamblia cysts given in capsules. Am J Hyg 59:209, 1954

47. Manson-Bahr PEC, Apted FIC: Amoebiasis, giardiasis and balantidiasis. p 143. In Manson's Tropical Diseases. 18th Ed. Ballière Tindall, London, 1982

48. Tomkins AM, Wright SG, Drasar BS, James WPT: Colonization of jejunum by enterobacteria and malabsorption in patients with giardiasis. (Abstract). Gut 17:397, 1976

49. Solomons NW: Giardiasis: Nutritional implications. Rev Infect Dis 4:859, 1982

50. Kacker PP: A case of Giardia lamblia proctitis presenting in a V.D. clinic. Br J Vener Dis 49:318, 1973

51. Beal CB, Viens P, Grant RGL, Hughes JM: A new technique for sampling duodenal contents: Demonstration of upper small-bowel pathogens. Am J Trop Med Hyg 19:349, 1970

18

Rectal Surgical Aspects of Sexually Transmitted Diseases and Sexual Trauma

Norman Sohn

There are several sexually related conditions of male homosexuals that will require attention by a surgeon. These include various traumatic affections, sexually acquired infections, complications in immunocompromised individuals, and premalignant and malignant conditions.

It is very important in assessing the patient with rectal trauma or one who is suspected of having a rectal manifestation of a sexually transmitted disease to ascertain the nature and type of the patient's sexual preferences. Appearance, occupation, and mode of dress can be misleading, and the patient must be questioned directly as to the type and frequency of rectal sexual experiences.[1]

In general, proctogenital intercourse is not associated with any significant rectal trauma. Digital rectal examination in many male homosexuals, who frequently engage in proctogenital intercourse, will reveal diminished anal sphincter tone. In reality this represents voluntary cooperation of the patient with the physician in order to facilitate examination. Incontinence is rarely associated with this finding except where there is overt evidence of prior traumatic disruption of the anorectal sphincters. The "O" sign is used to describe the patient who is able to voluntarily maintain his anus in a dilated position. This generally occurs only in patients who have engaged in frequent anal intercourse.

SYMPTOM ANALYSIS

Rectal pain is a common symptom. This can be due to hemorrhoids, fissures, and abscesses. Hemorrhoid pain typically is worse at the onset, and then progressively diminishes. Pain due to a fissure commonly has its onset following defecation, lasts for several minutes to several hours, and then subsides until the next defecation. The abscess pain pattern is one of continuously increasing rectal pain until the abscess is drained or drains spontaneously. These pain patterns are characteristic and frequently point to the correct diagnosis even prior to actual examination of the patient. In the male homosexual, gonococcal proctitis, anal herpes simplex, cytomegaloviral diseases, anorectal candidiasis, and lues also are causes of rectal pain.

Rectal bleeding can be caused by anal fissures, hemorrhoids, benign and malignant neoplasms, or specific or nonspecific inflammatory bowel disease. It can also be due to minor trauma incident to participation in rectal sexual activity. Proctocolitis of several possible etiologies can be a source of significant rectal hemorrhage. The acquired idiopathic thrombocytopenic purpura syndrome can also accompany any of these possible etiologies of rectal bleeding. These patients should all be investigated for coagulopathies. In particular, rectal biopsies should not be obtained until these bleeding parameters have been investigated.

Major bleeding rarely follows proctogenital intercourse. Fist fornication, however, is more commonly associated with significant bleeding. This can be immediate or delayed. Heavy rectal bleeding can also occur following diagnostic rectal biopsy. Other cases have been caused by trauma secondary to the use of rectal foreign bodies.

Since much of the bleeding thus far discussed occurs from within the distal portion of the colon and rectum it lends itself to rapid and easy correction. Direct pressure with a cotton-tipped applicator, which may be soaked with a dilute epinephrine solution, often will stop minor bleeding but usually will not be effective for major bleeding. Electrocoagulation can often be effectively used. A mucosal bleeding site can often be rubber band-ligated with a hemorrhoid ligator.

Local anesthesia will permit the use of rectal retractors permitting direct suturing of bleeding sites. Local anesthesia can be administered by injecting subcutaneously and submucosally $\frac{1}{2}$% bupivicaine, usually with epinepherine 1:200,000. Hyaluronidase, 150 units per 10–15 ml of anesthetic solution is added to the anesthetic solution. Transanal suturing is effective for bleeding up to the 7- to 8-cm level above the anal verge. Hemostatic staples also can be applied with a specially designed applicator through a sigmoidoscope.[2]

FIST FORNICATION

Fist fornication can result in either anorectal trauma or in colonic or intraperitoneal rectal trauma.[3] The anorectal trauma usually occurs in novices in this activity and has been known to occur in patients subjected to "fist rape." Mucosal injuries as well as sphincter injuries can occur. Hemorrhage must be controlled, infection must be controlled or prevented, and sphincter injuries must be repaired either as a primary procedure or at a later date. The same techniques mentioned above for control of rectal bleeding in general can be applied to traumatic mucosal lacerations due to fist fornication. Often the introduction of local anesthesia with direct suturing of the bleeding site and mucosa is performed. It is not necessary to repair the mucosal defect, as spontaneous healing is likely to ensue. Suturing may be required around the borders of the mucosal laceration in order to control bleeding. Management of sphincter lacerations will be described below.

Intraperitoneal rectal perforations or colonic perforations also are well-known complications of fist fornication. Recurrent fist fornication perforations of the colon have also been seen on a number of occcasions. The frequent concomitant use of drugs, or the fear or anxiety of presenting himself to the medical community as a result of this embarrassing complication, can result in delay of presentation. Delays of 24–36 hours have been known to occur. These patients require a prompt laparotomy. A delay in order to correct overt fluid and electrolyte imbalances may be necessary. The patient should be started promptly on broad-spectrum antibiotics. The most effective way of managing this intraperitoneal laceration has been found to be resection of the involved segment without reanastomosis. The proximal end of the bowel is brought out as a sigmoid colostomy, and the distal end either can be brought out as a sigmoid mucous fistula or, as is more common when the laceration occurs too distal to facilitate exteriorization, it can be stapled or oversewn as a Hartmann pouch. The abdomen should be drained and broad-spectrum antibiotics continued.

We generally defer reoperation for restortation of intestinal continuity for a minimum of three months. It is anticipated that the infection would be controlled, the patient's general homeostasis will be restored, and the reoperation, which can be technically trying, can be undertaken in a healthy patient.

A simplified technique for reestablishment of intestinal continuity with the use of an end-to-end anastomosis staple device has been described.[4] In the initial operation it is important not to mobilize the rectum from the sacrum unless this is necessary to complete closure of the Hartmann pouch. At a subsequent reoperation the rectal segment can easily be found immediately anterior to the sacrum. Various devices and techniques have been described to facilitate its identification, but these have been found not to be necessary if the surgeon merely looks anterior to the sacrum. Most of the difficulties in that operation are due to small bowel adherent in the pelvis usually to the sutured cut end of the rectum.

Hand infections in the patient administering the fist fornication secondary to stool-contaminating previous lacerations have also been seen, and this can result in a nasty infection.

A syndrome of pelvic cellulitis following rectal sexual trauma, usually fist fornication, has been described.[5] The patient presents two or more days following such an episode with fever, rectal pain, lower abdominal tenderness, or rectal discharge. Examination reveals rectal tenderness, mild proctitis, and no evidence of a perirectal abscess.

This syndrome is felt to be due to pelvic cellulitis secondary to microperforations about the rectum. These patients generally respond to broad-spectrum antibiotics. Depending on the severity of the clinical presentation, hospitalization for intensive broad-spectrum antibiotics and careful observation to assess the need for laparotomy is often required.

It may be difficult to distinguish between pelvic cellulitis as described above, which would be expected to respond to nonoperative treatment, and intraperitoneal perforation, for which laparotomy is mandatory. The first patient with this syndrome that we cared for was taken to the operating room; after 48 hours of intensive intravenous antibiotics, with continued fever and suspected sepsis. At the time of operation retroperitoneal edema on the right and left side was identified. A sigmoid colostomy was performed, and the pelvis was drained. This patient's condition rapidly improved. In view of the findings, the subsequent patients were managed nonoperatively and all successfully.

A supralevator abscess or infection in the supralevator space is probably responsible for the frightening signs of pelvic peritonitis. This entity must be sought, for if a supralevator abscess is identified, then drainage is indicated. This condition must be distinguished from nonspecific or specific proctocolitis, which can give the sigmoidoscopic picture of inflammation and purulent discharge. The signs of pelvic peritonitis usually are absent.

FOREIGN BODIES

Foreign bodies of various types are utilized by the male homosexual for sexual gratification. In my personal series of over

175 patients with retained rectal foreign bodies, 2 were females, 2 were heterosexual males, and the remainder were all male homosexuals.

The patient usually presents with information that there is a retained foreign body which he is unable to spontaneously pass per rectum. My protocol for management includes initial assessment for the possibility of intraperitoneal perforation. In the usual situation in which there is no suspicion of an intraperitoneal perforation, which may be confirmed by physical examination or x-ray of the chest and abdomen, digital rectal examination is performed.[6] The foreign body can usually be palpated in the midrectum. At this point there is an angulation of the anorectum, which prevents further passage of the foreign body. If the foreign body is not palpated, the patient is generally hospitalized, where peristalsis usually carries the foreign body to the point described above.

When the foreign body is palpated, local anesthesia is administered (see above for technique). A suitable retractor is placed in the rectum and the foreign body is grasped, deflected anteriorly, and removed. Sigmoidoscopy is then performed to determine the possibility of mucosal or transmural trauma to the rectum.

Using this protocol, of 175 cases, 172 were successfully removed, usually on an ambulatory basis. In 3 patients transanal removal could not be effected. In 2 cases a transanal removal was possible under general anesthesia. One was a large yam, which had absorbed fluid in the 24 hours that it was in place before the patient presented to the physician. The yam was carved up into small pieces utilizing an operating proctoscope and a uterine curette. When it was whittled away sufficiently it could be removed transanally. The other foreign body that required general anesthesia was in a patient who had twice been resected for fist-induced perforations of the rectosigmoid. During one of the operations the spleen was removed. The foreign body was a large latex dildo, which was fixed to the splenic flexure. When it would be retracted toward the rectosigmoid it was repeatedly "sucked" up back toward the splenic flexure. A female surgeon with a small hand was able to insert her entire hand into the anus, grab the foreign body and thereby remove it.

The only patient who required laparotomy was one in whom a 4-inch stainless steel ball bearing was stuck in the sigmoid. There was edema distal to it and this prevented its passage toward the rectum. At laparotomy the foreign body was milked toward the anus where it was easily removed.

Other foreign bodies which have been identified in this population include penile rings in which a ring is placed through the full thickness of the penile urethra. In the few patients we have seen, this has been a harmless occurrence.

There are other unusual surgical manifestations of sexually related diseases that will present to the surgeon. One of these is prepuce fixation.[7] Four cases in non-Jewish, nonpsychotic male homosexuals have been described in which the fixation with the prepuce led to a foreskin reconstruction by plastic surgical technique. Fournier's gangrene of the perineum has also been recognized as a complication of homosexual activity.[8] This can be a very dramatic life-threatening infection. Gangrene or gas gangrene occurs in the perirectal, perineal, and scrotal tissues. This requires broad-spectrum antibiotics and radical debridement. Liver abscesses have also been described in the male homosexual population both with and without amoebas present.[9]

Incontinence in the male homosexual can be due to sphincter injuries, usually secondary to a fist injury or foreign body injury to the muscles of the lower rectum. Sphincter injuries consequent to operations performed for the treatment of anal fistulas also occur.

Traumatic sphincter injuries that occur following sexual activity, if recognized early and the patient's general condition is satisfactory and there is limited amount of contamination, lend themselves to primary repair. The patient can be taken to the operating room, the bowel evacuated, cleansed, and prepared, allowing a primary repair by direct suture of the cut ends of the sphincter to be attempted. More commonly this repair is best left for another date. The patient can be maintained on hyperalimentation in an effort to get the cut edges of the wound to heal and then can be taken to the operating room where secondary repair can be attempted.[10] When attempts at repair by direct suturing of the cut ends of the sphincter either directly to itself or in vest-over-pants fashion have failed, the possibility of fully restoring continence is impaired. A gracilis muscle transplant can be utilized or a Thiersch wire can be inserted. In general, the gracilis muscle is preferred, particularly in a young patient. In the patient over the age of 50, where the results of gracilis muscle transplants are less satisfactory, the Thiersch procedure can be attempted. A Thiersch procedure involves merely the insertion of a circumanal wire. This is a very simple operation, which can enhance continence with minimal potential for its exacerbation.

Rectal prolapse is also seen in the male homosexual population. Most of these occur in patients who have had a trauma to their sphincter mechanism. This trauma, perhaps as a result of associated infection, can result in prolapse. It has also been seen to occur in patients who have had extensive surgery for anal fistulas. Prolapse can be repaired intraabdominally by means of a Ripstein procedure. In this operation a sling of Marlex or Teflon is placed around the rectum and this is then utilized to anchor the rectum to the sacrum. Perineal repairs also can be accomplished particularly by means of a Thiersch procedure or modified Thiersch procedure. If incontinence is associated with this problem a perineal repair directed toward correction of any sphincter defect is indicated if there is no obvious anatomic defect in the sphincters its correction is more difficult and probably would depend on the Thiersch operation or one of its modifications.

HEMORRHOIDS, FISSURES, FISTULAS

Contrary to other reports which have appeared in the literature, the author has observed no increase in symptoms due to hemorrhoids in the male homosexual population.[11] It is further apparent that there are fewer problems with hemorrhoids and with anal fissures in this population. Indeed the popularity in some centers, for the treatment of hemorrhoids by means of maximal anal dilatation, and its reputed efficacy would indicate that rectal dilatations might prevent hemorrhoidal problems from occurring. Likewise anal dilatation, while usually not the preferred technique for treating anal fissures, is yet a well-recognized effective treatment for them. Thus the clinical observation of lack of hemorrhoidal problems or anal fissures in the male homosexual has a theoretical basis in fact.

Rectal abscesses and fistulas appear to occur more frequently in the male homosexual. These infections are believed to arise as intermuscular (intersphincteric) abscesses.[12] Infection occurs in the anal glands which empty into the crypts of Morgagni and thereby gain access to the intermuscular space. The abscess here can then progress and extend and result in characteristically located perirectal abscesses and fistulas. Mere drainage of the perirectal abscess can convert it into an anal fistula. Definitive treatment of an anal fistula requires adequate drainage of the intermuscular component. Gonococcal proctitis is often seen to cause purulent infection in the crypts of Morgagni. It may be the gonococcal rectal infection that predisposes the male homosexual to rectal abscesses and fistulas.

CONDYLOMA ACUMINATA

Condyloma acuminata can usually be easily diagnosed on visual inspection of the perianal region or the lower anus. The warts appear as a velvety type of growth either flat or appear as a "sessile polyp." Biopsy of the warts can often unmask other associated pathology. Biopsy of all patients with warts should be considered particularly if the warts have an unusual appearance or occur in the absence of anal intercourse or are present in patients over the age of 45.

Warts can be divided into perianal and intraanal. Most patients have intraanal lesions, either alone or in combination with perianal lesions. In only about 5% of the male homosexual population are the warts solely perianal in location. Treatment of warts is difficult as frequent recurrences are common. Initial therapy directed toward the perianal warts consists of the topical application of podophyllum. Podophyllum either as 25% or 50% solution, in tincture of benzoin, is applied directly to the wart. Care is taken to avoid contaminating the surrounding normal skin with podophyllum. The patient is instructed to wash thoroughly 4 to 8 hours after the application in order to avoid severe perianal ulceration due to the podophyllum. After the podophyllum is in place a bland talcum powder or cornstarch is applied over it to avoid contact of the contiguous areas of the skin with the it. Failure to wash off the podophyllum or its intraanal use can be associated with very painful ulceration.

Those perianal warts which fail to respond to podophyllum, or those which are intraanal in location, can be treated by chemical cauterization utilizing topical bichloracetic acid.[13] Bichloracetic acid is applied directly to the wart, care being taken to avoid its application in normal skin.

Within a matter of 15 to 45 seconds the treated tissue turns white.

Treatments are given at intervals of one to three weeks depending on the amount of post treatment pain which is anticipated. Podophyllum therapy tends to be less painful than bichloracetic acid therapy thus permitting more frequent treatments. Those warts which fail to respond to the bichloracetic acid are treated by means of electrocauterization.

The area to be electrocoagulated is first infiltrated by inserting a needle through normal skin and mucosa adjacent to the wart and infiltrating lidocaine or other suitable local anesthetic. A metal ball tip coagulating electrode is then utilized to apply a current to the wart. After it is destroyed it is generally curetted and the area is electrocoagulated again. This form of therapy tends to be the most painful. When severe posttreatment pain is anticipated or when there are other associated rectal conditions which require surgery, the treatment may be best performed on an inpatient basis. This facilitates postoperative care. Since there is nothing uniquely available in a hospital operating room for the wart patient, this approach is generally discouraged and patients are almost always treated in the office.

Warts which persistently recur are then treated with topical 5-fluorouracil [5-FU (Efudex)] cream. This is applied with a finger cot, between once a day and once every three days beginning a few days after the local destructive therapy is administered. The 5-FU is commenced when it can be reasonably well tolerated.

Laser photocoagulation has been attempted and has been found to offer no advantages over electrocoagulation and is considerably more expensive.[14] Cryosurgical destruction of the warts has also been utilized and has been found to be more time-consuming, just as painful and associated with an inordinately high number of recurrences in anal warts. It has also declined in popularity.

Occasionally a wart will behave as a locally agressive invasive carcinoma analagous to a basal cell epithelioma. This entity is known as a Buschke-Lowenstein tumor and is treated by wide local excision.[15]

Condyloma acuminata can be associated with Bowen's disease or squamous carcinoma. Bowen's disease is quite common in the male homosexual population. There are two forms; Bowenoid papulosis which is intraepithelial carcinoma occurring in patients who have had condyloma acuminata. Long follow-up of these patients has revealed a minimal propensity for the conversion of these lesions into frankly invasive carcinoma. These are treated by means of local excision or topical 5-FU therapy.

The other type, true Bowen's disease or intraepithelial carcinoma, has also been found to occur more frequently in the male homosexual population. This is treated by total excision. This can usually best be accomplished in two stages performing what is in effect two extensive hemorrhoidectomies. The interval between the two operations is in the range of 3 to 4 months in order to permit complete healing. The residual skin is easily identified adjacent to the new scars and can be excised. Alternative means of treating this by means of a single excision with split thickness skin grafting also can be performed but this results in more prolonged hospitalization, more prolonged morbidity with no improvement in the overall results. Bowen's disease is associated with degeneration to squamous carcinoma and with remote site carcinomas.

An increased number of squamous cell carcinomas has been seen in the male homosexual population. These may be related to the condyloma acuminata or to undefined factors including immunosuppression or other viral infections. Squamous carcinoma is treated by combination of chemotherapy and radiation therapy with surgical excision or abdominoperineal resection reserved for failures.[16]

The patient is admitted and on day one he is given mitomycin C and a continuous intravenous infusion of 5-FU is commenced. He is also given radiation therapy consisting of 3,000 R commencing on day one. He is readmitted on day 28 for an additional course of 5-FU and then approximately two weeks later the site of the carcinoma is excised. If there is no residual carcinoma nothing further is done except for periodic observation. If carcinoma continues to be present abdominoperineal resection is generally recommended. Studies with alternate forms of chemotherapy in the initial failures are also under way.

Cloacogenic carcinoma also has been noted in the homosexual population.[17] The protocol of combination chemotherapy and radiation therapy with deferred surgery described above for squamous carcinoma originally was introduced for cloacogenic carcinoma and this same protocol is generally applied. True adenocarcinoma of the rectum also can occur in male homosexuals but and there are statistics which show that their risk is increased.[18]

Some homosexual patients will require a proctectomy or a panproctocolectomy during the course of treatment of anorectal neoplasms or in the management of inflammatory bowel disease, specific or nonspecific. Many homosexual patients can be rehabilitated and will adjust to living with the stoma. However, many patients have been seen in whom this adjustment has been impossible. The unusual dependence of the male homosexual patient on his rectum for sexual gratification can evolve into a severe depression and emotional trauma when the rectum has to be surgically excised. Consequently, the avoidance of a permanent stoma should be absolutely attempted wherever this can possibly be performed without compromising the chances of curing the condition for which the stoma is being recommended. For carcinomas of the anus or lower rectum, the approach of chemotherapy and radiation therapy described above can result in preserving the anus and rectum. Electrocoagulation or intracavitary radiation therapy also may be applicable for the patient with a rectal carcinoma.[19,20] Sphincter-saving techniques incorporating low anterior resection, restorative operations involving the newer intestinal stapling devices, abdominotranssacral resections, abdominotransanal resections, or pull-through operations have to be strongly considered in the male homosexual population.

The sphincter saving approach to the patient with ulcerative colitis is particularly relevant to the male homosexual patient.[21] An operation can be performed in which the colon is removed, the rectal mucosa is excised and the seromuscular coat and sphincter muscles of the rectum can be preserved. This operation is effective for patients with ulcerative colitis. It effects total eradication of the diseased tissue, yet preserves the important mechanism for sphincter control and continence.

Kaposi's sarcoma occurs with increased incidence in the male homosexual population with AIDS. Rectal involvement by the Kaposi's sarcoma or its initial presentation in the rectum is quite common. These lesions appear as submucosal, purple, spongy, irregularly shaped lesions. These are quite vascular and can bleed readily. In biopsying these, in order to avoid hemorrhage, it is often advisable to first grasp the site to be biopsied and withdraw it through the ligator drum of the hemorrhoid ligator and release the rubber band. This then ligates the mucosa at the base of this lesion and the lesion can then be biopsied without the risk of bleeding.

The AIDS patient will sometimes develop severely painful perianal ulcerations, usually due to cytomegalovirus or herpes. These lesions can also cause heavy rectal bleeding. Careful examination should be performed to exclude the possibility that the pain is due to an abscess. Treatment is symptomatic. The usual remedies directed toward relief of rectal pain can be offered. The author has found that Stomahesive powder, liberally applied to the perianal regions, can result in pain relief. Persistent bleeding should be treated by examination under local, regional or general anesthesia and suture ligation of bleeding sites.

The AIDS patient heals rectal wounds poorly. This possibility should be considered in the male homosexual who is being evaluated for elective rectal surgery. In the performance of essential rectal surgery in the AIDS patient or in the patient in whom AIDS cannot be definitively excluded, the principles of rectal surgery in the Crohn's disease patient is particularly relevant here.[22] The partial internal anal sphincterectomy is useful in the treatment of fistulous abscesses because it utilizes a predominantly intrarectal incision and spares the external sphincter. Other approaches which avoid large perirectal wounds, which may not heal, are also useful.

REFERENCES

1. Sohn N, Robilotti JG Jr: The gay bowel syndrome. Am J Gastroenterol 67:478, 1977
2. Sohn N, Weinstein MA, Robbins RD: Anorectal disorders. Cur Probl Surg 20;1, 1983
3. Sohn N, Weinstein MA, Gonchar J: Social injuries of the rectum. Am J Surg 134:611, 1977
4. Robbins RD, Sohn N, Weinstein MA, Steichen FM: Simplified technique utilizing EEA suture device for re-establishing intestinal continuity following Hartmann's operation. Coloproctology 3:4, 1983
5. Weinstein MA, Sohn N, Robbins RD: Syndrome of pelvic cellulitis following rectal sexual trauma. Am J Gastroenterol 75:380, 1981
6. Sohn N, Weinstein MA: Office removal of foreign bodies of the rectum. Surg Gynecol Obstet 146:209, 1978
7. Mohl PC, Adams R, Greer DM: Prepuce restoration seekers: Psychiatric results. Arch Sex Behav 10:383, 1981
8. Bernstein SM, Celano T, Sibulkin D: Fournier's gangrene of the penis. South Med J 69:1242, 1976

9. Thompson JE Jr, Freischlag J, Thomas DS: Amoebic liver abscess in a homosexual man. J Sex Transm Dis 10:153, 1983

10. Sohn N, Weinstein MA: Use of total parenteral nutrition as a "medical colostomy" in management of severe lacerations of the anal sphincter: Report of a case. Dis Colon Rectum 20:695, 1977

11. Turell R: Sexual problems as seen by a proctologist. NY State J Med 75:697, 1974

12. Parks AG, Thompson JPS: Intersphincteric abscess. Br Med J 2:537, 1973

13. Swerdlow DB, Salvati EP: Condyloma acuminatum. Dis Colon Rectum 14:226, 1971

14. Billingham RP, Lewis FG: Laser vs. electrical cautery in the treatment of condylomata acuminata of the anus. Surg Gynecol Obstet 155:865, 1982

15. Balthazar EJ, Streiter M, Megibow AJ: Anorectal giant condyloma acuminata (Bushke-Loewenstein tumor): CT and radiographic manifestations. Radiology 150:651, 1984

16. Nigro ND, Seydel HG, Considine B, et al: Combined preoperative radiation and chemotherapy for squamous cell carcinoma of the anal canal. Cancer 51:826, 1983

17. Cooper HS, Patchefsky AS, Marks G: Cloacogenic carcinoma of the anorectum in homosexual men: An observation of 4 cases. Dis Colon Rectum, 22:557, 1979

18. Daling JR, Weiss NS, Klopfenstein LL: Correlates of homosexual behavior and the incidence of anal cancer. JAMA 247:1988, 1982

19. Hughes EP Jr, Veidenheimer MC, Corman ML, et al: Electrocoagulation of rectal cancer. Dis Colon Rectum 25:215, 1982

20. Sischy B: The place of radiotherapy in the management of rectal adenocarcinoma. Cancer 50 (Suppl 11):2631, 1982

21. Rothenberger DA, Vermeulen FD, Christenson CE: Restorative proctocolectomy with ileal reservoir and ileoanal anastomosis. Am J Surg 145:82, 1983

22. Sohn N, Korelitz BI: Local operative treatment of anorectal Chrohn's disease. J Clin Gastroenterol 4:395, 1982

19

Sexual Behavior in America: Implications for the Control of Sexually Transmitted Diseases

William W. Darrow

Three questions are raised in this chapter: (1) Are sexually transmitted diseases (STD) epidemic in the United States? (2) Has there been a sexual revolution in America? (3) What is the relationship between changing patterns of sexual behavior and changing patterns of STD?

EPIDEMIC SEXUALLY TRANSMITTED DISEASES

Of the three questions to be addressed in this chapter, the first is the easiest to answer because we have adequate data on two STD, syphilis and gonorrhea, and we have an operational definition of an epidemic. An epidemic is said to occur when the number of cases of a medical problem in an area clearly exceeds normal expectations.[1] Most of us look at annual trends and decide for ourselves whether or not there is an epidemic. For others, an excess of cases at least two standard deviations above the mean* might consititute an epidemic.[2] Cases of syphilis and gonorrhea have been reported from all states since 1919,[3] so we can look at available data and determine if the United States experienced an epidemic of venereal diseases during the past two decades.

Figure 19-1 shows a 10-year moving average of reported cases of gonorrhea, the 95% confidence limit above the mean, and the number of cases reported annually for civilian residents of the United States. The 10-year moving average was calculated for 1960 from reports for the period 1950–1959, for 1961 from reports for the period 1951–1960, and so on. Similarly, the upper limit of variation around the mean was calculated and shown to change over time. Reported cases exceeded the mean but not the upper

---

* Using weekly mortality reports, Serfling[2] set the epidemic threshold for influenza at 1.64 standard deviations above the trend line.

261

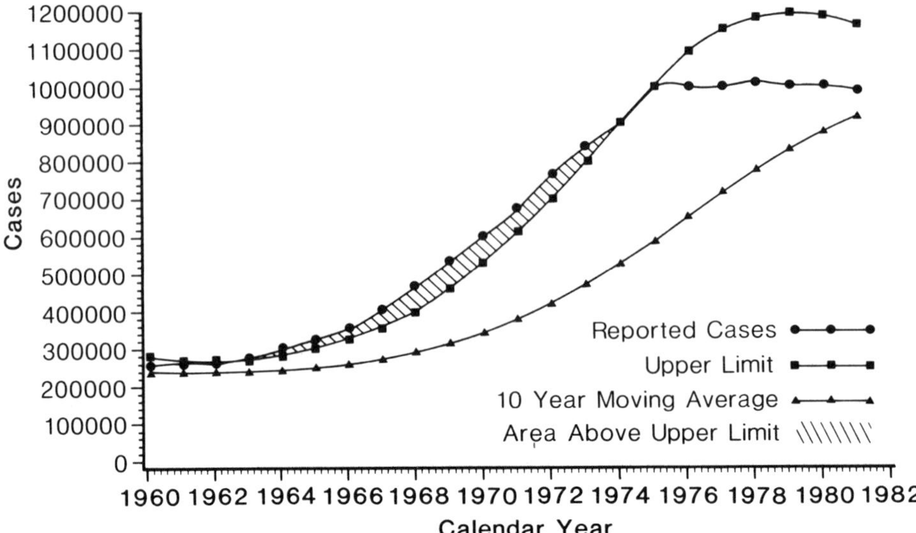

Fig. 19-1 Gonorrhea: United States, 1960–1982.

limit from 1960 to 1963, exceeded the upper limit from 1964 to 1974, and fell back within the upper limit after 1975. When we invoke the operational definition suggested earlier, we conclude that gonorrhea was "epidemic" in the United States for 11 years, from 1964 to 1974, but was not epidemic after that.

Figure 19-2 portrays trends for reported cases of infectious (primary and secondary) syphilis in the United States. The trend for expected cases rises in a fashion similar to the one portrayed for gonorrhea. The 95% confidence interval above the mean was found to fluctuate considerably. Interestingly, the number of cases of infectious syphilis reported in the United States exceeded the upper limit in two different periods: before 1963 and after 1980. Thus, we might conclude that infectious syphilis was

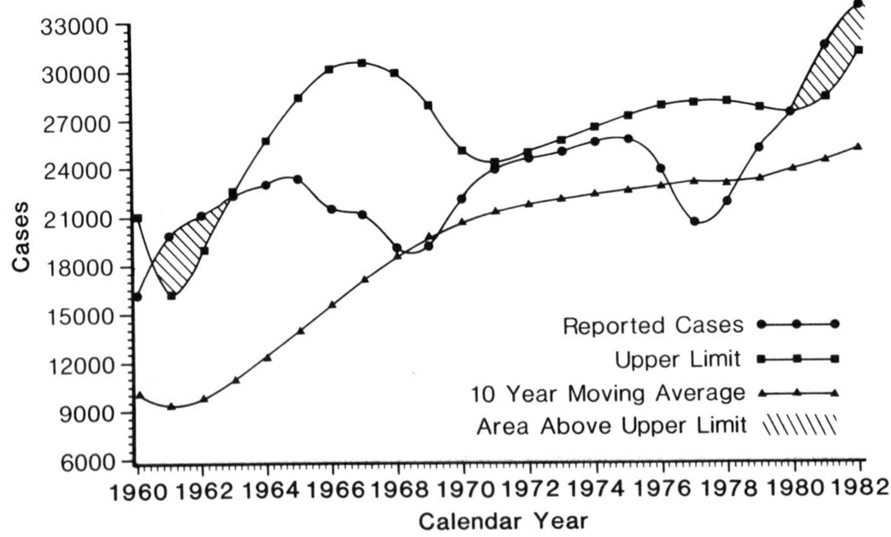

Fig. 19-2 Infectious syphilis: United States, 1960–1982.

epidemic for several years before 1963 and appears to be epidemic today. However, while gonorrhea was epidemic in America, infectious syphilis was not.

How shall we explain this intriguing finding? Those of us who worked so hard during the 1960s might argue that our efforts to eradicate syphilis kept the number of cases of infectious syphilis to a minimum during that decade.[4] When we shifted resources to control gonorrhea in the 1970s,[5] cases of infectious syphilis began to rise once again.

Even if we accept the argument that control programs have been successful in the United States, we imply that syphilis and gonorrhea are two different diseases that require two different control strategies. Furthermore, these two different diseases could occur in two different sexually active populations that are relatively independent of one another. In order to examine this hypothesis of different "social causes" for each of the STD, we must look at trends in sexual behavior in various segments of American society.

Unfortunately, data on trends in sexual behaviors do not go back in time as far as data on syphilis and gonorrhea. In fact, if it were not for the intellectual curiosity and courage of Alfred C. Kinsey,[6] we might not have any data on sexual behavior at all.

PROFESSOR KINSEY AND THE SEXUAL REVOLUTION

Professor Kinsey was a biologist at Indiana University who could readily explain the reproductive cycle of gall wasps, but could not answer the questions of his students regarding their own sexuality. As a scholar, he went to the library and read hundreds of articles about the sexual behavior of human beings. Few measured up to his scientific standards. So Professor Kinsey decided to gather his own data on the "sexual outlets" of his students, those who invited him to speak at their meetings,

and anyone else who voluntarily agreed to be interviewed.

His approach to human volunteers was like his approach to insects. He went into the field in order to gather and record information on those who happened to be in the same place at the same time. His goal was to interview 100,000 subjects, but he literally worked himself to death well before ever coming close to reaching his goal.

In 1948, ten years into his study, he published some preliminary findings on the sexual behaviors of 5,300 white men interviewed by himself and several colleagues.[7] The publication of the book, *Sexual Behavior in the Human Male,* turned out to be to the sexual revolution in America what "the shot heard around the world" was to a political revolution started 172 years earlier.[8] Kinsey, Pomeroy, and Martin[7] reported that 73% of American men had had premarital sexual intercourse by the age of 20 years, 69% had had some sexual experience with prostitutes during their lifetimes, and 37% had had some sexual experience with another male that had led to orgasm (Fig. 19-3). About 18% of the white men interviewed had had as much homosexual as heterosexual experience during a period of at least three years between the ages of 16 and 55, and 8% had been exclusively homosexual for at least three of their adult years.

A preliminary report on the sexual behavior patterns of 5,940 white women was published in 1953.[9] Males and females were compared (Fig. 19-4). Results showed that 20% of the women (compared to 73% of men) had engaged in premarital sexual intercourse by the age of 20, 20% of the women (compared to 37% of men) had had some homosexual experience, approximately 9% (8 to 11%) of the women (compared to 18% of men) had had equal amounts of homosexual and heterosexual experience for at least three years, and 4 to 5% of the women (compared to 8% of men) had been exclusively homosexual for at least three years. No women had had ex-

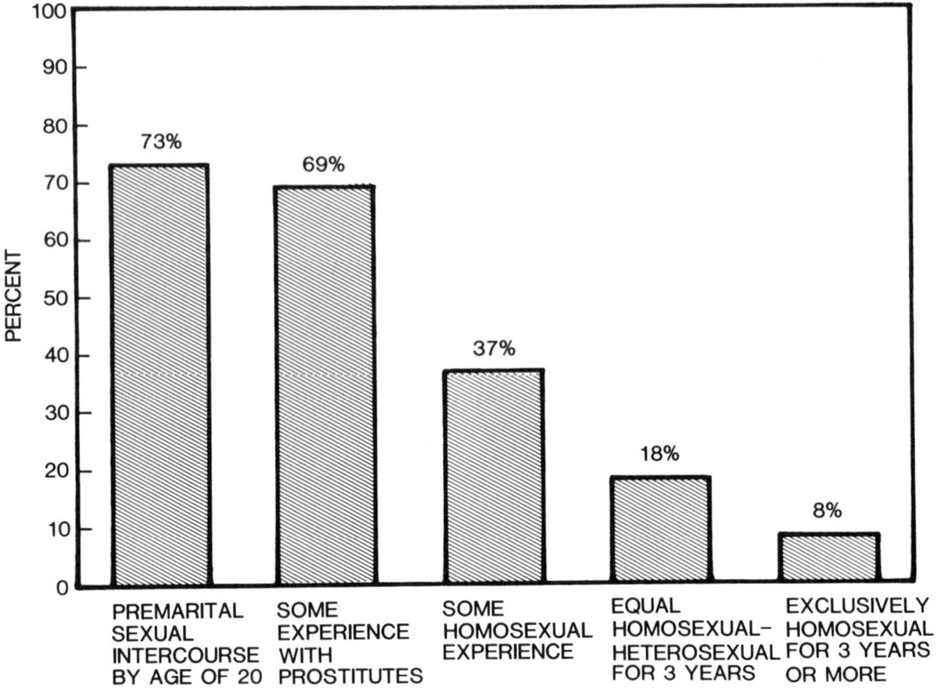

Fig. 19-3 Sexual behavior in American males. (Data from Kinsey AC, Pomeroy WB, Martin CE: Sexual Behavior in the Human Male. Saunders, Philadelphia, 1948.)

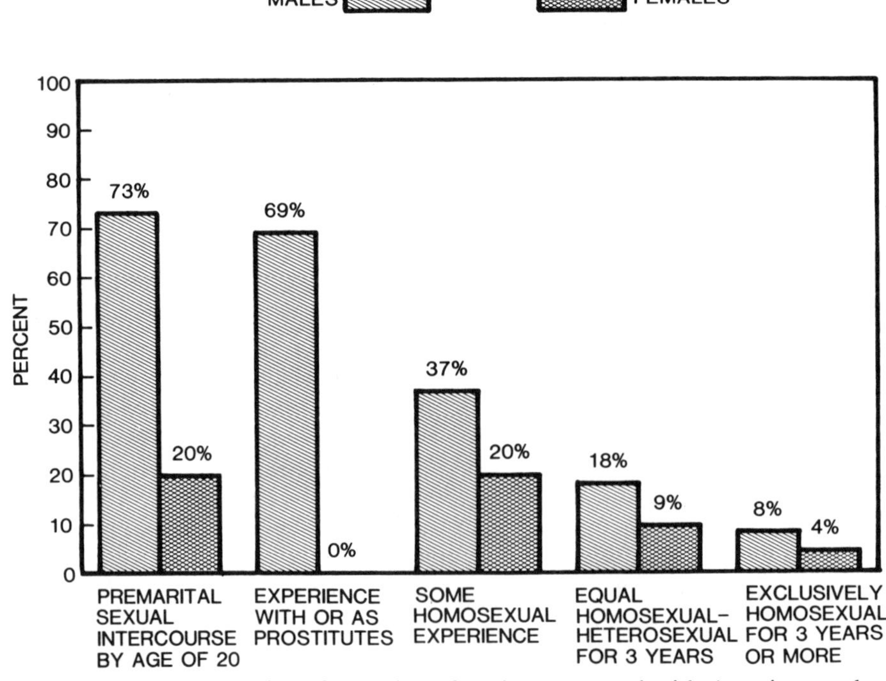

Fig. 19-4 Sexual behavior of American females compared with American males.

perience as prostitutes in this study because all who had been prostitutes were eliminated from the study sample.

These findings were attacked on ethical[10] and methodologic[11] grounds. Some said that Kinsey had no right to intrude into the bedrooms of the American people. Others said that his sample was unrepresentative of the population and his measurements, based on respondents' abilities to recall, were flawed. But no one could stop the impact his findings were having on Americans. Beliefs in premarital abstinence and marital fidelity were challenged with convincing evidence of frequent transgressions. New standards for sexual conduct were emerging in twentieth century American society.[12]

Alfred Kinsey suffered his first heart attack in 1953 and died three years later. Support for the type of research he was pursuing was curtailed. Although his Institute for Sex Research still exists, no one has completed the project he started in 1938.

Adolescents

Studies of representative samples of American adolescents have been conducted that permit us to trace their sexual activities during the 1970s. With grants from the National Institute of Child Health and Human Development and several private foundations, John Kantner and Melvin Zelnik gathered data from a national probability sample of 4,600 females aged 15 to 19 in 1971,[13] and another 2,200 in 1976.[14] Results showed that young women were more likely to have engaged in premarital sexual intercourse in 1976 than earlier, had larger numbers of different partners, and had sexual experiences without intense feelings of intimacy.[15]

Approximately 40% of never-married white women 19 years of age had had premarital sexual intercourse in 1971: twice as many as Kinsey and others reported in 1953 (Fig. 19-5). In 1976 the proportion that had

engaged in premarital sexual intercourse increased to 49%. Zelnik and Kantner also provided data on representative samples of young black women in the United States. The proportions of 19-year-old women engaging in premarital sexual intercourse were higher for blacks than whites: 76% for blacks (in contrast to 40% for whites) in 1971 and 84% for blacks (in contrast to 49% for whites) in 1976. Overall, 27% of unmarried women 15 to 19 years of age in the United States had had premarital intercourse in 1971 and 35% in 1976: an increase of 30% in five years.

Unlike Kinsey, Kantner and Zelnik have not been criticized by others on ethical and methodologic grounds.[16] Their findings have generally been accepted as valid.[17] However, they criticized themselves for failing to study the sexual behaviors of the male sexual partners of female adolescents. In 1979 they adjusted their sampling frame to include males as well as females.[18] To compensate for the addition of males, they restricted their study in 1979 to black and white adolescents living in households in metropolitan areas of the United States.

When 19-year-old never-married white women residing in metropolitan areas were considered, the proportion engaging in premarital sexual intercourse increased from 41% in 1971 to 54% in 1976, and to 65% in 1979 (Fig. 19-6). For 19-year-old black women residing in metropolitan areas of the United States, the proportions increased from 78% in 1971 to 84% in 1976, and to 89% in 1979. The proportion of never-married 19-year-old male residents of metropolitan areas engaging in premarital sexual intercourse in 1979 was similar for whites and blacks: 77% for 19-year-old white men and 80% for 19-year-old black men.

Data available from the Bureau of the Census[19] and studies by Kinsey, Kantner and Zelnik, and others allow us to estimate the number of sexually active 15- to 19-year-old women in the United States since World War II (Fig. 19-7). According to Kinsey and

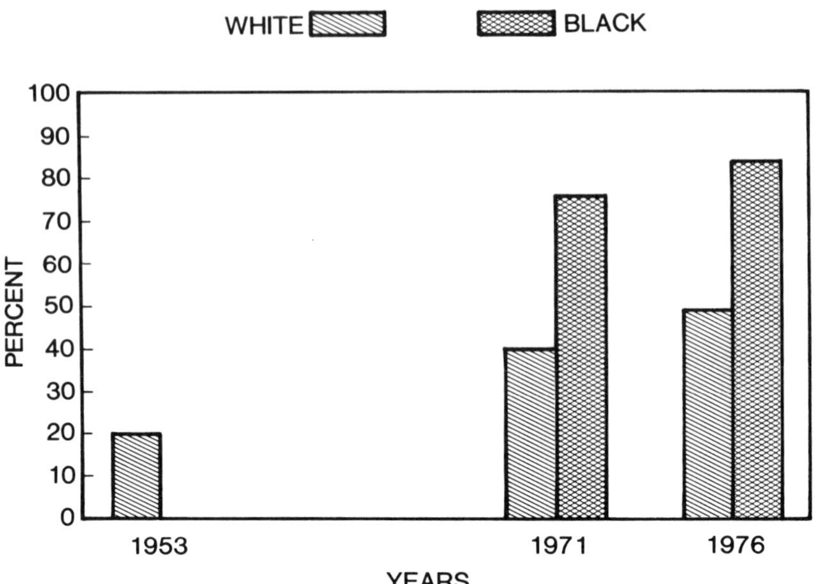

Fig. 19-5 Premarital sexual experience among black and white unmarried females 19 years of age and living in the United States.

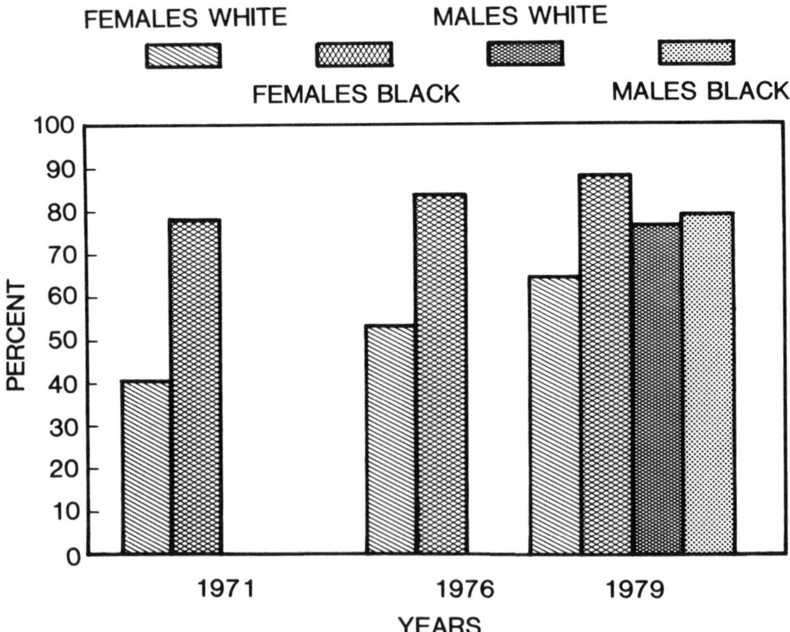

Fig. 19-6 Premarital sexual intercourse among never-married black and white adolescents 19 years of age and living in metropolitan areas of the United States.

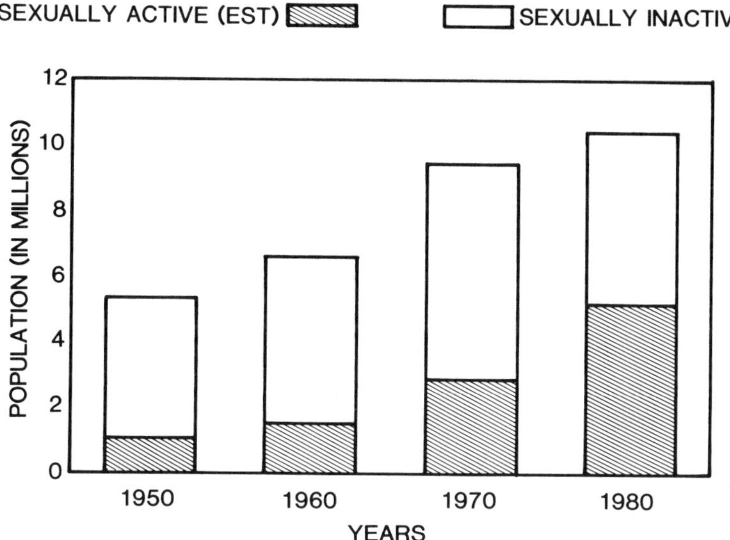

Fig. 19-7 Sexually active females 15–19 years old in the United States: 1950–1980.

his associates, about 20% of 5.3 million females 15 to 19 years old were sexually active in 1950. About 23% of 6.6 million females 15 to 19 years old were sexually active in 1960,[20] so the number of sexually active females 15 to 19 years old increased from about 1.1 million in 1950 to about 1.5 million in 1960. From the cross-sectional studies of Kantner and Zelnik, the number of sexually active females 15 to 19 years old in 1970 and 1980 can be estimated: 2.9 million in 1970 and 5.2 million in 1980. As the population of females 15 to 19 years old doubled from 5.3 million in 1950 to 10.4 million in 1980, the number of sexually active females 15 to 19 years old in the United States increased fivefold: from less than 1.1. million in 1950 to slightly over 5.2 million in 1980.

Kantner and Zelnik conducted a series of three cross-sectional studies instead of a single prospective study because they were unable to raise sufficient funds for a longitudinal study of adolescents. In 1976 Del Elliott and his colleagues at the Behavioral Research Institute (BRI) began a 5-year longitudinal study of the activities of adolescents 11 to 17 years of age.[21] Sexual ac-

tivities in the BRI sample of American youth can be compared with the Kantner-Zelnik sample of teenaged females by individual years of age. For those studied in 1976, Zelnik and Kantner showed an increase in the proportion of females who had ever had sexual intercourse from 2% at age 13, to 4% at 14, to 9% at 15, to 20% at 16, to 34% at 17, to 48% at 18, to 63% at 19. Thus, the number of sexually experienced females in 1976 would have included 34,000 13-year-olds, 76,000 14-year-olds, 193,000 15-year-olds, 408,000 16-year-olds, 702,000 17-year-olds, 1,000,000 18-year-olds, and 1,300,000 19-year-olds (Fig. 19-8). In 1976 Elliott and collegues[21] showed an increase in the proportion of all adolescents who were sexually active from 7% at 13, to 12% at 14, to 17% at 15, to 23% at 16, and to 33% at 17. When the results of these two independent surveys are examined, it appears that American males were more sexually experienced than females until age 17; then females became more likely to have engaged in sexual intercourse than teenaged males.

Data collected in the past 30 years on the

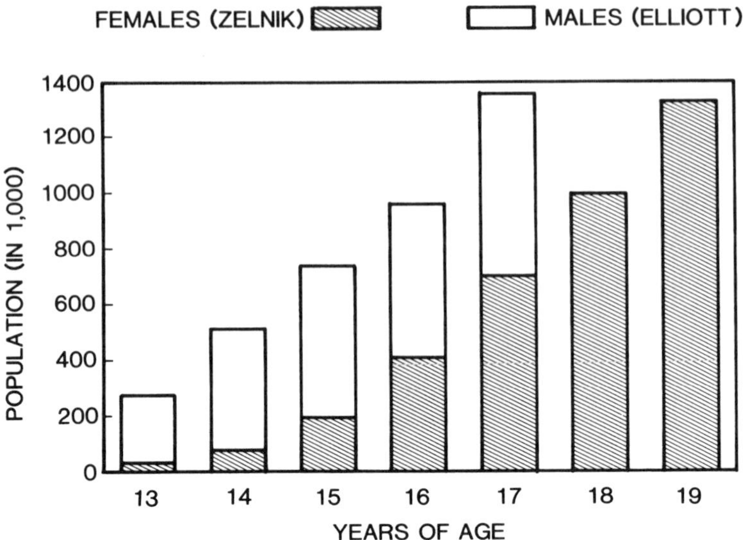

Fig. 19-8 Sexually experienced adolescents in the United States by years of age—1976.

sexual behavior patterns of American adolescents can be summarized as follows:

1. The number of Americans 15 to 19 years of age almost doubled from 10.7 million in 1950 to 21.2 million in 1980, as the total population increased only 50%, from 151 million in 1950 to 226.5 million in 1980.

2. The proportion of sexually active females 15 to 19 years old more than doubled from approximately 20% in 1950 to 50% in 1980; thus the number of sexually active females 15 to 19 years of age increased fivefold from one million in 1950 to over 5 million in 1980.

3. The proportion of sexually experienced 20-year-old males increased from approximately 73% in 1950 to 81% in 1980, and the number of sexually active males 15 to 19 years of age increased from about 2.7 million to 7.4 million; thus, there were about 9 million more sexually active teenagers in 1980 than in 1950.

4. Young sexually active females probably had more partners in 1980 than 1950. Kinsey and associates reported in 1953 that 47% of women who had had premarital intercourse had had multiple partners before marriage. In 1972 Hunt[22] found that 49% had had more than one sexual partner before marriage. However, Zelnik and Kantner reported that the proportion of sexually active females 15 to 19 years old with multiple partners increased even more dramatically: from 38% in 1971 to 50% in 1976.

5. Sexually active teenaged males may or may not have had more partners in 1980 than 1950. Kinsey and associates reported in 1948 that 45% of white males had had sexual intercourse with prostitutes by the age of 20, but many of these men had no more than a single experience or two with prostitutes. The frequency of intercourse with prostitutes among young men in the Kinsey survey was half as great as the frequency reported by older men. In the follow-up study conducted in 1972, Hunt[22] reported that only 3% of single white men under 25 years of age had had any experience with prostitutes in the past year.

Prostitution

Prostitution is not as common today as it was a century ago.[23] At the turn of the century in New Orleans, 230 brothels could be found in a 36-square-block area named after a city alderman, Sidney Story. A photographer named Ernest Bellocq took hundreds of pictures of the women who worked in Storyville, but most of his photographs and negatives were destroyed upon his death by his brother, a Roman Catholic priest.[24] During World War I, most houses of prostitution in urban areas of the United States were closed.[25] Prostitution has resurfaced in various forms since the 1920s, but now accounts for a relatively small proportion of the total sexual outlet. However, prostitution is still estimated to be a multibillion dollar a year business.[26]

No surveys with representative samples of prostitutes have ever been conducted, but the number of female prostitutes in contemporary American society has been estimated to be between 200,000 and 500,000. Most of the women who engage in prostitution cannot make a career of it, so they do it intermittently. The majority since World War II have been black and members of ethnic minority groups.[27] Most of the young women who work as prostitutes are streetwalkers, but some will take calls from steady clients and work in other ways as well.[28] Many are transient and move from city to city frequently.

The number of male prostitutes in contemporary American society has been estimated to be between 250,000 and 350,000.[29] Male prostitutes tend to be very young ("chickens") or muscular and handsome ("models"). In contrast to female prostitutes, most male prostitutes are white. Teenaged hustlers usually walk the streets, hang around public parks (or T-Rooms), or work out of selected bars. Male models tend to advertise in gay newspapers and take "out calls." While female prostitutes often work with a man ("pimp") or agencies that require fees, most male prostitutes work on their own.[30]

Homosexual Men

No surveys with representative samples of homosexual men have ever been conducted in the United States (or any other place). However, no evidence has been produced to suggest that the proportion of homosexual men in the population of the United States has increased. While the proportion of homosexual men appears to have remained constant in twentieth century America, the number of sexual partners these homosexual men have had apparently has increased.

Of the 1,402 white men who reported having had homosexual experiences in Kinsey's survey, 35% had had only one male partner, 22% had had more than 10 male partners, and 8% had had more than 100 male partners in their lifetimes. Among 873 white males with at least 50 homosexual experiences or 20 male partners, 6.5% had had only one partner and 64% had had 10 or more male partners.[31] When the number of different partners reported by the 873 "nondelinquent" white males with significant amounts of homosexual experiences (studied by Kinsey's Institute for Sex Research from 1938 to 1963) are compared with 4,212 homosexual men surveyed by Jay and Young in 1976,[32] we find that homosexual men tend to have more male partners today than a generation ago (Fig. 19-9). In 1976 only 2% had had one male partner and 81% had had 10 or more male partners in their lifetimes. In fact, the median number of partners in the *past year* (median = 9.6) reported by homosexual men in 1976 was larger than the median number of *lifetime* partners (median = 2.7) reported by men with homosexual experiences in the original survey conducted by Kinsey and his colleagues.

Caution must be exercised when Kinsey's sample of homosexual men is compared with the sample obtained by Jay and Young for at least three reasons: (1) the median age of the Kinsey sample (27 years old) was 4 years younger than the Jay-Young sample (31 years old); (2) all of Kinsey's respondents were interviewed in person, whereas all of the Jay-Young respondents mailed in self-administered questionnaires; and (3) only 8.3% of Kinsey's sample was

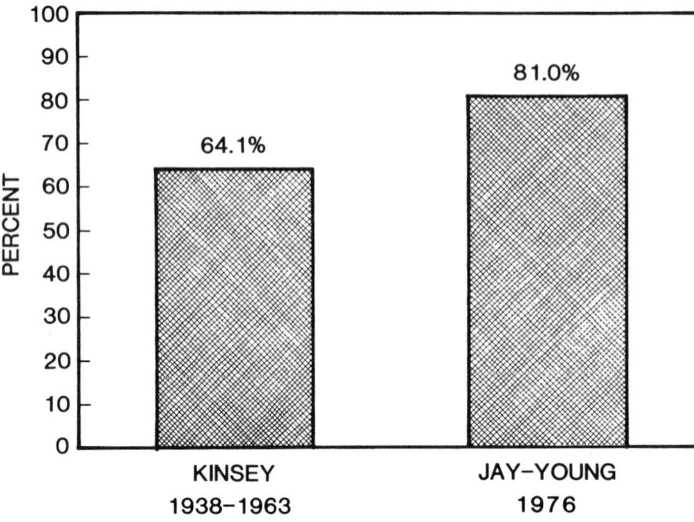

Fig. 19-9 Homosexual males with 10 or more male partners in lifetimes.

recruited from the Far West, while 25% of the Jay-Young sample lived in western states. More importantly, Kinsey sought diversity, while Jay-Young recruited members of homophile organizations. However, other samples of homosexual men suffer from similar or even more serious defects in size and recruitment.[33] Since other samples of homosexual men are smaller and biased in other ways, two additional comparisons of sexual activities between the Kinsey and Jay-Young samples might be worth making: the proportion of homosexual men with sexual contacts in bathhouses, and the proportion who had engaged in anilingus as active participants.

About 10% of the men with significant amounts of homosexual associations in the Kinsey sample had had sexual experiences with other men in steam baths, but less than 1% had significant amounts of homosexual contact in bathhouses.[31] In contrast, almost 60% of homosexual men responding to the Jay-Young survey had had sexual relations with other men in bathhouses (Fig. 19-10). Furthermore, 2% indicated that they had had *all* of their homosexual contacts in bathhouses, and about 25% of the homosexual men surveyed by Jay and Young in 1976 said that they went to bathhouses "frequently."

Kinsey and his colleagues found that 44% of homosexual men had engaged in anilingus as active partners, but only 16% had engaged in anilingus frequently. Jay and Young found that 74% had engaged in anilinctus actively, and 34% had done so frequently. Thus, it appears that the proportion of men with significant amounts of homosexual experience has remained stable at about 18% of the adult male population for the past 30 or 40 years, but the number of homosexual men increased due to increases in population, and their risks of acquiring venereal infections increased due to increased numbers of sexual partners and increased exposures to potentially infected (or infested) areas of the human body.

Dimensions of the Sexual Revolution

Before we examine the changing characteristics of STD in American society, we shall review some important dimensions of what is popularly called the "sexual revolution" in America:

1. The proportion of adolescents (particularly unmarried white women) engaging in premarital sexual activities increased dramatically after World War II. As the age of

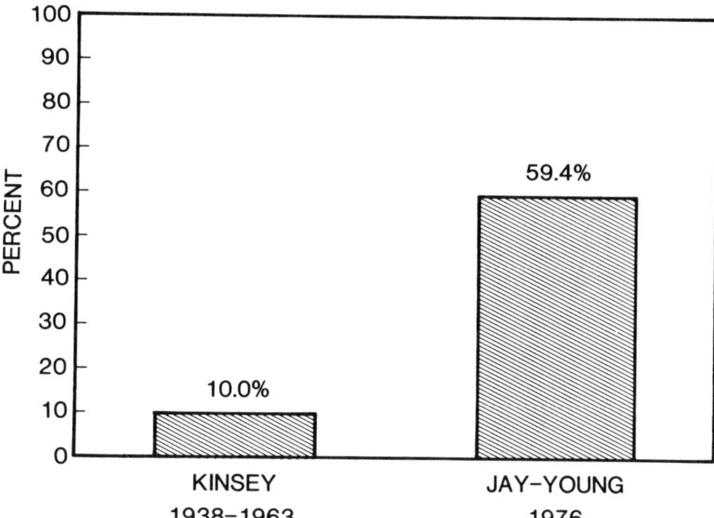

Fig. 19-10 Homosexual males with sexual exposures in bath houses.

first intercourse declined, the numbers of partners and sexual exposures before marriage increased.

2. Prostitution accounted for a relatively small proportion of the total sexual outlet of white men in the Kinsey survey of 1948, and the number of men having sexual contacts with female prostitutes has continued to decline since then. However, pockets of prostitution continue in large cities and in many other areas of the United States.

3. The proportion of homosexual men in the American population apparently has not changed since World War II, but now larger numbers of homosexual men tend to have larger numbers of different sexual partners, more sexual contacts in social settings such as bathhouses, and more sexual exposures (such as anilingus) that might facilitate the transmission of biologic agents from infected (or infested) hosts to susceptible sexual partners.

IMPLICATIONS FOR CONTROL OF SEXUALLY TRANSMITTED DISEASES

As noted at the outset of this chapter, cases of syphilis and gonorrhea have been reported to the Public Health Service since 1919. Although case definitions have changed with increasing knowledge and technical improvements in laboratory tests, it appears that rates of syphilis increased until penicillin therapy was introduced in 1943, and then declined. Gonorrhea followed a similar trend until 1957, then increased continuously for 20 years. When gonorrhea rates reached an all-time high in 1976, syphilis rates reached an all-time low.

When total syphilis cases are divided into primary and secondary (infectious), early latent, and other, we see that infectious syphilis began to increase in 1957—at about the same time that gonorrhea increased (Fig. 19-11). The abrupt increase in infectious syphilis was more dramatic than the increase in reported cases of gonorrhea for the period from 1957 to 1962. After 1962, rates of infectious syphilis tended to stabilize, while gonorrhea continued to increase at a rate of approximately 12% per annum.[34] Why did gonorrhea increase sharply as infectious syphilis cases remained relatively constant?

Gonorrhea among American Adolescents

Gonorrhea is an infectious disease with a relatively short incubation period of 3 to 5 days. The disease usually produces un-

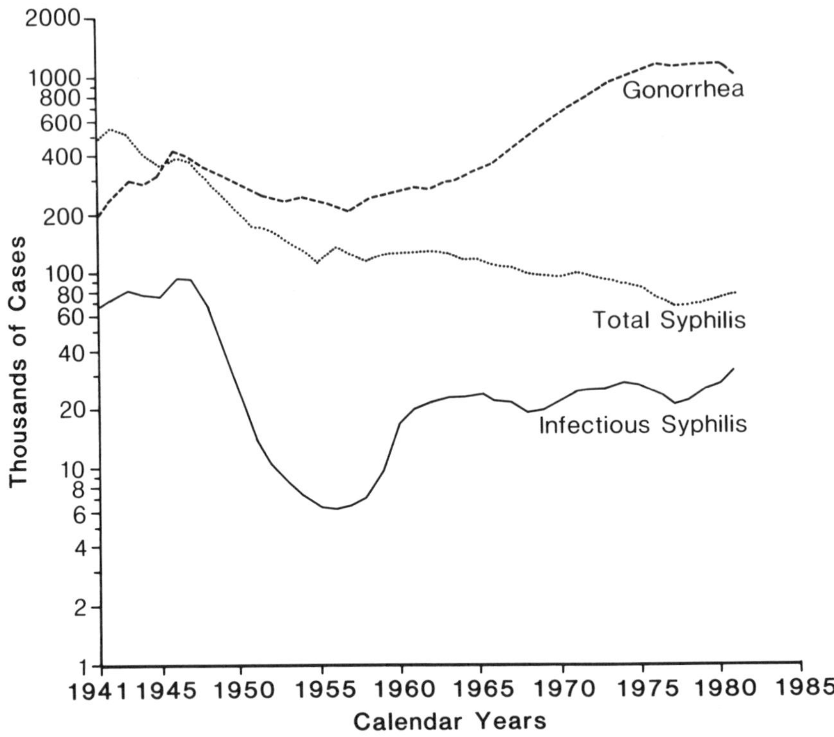

Fig. 19-11 Syphilis and gonorrhea: Reported cases by diagnosis—United States, calendar years 1941–1981.

pleasant symptoms in the urethra of the male, but less often causes discomfort in females. Therefore, sexually active heterosexual women are thought to constitute a major reservoir of asymptomatic (or "silent") gonococcal infections.[35] Now let me propose a simple hypothesis to answer the question about trends in gonorrhea: The fivefold increase in reported cases of gonorrhea from 214,000 in 1957 to over 1,000,000 in 1976 was due, in part, to the fivefold increase in sexually active adolescent women (especially white women) during this period, from about 1 million in 1953 to over 5 million in 1976.

In order to test this hypothesis, we need to examine reported morbidity for gonorrhea more closely to see if the rates of increase were particularly apparent for young white women as opposed to older white and other women. In addition, we need to see if the increases in gonorrhea are more closely tied to increases in sexual activity or to other factors, and we need to see if the ratio of male to female cases reflects an apparent decline in the "double standard."[36]

From 1960 to 1970, reported cases of gonorrhea increased most dramatically for white women 15 to 24 years of age. Cases among black women aged 25 to 39 hardly increased at all (Fig. 19-12). Reported cases of gonorrhea among young white women increased fivefold in the 1960s, and the numbers seem to fit an exponential curve. Evidence to this point certainly suggests a direct relationship between increasing premarital sexual activity among young white women and increasing rates of gonorrhea.

Cases of gonorrhea reported for women 15 to 19 years old from 1971 to 1976 are positively correlated with the increases in sexual activity reported by Zelnik and Kantner. However, cases of gonorrhea

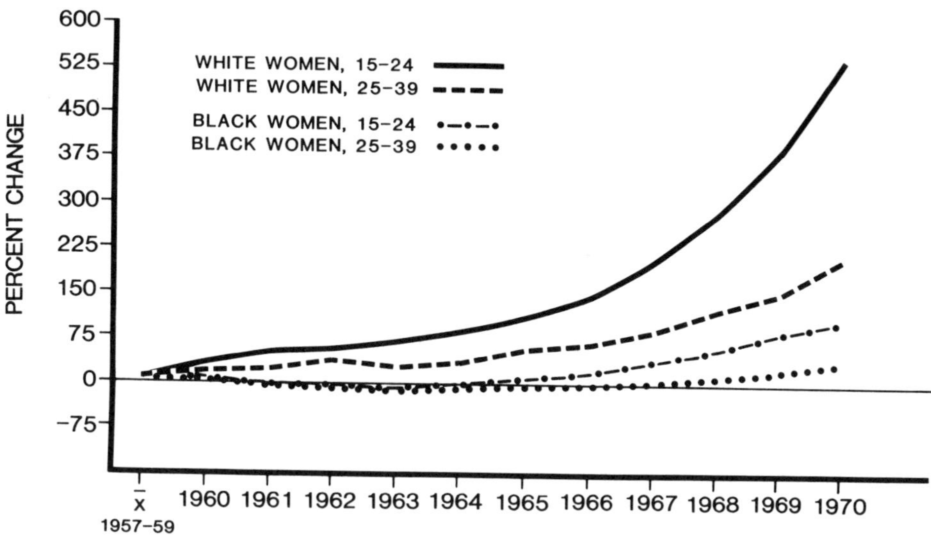

Fig. 19-12 Percent changes (based on the average number of cases reported 1957–1959) in reported cases of gonorrhea among black and white women, aged 15–24 and 25–39.

seem to be even more highly correlated with oral contraceptive use among 15- to 19-year-old females (Fig. 19-13). During the late 1960s and early 1970s large numbers of young unmarried women began using "the pill."[37] Oral contraceptive agents tended to be used by young women after they had in-itiated sexual activities[38] and instead of all other agents, such as condoms, contraceptive foams, and contraceptive jellies which might have prevented vaginal infections.[39]

Available data on reported cases of gonorrhea seem to reflect increasing numbers of sexually active teenaged women in the

Fig. 19-13 Percent changes in the number of American women 15–19 years of age who were sexually active, using oral contraceptives or condoms, and infected with gonorrhea: 1971–1976.

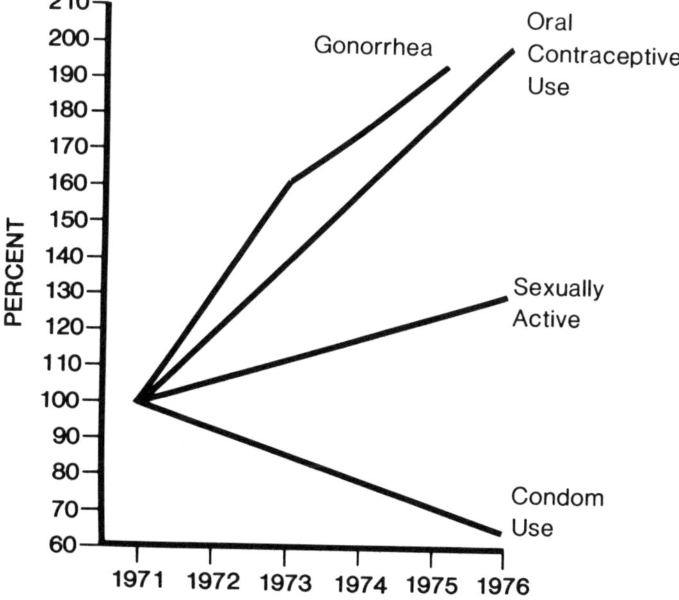

American population. From 1965 to 1979, the ratio of males to females reported with gonorrhea fell from 3:1 to 1.5:1. For 15- 19-year-olds, the sex ratio switched from 2:1 to 0.6:1. However, this reversal may have resulted primarily from increased screening by culture among young women during this period rather than from proportional increases in sexual activity.[40]

Age-adjusted rates of gonorrhea from 1967 to 1980 for white males and females show that the gap between males and females has closed slightly, but remains apparent. Rates for white females have followed rates for white males quite closely throughout this period of social change. Contrary to expectations, the continuing increase in sexual activities among white females from 1976 to 1979 apparently had no or very little affect on their rates on gonorrhea. Rates of gonorrhea declined slightly for white males and females from 1975 to 1980.[41] Therefore, one might speculate that coordinated efforts by national and local public health agencies to control gonorrhea offset pressures on the disease to increase even further.[42]

Kantner and Zelnik showed that rates of sexual activity are fairly constant throughout the United States, but slightly higher among teenagers in the West. Rates of gonorrhea are highest in the South, Alaska, Hawaii, and one other state in the West, Nevada. Nevada is the only state in the nation that has not made prostitution illegal.

Prostitution Spreads Sexually Transmitted Diseases

Although the prevalence of prostitution in the United States is believed to be quite small and the number of female prostitutes appears to be declining, female prostitutes are frequently infected with gonorrhea and other STD. They contribute more than their share to the transmission of STD. In Colorado Springs, 63% of 89 female prostitutes were infected with gonorrhea during 13 months of 1976–1977, 31% of all endocervical specimens taken from this group were positive by culture for *Neisseria gonorrhoeae,* and 75 episodes of pelvic inflammatory disease were diagnosed in these women.[43] In Fresno County, 21.7% of 512 female prostitutes first tested in 1976–1977 had gonorrhea, and 6.3% had syphilis.[44] In Atlanta, 19.8% of 237 women thought to be prostitutes and 14.7% of 34 men arrested for sexual offenses had gonorrhea when first tested in 1978.[45] In addition, 10.6% of the women had trichomoniasis, 3.4% had syphilis, and 2.1% had moniliasis; 14.7% of the men had syphilis and another 14.7% had nonspecific urethritis. In all, 29.3% of the women arrested for prostitution or related charges in Atlanta and 44.1% of the men were infected with one or more of the STD.

Data on the relationship between prostitution and STD were collected by the American Social Hygiene Association (ASHA) from World War I through 1971.[25] According to these historical data, female prostitutes have accounted for a disproportionate share of venereal infections. In the late 1960s, Winick and Kinsie[25] estimated that less than one half of one percent of women in the United States had ever engaged in prostitution, yet prostitutes accounted for 15 to 25% of syphilitic infections and were responsible for about 5% of gonococcal infections.[46]

Most of the data on prostitutes has been obtained from streetwalkers. Streetwalkers are more likely than house prostitutes to be infected with STD.[47] Data from Nevada suggest that the prevalence of gonorrhea in house prostitutes may be lower than in other sexually active women tested for gonorrhea.[48] The lower prevalence in house prostitutes is due to more frequent testing and treatment. However, the cumulative incidence of gonorrhea in female prostitutes who work in brothels may be 20 times higher than among other sexually active women tested for gonorrhea.[49]

The importance of female prostitutes as transmitters of gonorrhea has been stressed in investigations of outbreaks of penicillinase-producing *Neisseria gonorrhoeae* (PPNG) in the United States.[50] Some believe that PPNG was imported into the United States early in 1976 by military servicemen returning from the Far East.[51] Case-finding interviews with male patients showed that they often acquired PPNG from "hostesses" working in bars near military bases overseas and passed PPNG on to female prostitutes in the United States.[52]

The greatest number of cases of PPNG in the United States are found in California.[53] From the summer of 1980 to the summer of 1981, about 31% of the cases of PPNG in the United States were reported from Los Angeles County alone. Only 5% of the patients with PPNG in Los Angeles identified contacts overseas. About 14% of the 243 women infected with PPNG in Los Angeles during this period were prostitutes, and 19.4% of the 299 men with PPNG identified prostitutes as possible sources of their infections. PPNG control activities in Los Angeles focused on prostitutes and other possible transmitters with considerable success: the number of cases of PPNG reported per month fell from about 60 in August 1981 to only 5 or 6 per month in the summer of 1982.

During the peak of the outbreak in Los Angeles (October 1981), over half of the women infected with PPNG were considered to be prostitutes. Twelve months later no cases of PPNG were found among prostitutes. By October 1982, all of the cases of PPNG in Los Angeles could be related to sexual exposures to persons outside of the United States.

Infectious Syphilis among Homosexual Men

Trends for infectious syphilis do not follow trends for gonorrhea after 1963. As gonorrhea rates increased steadily from 149.2 per 100,000 in 1963 to 472.9 in 1975, rates for primary and secondary syphilis followed an erratic pattern. Infectious syphilis fell from 12.2 per 100,000 in 1965 to 9.6 in 1969, rose to 12.1 in 1975, and then fell again to 9.5 in 1977. For these differences to occur, one might hypothesize that the attempt to eradicate syphilis in the 1960s had some effect on the incidence of infectious syphilis, but no demonstrable effect on gonorrhea.

An alternative hypothesis might state that gonorrhea and syphilis were spread in two different groups that interacted infrequently: homosexual men and heterosexual couples, respectively. Although sexual activity increased among heterosexual adolescents in the 1970s, rates of infectious syphilis tended to decline in this population. However, rates of infectious syphilis tended to increase for homosexual men.

Evidence for the hypothesis of the transmission of two different venereal diseases in two distinct populations is provided in the data collected by the American Social Hygiene Association.[54] As the proportion of gonorrhea cases remained at or below 5% for homosexual men, the proportion of early syphilis cases among homosexual men tended to increase after 1966 (Fig. 19-14). Increases in reported cases of early syphilis among homosexual men continued through the 1970s.[55]

In fiscal year 1974, 26.4% of men with primary or secondary syphilis named only male sexual partners, and an additional 9.9% named both male and female partners.[56] Closer examination of unpublished data reveals that 55% of white men infected with primary or secondary syphilis named at least one male sexual partner in the period before they became infected, but only 27% of black men named one or more male sexual partners. Hence reported cases of infectious syphilis tended to increase for white men as they decreased for white women, but reported cases of infectious syphilis remained the same for men and women of other racial and ethnic groups.

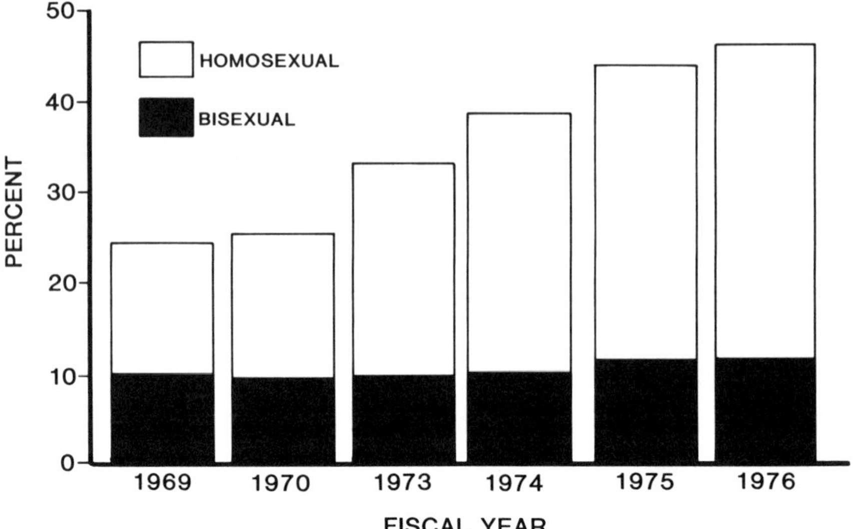

Fig. 19-14 Primary and secondary syphilis and early (less than one year) latent male patients by type of sexual contact—United States: Fiscal years 1969–1976.

A last piece of evidence for the hypothesis that syphilis and gonorrhea now travel in different companies is provided by age-specific rates for men and women. When primary or secondary syphilis is found in women, these infections are primarily in women under 25 years of age. Infectious syphilis, on the other hand, remains a problem for men 25 and older. Now the sex ratio for gonorrhea is almost 1:1. For primary and secondary syphilis, the sex ratio is 3:1.

Although gonorrhea appears to be more prevalent among heterosexual than homosexual men, homosexual men are infected with gonorrhea more often than heterosexual men. To untangle this apparent paradox, we need to look at the formula proposed by the British venereologist, R. R. Willcox, and some data from America. Willcox[57] argues that the risk of acquiring gonorrhea is equal to the number of sexual exposures, times the prevalence of disease in one's partners, times the risk of transmission per exposure. According to Hunt,[22] the average sexually active white heterosexual man 18 to 24 years old has 57 sexual exposures a year, the prevalence of gonorrhea in his seuxal partners is less than 1%,[34] and he has a 22% risk of acquiring gonorrhea from each sexual exposure with an infected female partner.[58] By the method of Willcox, about 10% of sexually active white heterosexual men 18 to 24 years old should acquire gonorrhea annually.

Now let us contrast this risk in heterosexual men with the hypothetical risk for homosexual men. The average sexually active white homosexual man, 18 to 24 years old, has 120 sexual exposures per year,[32] the prevalence of gonorrhea in his partners might be 2.5% (or higher),[59] and, depending on his sexual exposures, he could have a 50% chance of acquiring gonorrhea from an infected male partner. Thus, homosexual men may be 15 times more likely than heterosexual men to acquire gonorrhea. In fact, according to the formula proposed by Willcox, homosexual men who fit the description constructed above should be infected an average of 1.5 times per year.

CONCLUSIONS

Three interrelated questions were raised at the outset of this chapter:

1. Is there an "epidemic" of STD in the United States?
2. Has there been a "sexual revolution" in America?
3. What is the relationship between changing patterns of sexual behavior and changing patterns of STD?

These simple questions are very difficult to answer because longitudinal data are either severely biased or unavailable. Although unqualified answers cannot be given, available evidence can be assessed. We presented evidence that showed gonorrhea was "epidemic" when syphilis was not, sexual behavior patterns changed considerably in the past 25 years, and changing patterns of sexual behavior seem to be related to changes in the distributions of infectious syphilis and gonorrhea in different groups.

Cases of gonorrhea and syphilis have been reported since 1919 and show, paradoxically, that gonorrhea was "epidemic" when infectious syphilis was not, and, conversely, infectious syphilis was "epidemic" when gonorrhea was not. In a classical epidemiologic study of suicide, Durkheim[60] was confronted with similar evidence in the nineteenth century and concluded that there were different kinds of suicide, each with its own "cause" in the social environment. In twentieth century America, gonorrhea and infectious syphilis should be regarded as different diseases, each with its own "cause" in the social environment.

While data on STD may be biased, reliable data on trends in sexual behavior are simply not available. If it had not been for courageous scientists such as Alfred Kinsey, we might not have any data on sexual behavior at all. Although Kinsey's sample was not representative of the American population, his extensive findings on "sexual outlets" provide us with a baseline for measuring changes in certain groups within American society. Comparisons suggest that heterosexual adolescents increased in number after World War II, their numbers of different sexual partners before marriage also increased, and their use of contraceptive and prophylactic agents that might have reduced the risks of venereal infections decreased. Homosexual men increased in number due to natural increases in the population; their numbers of different partners increased and their chances of venereal infection also increased as a consequence of increasing frequencies of sexual exposures (such as anilingus) that could facilitate the spread of certain pathogens (such as *Entamoeba histolytica*). Prostitution is probably less prevalent today than before World War II, but it continues to offer opportunities for the introduction and transmission of new strains of gonorrhea and other STD in American communities. If we cannot safely conclude on the basis of this evidence that a "sexual revolution" has occurred, we can say that there have been significant changes in American society that should be reflected in reported cases of STD.

When data on changes in the distribution of STD are compared with data on apparent changes in sexual behavior, we find that trends in reported cases of gonorrhea seem to be most sensitive to trends in heterosexual relationships, trends in reported cases of infectious syphilis seem to be more sensitive to trends in the sexual relationships established by homosexual men, and that the emergence of new problems, such as PPNG, and the persistence of some old problems, especially in areas of low prevalence, may be related to the sexual practices of prostitutes and their clients. These differences in the ways in which different STD are cycled and recycled in different sociosexual communities should be taken into account when disease prevention and control program are designed, implemented, and evaluated.

Failure to gather and carefully analyze data on the characteristics of persons at risk for acquiring and disseminating STD have hampered public health efforts to control STD in the past. To better answer the three questions raised in this chapter, longitudinal studies of sexual behaviors and STD must be undertaken.

ACKNOWLEDGMENTS

Akbar Zaidi of the Centers for Disease Control, Center for Prevention Services, Division of Sexually Transmitted Diseases, compiled morbidity data and calculated 10-year moving averages for gonorrhea and infectious syphilis cases reported in the United States. Ruthie King and Sunny McKeon assisted in the preparation of the graphics.

REFERENCES

1. Benenson AS (ed): Control of Communicable Diseases in Man. American Public Health Association, Washington, DC, 1981
2. Serfling RE: Methods for current statistical analysis of excess pneumonia-influenza death. Public Health Rep 78:494, 1963
3. Brown WJ, Donohue JF, Axnick NW, et al: Syphilis and Other Venereal Diseases. Harvard University Press, Cambridge, MA, 1970
4. Baumgartner L, Curtis AC, Gray AL, et al: The Eradication of Syphilis. Public Health Service Publication No. 918. Government Printing Office, Washington, DC, April 1963
5. Henderson RH: Control of sexually transmitted diseases in the United States—A federal perspective. Br J Vener Dis 53:211, 1977
6. Pomeroy WB: Dr. Kinsey and the Institute for Sex Research. Harper & Row, New York, 1972
7. Kinsey AC, Pomeroy WB, Martin CE: Sexual Behavior in the Human Male. Saunders, Philadelphia, 1948
8. Sorokin PA, The American Sex Revolution. Porter Sargent, Boston, 1956
9. Kinsey AC, Pomeroy WB, Martin CE, Gebhard PH: Sexual Behavior in the Human Female. Saunders, Philadelphia, 1953
10. Geddes DR (ed): Reports on Sexual Behavior in the Human Male and Female. New American Library, New York, 1954
11. Cochran WG, Mosteller F, Tukey J: Statistical Problems of the Kinsey Report on Sexual Behavior in the Human Male. American Statistical Association, Washington, DC, 1954
12. Reiss IL: The sexual renaissance: A summary and analysis. J Social Issues 22:123, 1966
13. Kantner JF, Zelnik M: Sexual experience of young unmarried women in the United States. Fam Plann Perspect 4:9, 1972
14. Zelnik M, Kantner JF: Sexual and contraceptive experience of young unmarried women in the United States, 1976 and 1971. Fam Plann Perspect 9:55, 1977
15. Zelnik M, Kantner JF, Ford K: Sex and Pregnancy in Adolescence. Sage, Beverly Hills, CA, 1981
16. Chilman CS: Adolescent Sexuality in a Changing Society. DHEW Publication No. (NIH) 79-1426. Center for Population Research, Bethesda, MD, 1978
17. Clayton RR, Bokemeier JL: Premarital sex in the seventies. J Marriage Fam 42:759, 1980
18. Zelnik M, Kantner JF: Sexual activity, contraceptive use and pregnancy among metropolitan-area teenagers: 1971–1979. Fam Plann Perspect 12:230, 1980
19. U.S. Bureau of the Census: Census of Population: 1970. General Population Characteristics. Final Report PC(1)-B1. United States Summary. Government Printing Office, Washington, DC, 1972
20. Bell RR: Premarital Sex in a Changing Society. Prentice-Hall, Englewood-Cliffs, NJ, 1966
21. Elliott DS, Ageton SS, Huizinga D, et al: The Prevalence and Incidence of Delinquent Behavior: 1976–1980. The National Youth Survey Report No. 26. Behavioral Research Institute, Boulder, CO, 1983

22. Hunt M: Sexual Behavior in the 1970s. Playboy Press, New York, 1974
23. Bullough VL, Bullough BL: Prostitution: An Illustrated Social History. Crown, New York, 1978
24. Rose A: Storyville, New Orleans. University of Alabama Press, Birmingham, AL, 1974
25. Winick C, Kinsie PM: The Lively Commerce: Prostitution in the United States. Quadrangle, Chicago, 1971
26. Sheehy G: Hustling: Prostitution in our Wide-Open Society. Delacorte, New York, 1973
27. Federal Security Agency: 1944-5 Social Protection Division Series on Prostitution in America. Charts D105-44 to D119-45. Division of Social Protection, Washington, DC, 1945
28. Hall S, Adelman B: Ladies of the Night. Trident, New York, 1973
29. Lloyd R: For Money or Love: Boy Prostitution in America. Ballantine, New York, 1976
30. Hoffman M: The male prostitute. Sex Behav 2:16, 1972
31. Gebhard PH, Johnson AB: The Kinsey Data. Saunders, Philadelphia, 1979
32. Jay K, Young A: The Gay Report. Summit, New York, 1979
33. Weinberg MS: Homosexual samples: Differences and Similarities. J Sex Res 6:312, 1970
34. U.S. Department of Health, Education and Welfare: STD Fact Sheet, Edition 35. HEW Publication No. (CDC) 79-8195. Centers for Disease Control, Atlanta, GA, 1981
35. Washington AE, Wiesner PJ: The silent clap. JAMA 245:609, 1981
36. Smigel ED, Seiden R: The decline and fall of the double standard. Ann Am Acad Polit Social Sci 376:6, 1968
37. Scrimshaw SCM: Women and the pill: From panacea to catalyst. Fam Plann Perspect 13:254, 1981
38. Zabin LS, Clark SD: Why they delay: A study of teenage family planning clinic patients. Fam Plann Perspect 13:205, 1981
39. Cutler JC: Venereal disease prevention. Cutis 27:321, 1981
40. Henderson RH: Venereal disease: A national health problem. Clin Obstet Gynecol 18:223, 1975
41. Zaidi AA, Aral SO, Reynolds GH, et al: Gonorrhea in the United States: 1967–1979. Sex Transm Dis 10:72, 1983
42. Aral SO, Johnson RE, Zaidi AA, et al: Demographic effects on sexually transmitted diseases in the 1970s. Sex Transm Dis 10:100, 1983
43. Potterat JJ, Rothenberg R, Bross DC: Gonorrhea in street prostitutes. Sex Transm Dis 6:58, 1979
44. Jaffe HW, Rice DT, Voigt R, et al: Selective mass treatment in a venereal disease control program. Am J Public Health 69:1181, 1979
45. Conrad GL, Kleris GS, Rush B, Darrow WW: Sexually transmitted diseases among prostitutes and other sexual offenders. Sex Transm Dis 8:241, 1981
46. Fleming WL, Bowling FL, Buchanan CS, et al: Today's VD Control Problem. American Social Health Association, New York, 1968
47. Bess BE, Janus SS: Prostitution. p 594. In Sadock BJ, Kaplan HI, Freedman AM (eds): The Sexual Experience. Williams & Wilkens, Baltimore, 1976
48. Edwards WM: Vaginal prophylaxis. p 94. In Epidemic Venereal Disease: Proceedings of the 2nd International Venereal Disease Symposium. American Social Health Association, New York, 1973
49. Darrow WW. Prostitution and sexually transmitted diseases. In Holmes KK, Mårdh P-A, Sparling PF, Wiesner PJ (eds): Sexually Transmitted Diseases. McGraw-Hill, New York, 1984
50. Centers for Disease Control: Penicillinase-producing Neisseria gonorrhoeae—Los Angeles. MMWR 32:181, 1983
51. Perine PL, Morton RS, Piot P, et al: Epidemiology and treatment of penicillinase-producing Neisseria gonorrhoeae. Sex Transm Dis (Suppl) 6:152–158, 1979
52. Handsfield HH, Sandstrom EG, Knapp JS, et al: Epidemiology of penicillinase-producing Neisseria gonorrhoeae infections. N Engl J Med 306:950, 1982
53. Jaffe HW, Biddle JW, Johnson WR, Wiesner PJ: Infections due to penicillinase-producing Neisseria gonorrhoeae in the United States: 1976–1980. J Infect Dis 144:191, 1981
54. Fleming WL, Altman R, Anderson RS, et al: Today's VD Control Problem. American Social Health Association, New York, 1972

55. Fichtner RR, Aral SO, Blount JH, et al: Syphilis in the United States: 1967–1979. Sex Transm Dis 10:77, 1983

56. Henderson RH: Improving sexually transmitted disease health services for gays: A national perspective. Sex Transm Dis 4:58, 1977

57. Willcox RR: Society and high-risk groups. p 31. In Catterall RD, Nicol CS (eds): Sexually Transmitted Diseases. Academic, London, 1976

58. Holmes KK, Johnson DW, Trostle HJ: An estimate of the risk of men acquiring gonorrhea by sexual contact with infected females. Am J Epidemiol 91:170, 1970

59. Ostrow DG, Shaskey D, Steffen G, Altman N: Epidemiology of gonorrhea infections in gay men. J Homosex 5:285, 1980

60. Durkheim E: Suicide: A Study in Sociology. (First published in 1897). Free Press, New York, 1968

20

The Prevention of Sexually Transmitted Diseases

John C. Cutler

Sexually transmitted diseases (STDs) are an important element among the multiple causes of rising costs of health care. In 1980 Curran[1] reported that there were 850,000 episodes of pelvic inflammatory disease (PID) per year. These required 212,000 hospital admissions and 115,000 surgical procedures. The direct and indirect costs were estimated to be $1.25 billion in 1979. If there is no significant change in the national approach to this problem, Curran projects that by the year 2000 there will be at least one episode of PID for each female who reached reproductive age in 1970; 15% will have required hospitalization, and at least 10% will be sterile as a result of the disease.

The social, economic, and personal consequences of such projections are self-evident. The need to take action to stem the rising tide of STD's, as was done successfully in the past when medical knowledge and techniques were less complete and sophisticated than today, should lead to reexamination of those programs that made an important contribution to the control of sexually transmitted diseases—such as self-protective sexual behavior and prophylaxis. In addition, new, enhanced programs of effective case-finding and treatment, educa-

tion, and motivation of the individual must be instituted.

The current rise in STD rates began in 1957 following congressional action to cut back on appropriations needed to maintain the successful, well-planned, and highly integrated national program, which involved federal, state, local, and international health agencies, as well as private practitioners and voluntary agencies, and which encouraged case finding, epidemiologic practices, treatment, laboratory services, and research. The reason for the initial cutback in the 1955 appropriations was that the congressional committee took the stand that, since a single-dose, simple method of treatment for syphilis and gonorrhea, that is, long-acting penicillin, had proved to be effective, there was no further justification or need for continuation at the same level of funding. It was stated that treatment alone should be sufficient, and it was implied that much of this could be accomplished without the public health system.

The pattern of gonorrhea and syphilis rates alone since then reflect the adverse impact of that decision. Cutbacks in federal funds meant that less federal funding was available to support state and local efforts as well. No other sources of funding were

281

forthcoming from state or local levels, and the highly successful, integrated program was thus unable to continue to function. The gonorrhea rate per 100,000 population, which rose during the war years, peaked at 284.2 in 1947, was brought down to 147 in 1955, and reached a low point of 127.4 in 1957. The rise which started after 1957 peaked at 472.9 in 1975 and by 1982 had been reduced to 417.9. In terms of numbers, there were 214,496 cases reported in 1947, and by 1983 that number had almost quintupled. The number of cases reported, primarily from the official agencies and hospitals, represents only a part of the actual number. Thus, the magnitude of the problem, as indicated by this single disease, is self-evident and provides justification for revitalization of the national STD control program.

Of course, a number of factors, such as changes in patterns of sexual behavior and demographic shifts, are involved. But, it is probable that, in addition to the cutbacks in public health programs, the widespread popularity of oral contraceptives and IUD's has resulted in the loss of protection afforded by the condom and vaginal contraceptives, thus reducing the contribution of one of the elements, prophylaxis, of a successful control program. At the same time, the approach to management of STD's has concentrated on treatment, with little or no attention given to promotion of personal prophylaxis. The internationally accepted guide to infectious disease control of the American Public Health Association still recommends teaching methods of personal prophylaxis which may be used before, during, or after exposure.[2] This straightforward, simple recommendation should be implemented with greater emphasis.

A review of research on and public health experience with prophylactic and preventive measures will provide information on past experiences and recent research findings that may be more effectively utilized in current control efforts.

The relationship between sexual intercourse and certain diseases was recognized for centuries before the era of scientific medicine. Based upon observation and reasoning, measures were introduced, such as the imposition of a barrier—the condom (at the time, an animal caecum)—to prevent the transmission of disease. This innovation is credited to Fallopius in the sixteenth century. He is also credited with the introduction of the linen penile sheath for the same purpose.

During this same period, the value of certain mercury compounds for treatment of the symptoms of syphilis was recognized, as well as some of the adverse effects. Thus, the desirability of preventing the disease through the use of a condom—as unaesthetic and unsatisfying as such prevention devices were at the time—was epitomized by the aphorism: "You spend a night with Venus and the rest of your life with Mercury."

The advances in technology during the latter half of the nineteenth century led to improvements in the manufacture of both natural (animal) and rubber condoms, so that they were much more appealing aesthetically, less prone to rupture, and cheaper. Thus they played a highly significant role in VD control as well as in contraception. By 1950, about half the married couples in the United Kingdom and the United States were using the condom as a contraceptive method. However, with the introduction of oral contraceptives in the late 1950s, the use of the condom and of vaginal contraceptives declined rapidly. This change in contraceptive practice was accompanied by a rapid rise in rates of gonorrhea in countries where the reporting systems had long been in existence, that is, in the United States, the United Kingdom, and the Scandinavian countries.

The condom played a very important role in venereal disease control for the U.S. Army in World Wars I and II. The reason for such strong military efforts to control

VD through a program that epitomized the public health approach—treatment, prevention through prophylaxis, control of prostitution, cooperation with civilian health authorities and the voluntary sector, and educational programs—was that, until the discovery of penicillin, venereal disease was the leading or second single cause of absence from duty. (In World War I influenza was the first cause.)

A review of the military experience is highly interesting. The classic report by Moore[3] of his experience as consultant urologist in the U.S. Army in Paris, 1918–1919, epitomizes the problems of VD control and clearly demonstrates the value of prophylactic programs under conditions such as in the military where well-planned public health measures can be put into practice, including enforcement of compliance. While efforts were made to promote chastity, for obvious reasons, a program had to be set up to deal with a permanent U.S. Army population in Paris of 22,000 and an unknown but large number of transients, all having access to a large population of prostitutes. In addition to condom distribution and promotion, a program was organized through which a system of prophylactic stations was set up in Paris so that every building housing more than 50 troops also had a prophylactic station. Each station was manned by trained attendants, and each soldier who had had contact was required to report to the station for prophylaxis which consisted of (1) urination, (2) washing of gentalia with soap and water, (3) examination by station attendant for disease or discharge, (4) intraurethral injections of 2% protagol solution, and (5) application of a 33⅓% calomel ointment to the penis. These procedures were administered by attendants who staffed the stations.

The findings may be summarized as follows (gonorrhea, syphilis, or chancroid aggregated as "case of VD"): 1 case of VD per 274 exposures with prophylaxis; 1 case of VD per 37 exposures without prophy-

laxis. Numerous reports of the experiences in World War I further substantiated Moore's findings.[4]

However, then as today, the problems related to bringing about self-protective sexual behavior were very well recognized. The human factors, such as emotion, drug or alcohol use, shame, and overconfidence, influenced individual behavior. In addition, differences in opinions and recommendations among both civil and military health professionals as well as among civil and military administrators and politicians were evident then as today.

It is not possible to quantify the contribution of any single procedure utilized, but it seems evident that the institution of a "public health" approach that effectively integrated programs to promote and implement use of various specific contraceptive/prophylactic methods in a variety of settings proved to be highly effective in the prevention of disease. Such programs were of benefit to the war effort, as well as to veterans in postwar years, in that they were relieved of unnecessary costs of medical care.

The seriousness of the VD problem was such that continued research in prophylaxis as an element of the total VD control program, was carried out by the military, the U.S. Public Health Service, state and local health departments, and the academic community after World War I. The Venereal Disease Research Laboratory of the United States Public Health Service at Staten Island, New York was the focal point for prophylactic studies, particularly with syphilis, using the rabbit as the experimental model for both prophylaxis and treatment.

During this period, with the discovery of sulfonamides, as well as new, less toxic, and more easily administered arsenical preparations, numerous studies were made of prophylactic therapy, while these and many other new products were tested for local prophylactic value. One such preparation, Progonasyl, consisting of 1% O-iodobenzoic acid and 11% triethanolamine in a mineral-vegetable oil base, was marketed for topical therapy. This product was studied as a potential vaginal prophylactic by Porter and coworkers,[5] who carried out extensive laboratory studies, followed by a clinical study on a small volunteer group of prostitutes and males. Three males with acute gonorrhea had contact with six uninfected females, five of whom had a vaginal injection of the preparation before contact. Culture studies were not done, but microscopic studies showed that only the untreated female showed positive smears and symptoms. Obviously the study was criticized for its serious methodologic shortcomings, but the authors were convinced of the importance of their findings in "contributing to diminishing the incidence of venereal disease."

World War II gave rise once again to serious concern with prophylaxis because of the potential absence from duty of significant numbers of troops. In spite of the problems of noncompliance with recommended prophylactic practices, observed during World War I in both the military and the civilian populations at high risk, the importance of prophylaxis as an element of this total VD control program was fully appreciated, and aggressive measures were instituted to build upon advances in venereal disease prophylaxis, therapeutics, and control methodology.

A priority for the limited supply of latex was the manufacture of condoms, the use of which was actively promoted. Prophylactic stations for the troops in areas of high risk for infection were set up within the United States and abroad. The practice of personal chemical prophylaxis was promoted, utilizing both the classical 33% calomel ointment and newly developed preparations such as a single-tube preparation of 30% calomel and 15% sulfathiazole. The latter replaced the two-tube preparation for personal use, which consisted of calomel and various silver compounds. The silver compounds were irritating and stained the clothing, and the need to use two tubes was not conducive to widespread acceptance and use.

Evaluation of the experiences reported in the series of reports of programs of preventive medicine in World War II, indicates that, in spite of the problems of noncompliance, prophylactic programs were both important and effective elements of the total public health approach.[6] Since World War II, the development of long-acting penicillin preparations and other antibiotics, along with the continuing problems of motivation for self-protective behavior and other problems inherent in health education and motivation programs related to sexual behavior, have led to a loss of interest in prophylaxis within the public health community. Since the cost of prophylactic programs was high, as compared to the very low cost of therapy, this approach was discontinued in the military and civilian populations during the Korean war. It should be noted, however, that, in addition to local prophylaxis, chemoprophylaxis and antibiotic (penicillin), prophylaxis were utilized successfully under certain circumstances in large-scale VD control programs.

The continuing studies in prophylaxis by the United States Public Health Service–Venereal Disease Research Laboratories led to the finding by Mahoney and Arnold, as reported by Arnold and Cutler,[7] of the potential prophylactic value of an aqueous preparation that could be used as a post-coital douche or solution for washing the genitalia. An aqueous solution of 0.2% mapharsen and 1% alkyl aryl sulfate (Orvus) was found to be highly effective as a prophylactic against syphilis in studies on the rabbit. The studies also showed the effectiveness of certain other surfactants and antiseptics as well as of the 30% calomel ointment. These important studies showed the synergistic effect of the surfactants and mapharsen. The relative value of several agents used for prophylaxis in the rabbit is shown in Table 20-1.

Table 20-1. Relative Value of Prophylactic Agents in Rabbits

	Animals Exposed	Animals Infected	Animals Not Infected
Controls (all experiments)	289	261	28
Mapharsen 0.2% Orvus 1%	9	0	9
Calomel 30% Sulfathiazide 15%	17	2	15

Arnold RC, Cutler JC: Br J Vener Dis 32:24, 1956

Clinical studies based on these laboratory findings were carried out by Funes and Aguilar[8] in a group of prostitutes who were served medically by the Guatemalan Public Health Service. Six of the prostitutes volunteered to use the aqueous solution of 0.02% mapharsen and 0.2% orvus as a douche following each contact. In the six-month period prior to use when only cervical smears were examined, there were 11 positive smears for gonorrhea in the 6 women. In the subsequent six months, when the women douched with the preparation after each contact, during which both cervical smears and cultures were done, only one positive culture was found. No specific information was gathered through a contact log as to the number of contacts per woman during each 6-month period, but data available from their histories indicate they usually had at least three contacts per day seven days per week. During the second part of the study, while under prophylaxis, the women were examined and cultured twice a week when they reported to the clinic to pick up their prophylactic preparations. Cultures were not done during the intitial control period, as funds were not available at that time to cover the laboratory costs. However, the rate of culture positivity related to smear positivity, when cultures could be done on this group, indicated that the number of culture-positives would have been greater than the number of positive smears.

A study by Edwards[9] using Progonasyl, 1% orthoidobenzoic acid in an oil base, was carried out in Nevada (where prostitution is legally controlled) with a group of vol-unteer prostitutes who used the preparation as a vaginal installation once per day. One positive culture was found among the 163 users of the preparation, and among the 322 nonusers, 9 positive cultures were found. While questions have been raised as to the methodology, a significant degree of protection seemed to exist.

The potential value of a single agent in providing protection against both vaginal infection and pregnancy was recognized by Johnson and Masters,[10] who developed a method of artificial coition for evaluating germicidal contraceptives. Studies using Progonasyl showed potential for both contraceptive and therapeutic purposes.

In 1958, a study by Ohno and coworkers[11] with a group of prostitutes practicing daily insertion of a vaginal foaming tablet containing either penicillin, chlortetracycline, chloramphenicol, or oxytetracycline, demonstrated protection against infection. The test group of 10 who used penicillin tablets had one case of gonorrhea in the month of use, while the control group of 20 had 9 cases during this same period. Similar studies, using chloramphenicol and oxytetracycline, showed a significant reduction in the rate of infection with gonorrhea. However, the concern for such use of antibiotics that can be combined with contraceptive agents is that widespread use could further contribute to the development of antibiotic resistance in the gonococcus.

A recrudescence of interest in the potential public health significance of a combined prophylaxis-contraceptive approach led by Dr. R. T. Ravenholt, Director, Office of Population of U.S. AID resulted in the availability of financial support for further investigation. The potential prophylactic value of all currently marketed vaginal contraceptive preparations was determined through laboratory studies by Singh and coworkers[12] (Tables 20-2, 20-3). A clinical study was carried out by Cutler and coworkers[13] in cooperation with the Venereal Disease Program of the Allegheny County Health Department to determine the possible value of a vaginal product used as directed for contraceptive purposes for prevention of reinfection with gonorrhea in women presenting at the VD clinic for treatment. In selecting the product for study, consideration was given to laboratory studies of antibacterial properties, packaging, and other characteristics that might influence the use of the preparation by the women at risk of infection. The product selected for use was Conceptrol the single-dose package of Delfen Cream, the active ingredient of which is 5% nonoxynol 9. The volunteers were clinic patients who had received treatment for gonorrhea and were using an IUD or oral contraceptive. No placebo was used because the chemicals used in manufacturing vaginal creams and gels, the emulsifiers themselves, have antibacterial properties. Although only limited studies have been done on this,[7,12] it was felt desirable not to use any potentially germicidal preparation as a placebo. Thus, the control group, randomly selected, used no vaginal preparation and returned to the VD clinic for scheduled visits for the purpose of examination only. In contrast, the study patients were given a new supply of the preparation under study as well as being examined. But both groups were equally reimbursed for their time and travel expenses, and contact history and other relevant data were secured in interviews with the study staff. In the six-month period with 22 study and 20 control females, the number of infections per patient months in the control group was 6.14, as compared to 0.67 in the group using the product as directed for contraception. As noted, compliance with the study protocol called for weekly visits to the clinic for culture and replenishment of the study preparation. After the first six months following treatment for the infection which brought the patient into the study, many participants failed to return to the clinic for follow-up. This meant that patients were no longer under protection, and attempts to reach them through follow-up procedures were often unsuccessful, since many had moved and left no forwarding address or

Table 20-2. Dilutions of Contraceptives Required to Immobilize *Treponema pallidum* (Suspension Within 1 to 1.5 Minutes) *

Group	Contraceptive	Concentration (%)	No. of Contraceptives	pH Range
A	Emko Concentrate + B, Ortho Cream	1	2	6.2–7.1
B	Certane Vaginal Jelly, Contra Foam, Cooper Creme, Delfen Cream, Delfen Foam, Emko Concentrate, Emko Concentrate + A, Finesse, Immolin Vaginal Cream-Jel, Lorophyn Suppositories, Ortho Gynol Jelly, Preceptin Gel	10	12	4.5–7.5
C	Contra Creme, Lanesta Gel, Ramses Vaginal Jelly	20	3	5.5–6.9
D	Koromex A Vaginal Jelly, Milex, Crescent Jelly	50	2	5.5–5.6

* Control from pH 3.5 to 9.4 did not immobilize spirochaetes in 5 minutes.
From Singh B, Cutler JC, Utidjian HMD: Studies on the development of a vaginal preparation providing both prophylaxis against venereal disease and other genital infections and contraception, Br J Vener Dis 48:57, 1972, with permission.

Table 20-3. Highest Dilution of 20 Contraceptives Required to Inhibit the Growth of *Neisseria gonorrhea* by Two Methods[a]

No.	Contraceptive	Time-Exposure Method					Plate-Dilution Method		
		Concentration percent[b]	pH	Growth after exposure (min) 1	5	10	Concentration percent	pH[c]	Growth[d]
1	Certane Vaginal Jelly	10	4.6	+	−	−	10	7.5	−
2	Contra Creme	50	6.9	+	+	−	10	7.5	−
3	Contra Foam	10	7.6	+	−	−	10	7.5	−
4	Cooper Creme	1	6.7	−	−	−	10	7.6	−
5	Delfen Cream	20	5.2	+	+	+	10	7.6	−
6	Delfen Foam	50	4.9	−	−	−	20	7.6	−
7	Emko Concentrate	50	7.4	−	−	−	20	7.5	−
8	Emko Concentrate + A	50	7.1	−	−	−	20	7.2	−
9	Emko Concentrate + B	50	7.2	−	−	−	20	7.2	−
10	Emko Concentrate + Spermicide	20	7.0	+	+	−	20	7.3	−
11	Emko Foam	10	7.3	−	−	−	10	7.4	−
12	Immolin Vaginal	50	4.9	−	−	−	10	7.5	−
13	Koromex A Vaginal Jelly	10	6.0	+	−	−	50	7.5	−
14	Lanesta Gel	10	5.6	+	−	−	10	7.5	−
15	Lorophyn Suppositories	10	5.7	+	−	−	10	7.5	−
16	Milex Crescent	10	5.7	−	−	−	10	7.5	−
17	Ortho Creme	1	6.2	+	−	−	1	7.4	−
18	Ortho-Gynol Jelly	10	5.5	+	−	−	10	7.4	−
19	Preceptin Gel	1	5.6	−	−	−	1	7.4	−
20	Ramses Vaginal	50	6.7	+	+	−	50	7.5	−

[a] Bacterial suspension for these experiments contains about 10 CFU per 0.1 ml, the inoculated Thayer-Martin selective medium plates were incubated at 37°C in CO_2 incubator.
[b] Only 50, 20, 10, and 1% dilutions in physiologic saline solution were tested.
[c] pH of media after adding the contraceptive at different concentrations.
[d] Results from duplicate plates.
From Singh B, Cutler JC, Utidjian HMD: Studies on the development of a vaginal preparation providing both prophylaxis against venereal disease and other genital infections and contraception. Br J Vener Dis 48:57, 1972, with permission.

would not respond to attempts by the research staff to encourage them to visit the clinic. But in spite of the problems involved in securing patient compliance—problems that must be dealt with in any type of self-protective public health approach—the findings did indicate a high level of prophylactic value of the contraceptive agent when properly used.

Two studies have been done using a vaginal-suppository contraceptive, Lorophyn, the active ingredient of which is phenylmercuric acetate (PMA). It should be noted, however, that PMA is no longer approved by the Food and Drug Administration.

Cole and associates[14] studied reinfection rates of VD clinic patients in two separate VD clinics in Tampa and Orlando, Florida. One group of patients was provided with the preparation to be used as directed for contraception. In the 1,245 women studied, the reinfection rate was 40% in the control group and 19% in the group using the suppository as directed for contraceptive purposes—a significant difference.

Rendon and coworkers[15] studied 138 women prostitutes in a public health clinic in Nuevo Laredo, Mexico, using suppositories of three types: Lorophyn with phenylmercuric acetate, a formulation with nonoxynol-9, and a placebo. In the 77 women who completed the six-month study, 14 cases of gonorrhea were observed—2 in users of the PMA suppositories, 4 in the nonoxynol-9 users, and 8 in the placebo group. There was a significant reduction in infection rates in the phemylmercuric acetate users.

The study of gonorrhea rates of the 280,000 member Group Health Cooperative of Puget Sound by Jick and associates[15] in 1980 provides significant findings with respect to infection rates in the group of women members who chose their preferred method of contraception. This group obviously differed from those attending a conventional health department VD clinic. While a variety of vaginal contraceptives was used, it was found that a 75% higher protective rate was provided for users of vaginal spermicides as a category. The authors are aware of methodologic problems inherent in this and other studies of potential prophylactic effects of vaginal preparations, but concluded that all of their studies favor the concept that vaginal contraceptive preparations prevent venereal disease in a significant number of users.

While the value of the condom as a prophylactic has long been known, it is of interest to note one of the recent studies carried out in Paris by Siboulet,[17] which provides striking confirmation and is particularly relevant because of the age of the males involved: age 16 to 22. Of the 302 condom-users who had contact with 142 females with proven gonorrhea and 142 with *Trichomonas vaginalis,* there were only 2 male cases of gonorrhea and 6 of *T. vaginalis* urethritis. In contrast, 464 of the 480 non-condom-users who had contact with females with gonorrhea were infected. Of the 104 contacts from this same group with *T. vaginalis,* 89 males were found to be infected. These findings reconfirm the protective value of the condom.

It should be noted that the development of oral contraceptives and IUD's led to diminished use of condom, chemical, and chemical/diaphragm contraceptive methods. It has been suggested that the rise in VD rates in both the United States and Europe may be related, in part at least, to the loss of the prophylactic effects of these contraceptive methods.

Before the discovery of specific, easily administered treatment for gonorrhea or syphilis, the importance of promoting prophylaxis, whether by local chemical or barrier methods, was recognized and appreciated, even though it was recognized that no single method was completely effective. It is also well known that the patterns of compliance with self-protective procedures, such as use of the condom, self-administerd local prophylactic or prophylactic-therapeutic preparations, or compliance with organized programs such as reporting to military prophylactic stations, are related to patterns of human behavior influenced by such factors as sexual arousal, alcohol or drug use, etc. In my experience as a Coast-Guard ship's physician during World War II, prophylaxis was administered to all men returning from shore leave "for recreational purposes" in foreign ports where prostitutes were freely available. A significant number of men were brought back to the ship completely drunk, assisted by their shipmates, and with no recollection of their sexual contacts. Under these conditions, station-administered prophylaxis can be considered good public health practice. Under circumstances where no such prophylactic procedures are available, such individuals cannot be expected to practice self-administered prophylaxis, thus the only methods of control available are prophylactic methods used and controlled by the female, such as vaginal preparations and long-term penicillin injections or oral antibiotics.

It should be kept in mind that many factors influence the patterns of sexual behavior, contraceptive practices, and self-protective or prophylactic behavior, and no attempt will be made to discuss these factors in detail. However, several other examples of this problem may serve to illustrate the complexity, and the resultant difficulties, in even carrying out carefully designed scientific studies of prophylaxis.

Samame[18] carried out a study of prophylaxis using a long-acting penicillin injection (PAM) in prostitutes in Tijuana, Mexico, serving primarily the U.S. military on the other side of the border. While this prophylactic penicillin therapy protected the female, difficulty was encountered in securing continued compliance with the regime. One of the reasons was that the women were becoming pregnant, presumably as a result of the treatment of chronic cervical infections which had resulted in pathologic sterility. Pregnancy interfered with their professional practice and cut off their income; thus some did not want to continue to receive penicillin and refused to comply with the prophylactic treatment regimen.

In spite of the problems of compliance there was evidence of success in reducing infection. In a group of 680 prostitutes who were to be given weekly injections of 300,000 U of procaine penicillin G with aluminum monostearate (PAM), 400 appeared regularly for injection and examination, 93 were irregular, and 187 dropped out. Prior to the study, the group had been found to have 111 culture-positive cases of gonorrhea, and 2 early and 9 early-latent cases of syphilis. In the 8 months of the study there were only 38 cases of gonorrhea and no new cases of syphilis.

Of particular significance, and obviously a better marker, is the monthly average of cases of VD in the 11th Naval District, treated in San Diego, California, with Tijuana, Mexico as the point of contact. Prior to the prophylactic therapy program for the prostitutes there were 87 cases per month. After the study started, there were 47 cases per month seen in the clinic. In this study,

as in others, problems of experimental design and implementation are evident, but the outcome of the program was a significant reduction in number of the military receiving treatment in one clinic. It can be assumed that the civilian clients also benefited.

A similar problem was recently encountered in a study begun on a group of prostitutes in Bangkok, Thailand. A vaginal contraceptive was being studied with respect to its prophylactic value, under a protocol designed to deal with the criticisms of various recent studies of prophylactic use as described in studies reported above.[13–15] The study was terminated because of two factors that influenced the pattern of compliance by the prostitutes. First, many of the professional prostitutes were married and, because such use would suggest that the husband might be infected, it was culturally unacceptable; they would not use the preparation in marital contact. Second, many of their clients were repeat customers, often slow to ejaculate. Since the prostitute's income depends on the number of customers per working day, and since she knew that increased lubrication provided by vaginal preparations further delayed ejaculation, the study subjects would not follow the study protocol with these clients. Therefore the study was terminated and never reported.

These two examples are indicative of the problems involved in carrying out the type of study required with respect to the questions raised as to the validity of the findings regarding recent studies reported and analyzed in the editorial by Cates and coworkers.[19] The design and implementation of a study which would be scientifically ideal posed many problems because of the social attitudes toward studies related to sexual practice. Thus, decisions may have to be made on the basis of analyses of a number of similar studies, each of which may provide a few of the necessary facts.

The existence of a degree of immunity to

reinfection, based upon a history of previous infection, whether accompanied by serologic evidence provided by standard, existing diagnostic tests or not, was shown by studies on human volunteers by Mahoney and coworkers[20] for gonorrhea and Magnuson and associates[21] for syphilis. The interest in immunization as a method of control has centered on gonorrhea, regrettably with little interest or financial support for such studies until very recently. However, a recent study by Brinton and colleagues[22] proves the existence of vaccine-produced immunity and suggests the potential for development of a vaccine against gonorrhea. The potential contribution of immunization against gonorrhea to STD control programs is obvious. However, it must be recognized that public attitudes, particularly parental attitudes with respect to what immunization they will permit their children to receive or what they will permit them to be taught in this highly emotional area of sexual behavior, will influence immunization programs against gonorrhea.

The extensive research studies done to date, with respect to immunization and the problems yet to be overcome, are described in detail in the report of a WHO consultative group on the development of a gonococcal vaccine.[23] It appears that there is no prospect for incorporation of immunization as an element of programs of prevention in the near future.

The use of therapeutic prophylaxis or prophylactic treatment for gonorrhea and syphilis has long been practiced. The level of usage has varied with the types of populations at risk, current medical knowledge and practices, and therapeutic agents available. However, prophylactic therapy for syphilis, when the usual treatment with arsenicals required two years, posed quite a different question of choice for physicians and contacts than a single-injection curative dose of antibiotic does today. Prophylactic administration of sulfonamide preparations was an element of VD control programs during World War II.[6] Various civilian and military programs have carried out limited research or control programs utilizing prophylactic antibiotic procedures with both oral therapy and injections of long-acting agents.[18,24–26] While such prophylactic measures have been shown to be effective under certain circumstances, particularly where there is good medical management, the serious medical/public health problems of potential development of drug resistance resulting from noncompliance with standard procedures must be faced.

Sulfonamide-resistant gonococcus was a serious problem, particularly in the military, by the time penicillin became available. Subsequently, the misuse of antibiotics for both prophylaxis and therapy caused a significant increase in the penicillin-resistant gonococcus, commonly seen today.

There are circumstances under which such prophylactic therapy represents the optimal practice of medicine, but this method should play only a minor role in control efforts, and then only under medical supervision that assures adequate curative doses. Fortunately, thus far there is no evidence of development of penicillin resistance by *Treponema pallidum*.

The history of concern for the civilian population and of effective action to cope with the problem is perhaps best reflected in the national program instituted by the U.S. Public Health Service, beginning with the Chamberlain-Kahn Act of 1918. This program was revitalized and enlarged under the leadership of Surgeon General Thomas Parran when funds became available in 1936. As part of the cooperative program involving federal, state, and local health agencies, with strong support from the academic community and the private and voluntary sectors of medicine, attention was paid to prevention of the spread of disease. This was accomplished by the institution of the case-finding program through contact tracing, screening measures such as premarital blood tests, testing pregnant women, and many other highly effective procedures. Existing prophylactic methods—the condom, chemicals systemic therapy—as well as health education were promoted.

What is of particular significance from these experiences, with respect to the problem of control today, is that the leaders in the field effectively used a variety of methods of control in a well-integrated and co-ordinated classic public health program. In addition to trying to promote responsible sexual behavior through efforts of the church, voluntary agencies, and other sectors of society, the program leadership recognized that there was no single approach that could effectively reach all individuals at risk or actually infected. Thus, even at a time when treatment depended upon arsenic bismuth and sulfonamides and required days, weeks, or years of therapy, the total public health approach encompassed case-finding, treatment, and prophylaxis, thereby achieving major advances in control.

One example of the importance of social attitudes and the problems they pose in the development and implementation of VD control programs is exemplified by the history of funding of the research in patterns of sexual behavior by the Kinsey group, which began in 1938.[27]

Although knowledge of sexual behavior was necessary for planning the Public Health Service VD control activities, particularly for case finding, contact identification, and management, the issue was so politically sensitive that federal VD control funds could not be used for such studies. After some initial small-scale funding, later discontinued because of the political sensitivity, the landmark Kinsey studies were supported completely by private funds, largely from the Rockefeller Foundation. These studies provided critically important data for program planning and development as well as for development of methodology for future studies. These ''baseline data''

permit a better understanding of the current status of the STD's.

There are several factors related to human behavior that are important in understanding the reasons for the present STD problem and in developing methods of control. The lower age at which an increasingly large segment of the population initiates sexual intercourse, increasing break-up of marriages, increasing sexual freedom and activity of the female, a pattern that was formerly considered predominantly male, are all factors that increase the risk of acquiring or transmitting STD's in addition to the related risks of unplanned pregnancy. A substantial proportion of the population is starting sexual activity before marriage, and there is a significant time lapse between onset of intercourse and initiation of contraceptive practice.

A recent study by Zelnik and Shah[28] reports findings of great relevance to current STD control programs. In the metropolitan areas studied, 50% of females 15 to 19 years of age, and 70% of males 17 to 21 years of age had had intercourse. Of particular interest is the finding that 19% of the white and 37% of the black females and 32% of the white and 65% of the black males had had first intercourse at age 15 or earlier. Since the pattern of contraceptive usage at first intercourse offers important insight with respect to STD control methods, it is important to note that only 49% of white females and 44% of white males used any contraception, as compared with only 41% and 30% of black females and males, respectively. There was a difference in self-protective (contraceptive) behavior related to whether the first intercourse had been planned or unplanned. Up to 35% of the white males and 20% of the black males used the condom at the first intercourse. These findings, with respect to family planning, have great relevance to STD control activities, and in spite of the high rates of noncontraceptive practice, progress has been made. To quote Zelnick and Shah, "the data presented here . . . clearly demonstrate the the problem of adolescent pregnancy would be considerably greater than it is if there were no organized family planning programs to deal with the problem."

Even if one is using a method for contraception, the effectiveness of the method depends in part upon proper use of the method. One of the advantages of the IUD or oral contraceptives is that the procedure is not related to the act of intercourse; thus there is a higher degree of compliance with lower failure rates. However, from the public health point of view one must make the best use of available knowledge and resources and work toward improvement. The range of failure of contraceptives within the first year of use (mostly due to noncompliance) by American women is as follows: oral contraceptives, 2%; IUD's, 5%; the condom, 10%; foam, 18%; diaphragm, 19%, and fertility-awareness methods (cervical mucus, basal body temperature, etc.), 24%. In spite of these failure rates, the net effect of the use of a variety of methods has been a reduction in unplanned pregnancy. The same range of failures, but overall beneficial effects, can be postulated for prophlactic measures.

The rise in gonorrhea rates, particularly asymptomatic male urethritis, the cause of which is still unexplained, plus the increasing number of women with pelvic inflammatory disease of various etiologies, in particular gonococcal/chlamydia, have resulted in major increases in health care costs and resultant social concerns. The potential value of a revitalized and strengthened public health approach is well stated by Wiesner and Parra,[30] who reviewed the role of prevention in reducing social and economic costs of STD's, which are continuing to increase despite current public health and medical knowledge and efforts. A model of the potential effect of the use of a less than absolutely effective method of prevention of transmission of infection by various proportions of the population at risk

was developed by Lee and coworkers.[31] The use of a preparation only 50% effective by as few as 25% of the population at risk could theoretically result in a reduction of about 80% per year in the number of cases expected in an unprotected and otherwise untreated population. These projections are theoretical, but the magnitude of the potential impact is in keeping with that reported in some past military experiences such as those of Moore.[3]

Current VD control programs take into account the fact that the female at risk has only one method of protection over which she has some control, other than to say "no," and that is systemic prophylactic therapy. The need for women to take an increasingly independent role in maintaining their health and the methods by which they can accomplish this through self-care as in the prevention of unplanned pregnancy or VD through various methods is being made known by groups such as the Boston Women's Health Book Collective. Their publication, *Our Bodies, Ourselves*[32] provides easily understood and practical means for women to protect and improve their health, particularly reproductive health.

A similar approach for both men and women is exemplified by the instructional pamphlet prepared and widely distributed by the American Foundation for the Prevention of VD.[33] Emphasis is placed on self-protective sexual practice through existing methods by which both the male and female may avoid infection.

On the basis of the experiences summarized in this chapter, it seems obvious that the concept and practice of prophylaxis—self-administered or applied—must once again be strongly promoted as an element of STD control programs. Contraceptive technology, race, education, and so on, will play an important role in usage following initiation of sexual activities. Absolute compliance with prescribed patterns of usage cannot be realistically expected, but usage will take place in varying degrees if the concept is promoted, with a resultant lowering of the rates of infection. While the attainment of the highest levels of use and effectiveness of any health protective or promotive procedure is the ideal goal of a public health worker, one must keep in mind the old Spanish proverb "the perfect is the enemy of the good." We should learn from past successes of the well-planned and well-administered "good" in VD diagnosis, treatment, and prevention before the "perfect" penicillin, for instance, ever existed; then we must revitalize the prophylactic element of control programs while taking other necessary actions to rebuild the total STD control program.

REFERENCES

1. Curran JW: Economic Consequences of pelvic inflammatory disease in the United States. Am J Obstet Gynecol 138:848, 1980
2. Benson AS (ed): A.P.H.A. control of communicable diseases in man. 12th Ed. American Public Health Association, Washington, DC, 1978
3. Moore JE: The value of prophylaxis against venereal diseases. JAMA 75:911, 1920
4. Stokes JH, Berman H, Ingrahm NR: Modern Clinical Syphilology. 3rd Ed. p 1226. Saunders, Philadelphia, 1944
5. Porter HS, Witcher RB, Knoblock C: Social disease at the crossroads. J Okla State Med Assoc 32:54, 1939
6. Sternberg TH, Howard EB: Prophylaxis, preventive medicine in World War II. Commun Dis Office of the Surgeon General, Department of the Army, 196, 1960
7. Arnold RC, Cutler JC: Experimental studies to develop a local prophylaxis of gonorrhea in women. Br J Vener Dis 32:24, 1956
8. Funes JM, Agular CL: Mapharsen-orvus solution in the prophylaxis of gonorrhea in women. Bull Pan Am Health Organ 33:121, 1952
9. Edwards WM: Vaginal prophylaxis. p 94. Epidemic venereal disease proceedings of the 2nd international VD symposium, St. Louis, 1972. American Social Health Association, Pfizer Laboratories, New York, 1973
10. Johnson VE, Masters WH: A product of dual import: Intravaginal infection control and conception control. Pacific Med 73:269, 1965
11. Ohno T, Kato K, Nagata M, et al: Prophylactic control of the spread of venereal disease through prostitutes in Japan. Bull WHO 19:575, 1958
12. Singh B, Cutler JC, Utidjian HMD: Effect in vitro of vaginal contraceptive and noncontraceptive preparations on T. pallidum and N. gonorrhea. Br J Vener Dis 48:57, 1972
13. Cutler JC, Singh B, Carpenter U, et al: Vaginal contraceptives as prophylaxis against gonorrhea and other sexually transmissible diseases. Adv Plann Parent 12:45, 1977
14. Cole CH, Lacher TC, Bailey JC, Fairclough DL: Vaginal chemoprophylaxis in the reduction of reinfection in women with gonorrhea. Br J Vener Dis 54:314, 1980
15. Rendon AL, Covarrubias J, McCarney KE, et al: A controlled comparative study of phenylmercuric acetate, nonoxynal-9, and Placebo vaginal suppositories as prophylactic agents against gonorrhea. Curr Ther Res 27:780, 1980
16. Jick H, Hamman MT, Stergadris A, et al: Vaginal spermicides and gonorrhea. JAMA 248:1619, 1972
17. Siboulet A: Maladies sexuelles transmissibles interêt des traitments prophylactiques. Prophylaxis Sanitaire it Morale (France) 44:155, 1972
18. Samamé G: Systemic antivenereal prophylaxis, preliminary report on the study in Tiajuana, Mexico. Bull Pan Am Health Organ 30;42, 1951
19. Cates WJ, Wiesner PH, Curran SW: Sex and spermicides: Preventing unintended pregnancy. JAMA 248:1636, 1982
20. Mahoney JF, Van Slyke CJ, Cutler SC, Blum HL: Experimental gonocci urethritis in human volunteers. Am JSCVD 30:1, 1946
21. Magnuson HJ, Thomas EW, Olansky SJ, et al: Inoculation syphilis in human volunteers. Medicine (Baltimore) 35:33, 1956
22. Brinton CC, Brown A, Rogers K, et al: Preparation, testing, safety, antigenicity, immunogenicity, and serologic specificity of a

purified gonococcal pilus vaccine for gonorrhea. p 140. In Weinstein L, Fields B (eds): Current Chemotherapy and Infectious Diseases. Vol IV, Bacterial Vaccines. Thieme-Stratton, New York, 1981

23. WHO Consultive Group on Development of a gonococcal vaccine; current status and recommendations for further research. Montreal, Aug. 7, 1982. WHO/VDT/83.434, WHO/VDT/RES/GON/83.140

24. Greenberg JH: Venereal disease in the armed forces. Med Aspects Hum Sex 6:165, 1972

25. Harrison WO: Prophylaxis against gonorrhea: Is an ounce of prevention worth the cost? Milit Med 146:9, 1981

26. Hume J: On reports and rapport in VD control. JAMA 70:946, 1980

27. Kinsey AC, Pomeroy WB, Martin CE: Sexual behavior in the American male. Saunders, Philadelphia, London, 1948

28. Zelnick M, Shah FK: First intercourse among young Americans. Fam Plann Perspect 15:64, 1983

29. Tyrer LB, Duarte J: The state of the contraceptive art. Plann Parent Rev 3:5, 1983

30. Wiesner PH, Parra WC: Sexually transmitted diseases: Meeting the 1970 objectives—a challenge for the 1980s. Public Health Rep 97:409, 1982

31. Lee TY, Utidjian HMD, Carpenter U, Cutler JC: Potential impact of chemical prophylaxis on the incidence of gonorrhea. Br J Vener Dis 48:376, 1972

32. Boston Womens' Health Book Collective: Our Bodies, Ourselves. 2nd Ed. Simon & Schuster, New York, 1979

33. American Foundation for the Prevention of VD: The New Venereal Disease Prevention for Everyone. 10th Ed., rev. 1983.

21

Gardnerella and Trichomonas Vaginitis

Michael R. Spence

One of the most common reasons that a woman visits a gynecologist today is because of an abnormal vaginal discharge. It has been estimated that approximately one third of all office visits are for this indication.[1] Upon evaluation of the patient, the question that is usually asked is, "Do you have a discharge?" The answer to this question is almost uniformly "yes." However, a more appropriate question would be, "Do you have an abnormal vaginal discharge?" All women have a physiologic vaginal discharge, and what is normal for one woman may be considered abnormal for another and vice versa. Additionally, when a clinician identifies a patient with a discharge, rather than initiate what may be inappropriate diagnostic evaluations or therapy she should be asked what is abnormal for her.

The causes of abnormal vaginal discharge are physiologic, noninfectious, and infectious. The infectious etiologies can further be subdivided into those secondary to cervicitis and those caused by vaginitis. These phenomena will be more thoroughly described in this section.

Each month, in the ovulating woman, midcycle is marked by an increased production of cervical mucus. This is frequently perceived by the patient as being an increase in her vaginal discharge. It is usually white and is often associated with mild itching. If, at this time, the patient has midcycle spotting, a discharge can appear brown or brownish-green due to blood breakdown by-products. It can also have a disagreeable odor. This can result in the patient seeking immediate medical attention. Therefore, when a patient is encountered with an abnormal vaginal discharge, it should be determined where she is in her menstrual cycle. Another form of physiologic discharge is associated with the loss of estrogen stimulation to the vaginal epithelia. This is most often seen in older women who have reached menopause, have undergone ovarian failure, and have not received exogenous estrogen supplement. This "senile vaginitis" is associated with a watery, serosanguineous discharge, and discomfort with intercourse. The vaginal mucosa appears pale and thin, and the trauma from pelvic examination is often enough to initiate bleeding. Microscopic examination of a specimen from the discharge reveals red blood cells and parabasal cells. Large squamous epithelial cells are rare.

Another cause of "senile vaginitis," especially in the premenopausal woman, is pelvic surgery. Patients who are surgically castrated must be provided with supplemental estrogen. Otherwise, they will develop "senile vaginitis" as described above.

Other noninfectious causes of abnormal vaginal discharge include trauma secondary to a foreign body, and a reaction to a noxious chemical agent. Foreign bodies that have been removed from the vagina include buttons, safety pins, pens, implements of masturbation, condoms, and diaphragms. However, the most common foreign body is the tampon. This is usually not found in the young patient who has just started menstruating, but is more commonly encountered in a woman between the ages of 20 and 30. The patient usually presents complaining of an offensive body odor. She often will give a history of using many feminine sprays, deodorants, and douches to no avail. She will also frequently be fearful that she has contracted some sexually transmitted disease. Upon examination, it is readily confirmed that the odor that she has is offensive. On speculum examination, the presence of the foreign body is readily apparent. The condition can be cured by the simple removal of the foreign body. However, when this is done, efforts should be made to put it into a sealed container such as a baggie, or into a couple of inverted gloves in which the wrist portion has been tied off so as to preclude the continual effusion of the odor. Upon inspection of the vaginal mucosa after removal of the foreign body, it is usually erythematous and sometimes eroded. There is no need to initiate therapy with an antimicrobial cream or systemic agent. If the patient is reevaluated within 72 to 96 hours, the areas of erythema and erosion have spontaneously disappeared. These patients are quite often embarrassed as well as relieved once the diagnosis is made.

Many of the currently marketed feminine hygiene sprays, deodorant suppositories, and spermicidal foams and jellies can be associated with an allergic reaction and the development of an abnormal vaginal discharge. Likewise, many of the rubber products, including condoms and diaphragms, can give a similar reaction. Reports will undoubtedly soon be demonstrating a similar problem with the contraceptive sponge. These are allergic phenomena and usually removal of the offending agent is all that is necessary to cure the condition.

Infectious causes of abnormal vaginal discharge include infections of the cervix and vagina. It is beyond the scope of this chapter to describe all the agents that are associated with the abnormal vaginal discharge that are infectious in nature. In subsequent sections, two agents that are known to be associated with vaginal infection (vaginitis) will be discussed.

GARDNERELLA VAGINALIS VAGINITIS

History

In February 1953 Leopold[2] reported that he had isolated an organism from the genitourinary system that he felt had not been previously described. This organism was a gram-negative, nonmotile, nonencapsulated, pleomorphic rod approximately 0.5 μm wide and from 0.5 to 2 μm long. He described the colonial morphology of the organism, and also the growth characteristics. Additionally, he noted that it was associated with clinical symptoms in the patients from whom it was isolated. The men from whom he obtained the organism showed signs of a mild to moderate prostatitis, which was found both with and without urethritis. He noted in many that the prostatitis was detected by physical examination after the laboratory reported the presence of the organism in the urine, indicating that this condition was mildly symptomatic or asymptomatic. The women from whom the organism was isolated were diagnosed as having cervicitis. Many of the women were without symptoms. He was unable to isolate this organism from the upper genitourinary tract by ureteral catheterization.

Leopold's report went unnoticed for approximately two years. In 1955 Gardner and Dukes[3] published their report: "A Newly Defined Specific Infection Previously Classified 'Non-specific' Vaginitis." They, like Leopold, described a gram-negative rod of similar morphology. Also, like Leopold, they believed that this organism was a member of the family *Haemophilus*. The name *Haemophilus vaginalis* was assigned to this new agent. Their report included the clinical observations H. L. Gardner made in evaluating 1,181 patients in his practice. The report described a symptom complex associated with the organism that was differentiated from symptom complexes associated with other known pathogens. The "clue cell" was also first described. The "clue cell" was thought to represent an epithelial cell that had been virtually covered in the entirety of its surface with the organism thought to be causative of this condition. Attempts were made to fulfill Koch's postulates. Two methods were undertaken. Pure cultures of the organism in question were inoculated into the vaginas of 13 volunteers. Only one of the patients developed the typical signs of the condition. The reason for the inability to initiate the infection was based on the difficulty in maintaining the organism owing to its extreme fastidiousness. They noted that the organism was easily lost in serial passage.

In an additional 15 patients demonstrated to be free of the infection, inoculation was made from material taken from the vaginas of infected patients. Subsequently, 11 of the 15 developed the clinical manifestations seen in the donors. Although this experiment did not fulfill Koch's postulates in the strictest sense, the results strongly implied an interrelationship, and the interpretation

was that the organism *Haemophilus vaginalis* was causative of the condition. Further work by Criswell and coworkers,[4] utilizing different strains of the same microorganism in 29 volunteers, resulted again in only a minimum of patients acquiring the infection. The authors were able to demonstrate that the infections were derived from specific strains. This may indicate that there are strain variations with regard to infectivity.

When first identified and described by Leopold, and subsequently by Gardner and Dukes, the organism was named *Haemophilus vaginalis*. Subsequently, Zinnemann and Turner,[5] on evaluating the growth characteristics of the organism, proposed that it be placed in the *Corynebacterium* genus. In 1980 Greenwood and Pickett[6] felt that the organism did not meet the criteria necessary to be classified in the genus *Haemophilus* or the genus *Corynebacterium,* and they have proposed that a new genus *Gardnerella* be established. This has been accepted and is now the terminology employed for describing this organism. In the text of this article *Gardnerella vaginalis* will be the predominant name used to signify the organism that has previously been described as *Haemophilus vaginalis* and/or *Corynebacterium vaginale*. It is thought that these names for this organism are synonymous and describe flora associated with a specific syndrome.

The aforementioned work has resulted in a controversy that has yet to be resolved. The role of *Haemophilus vaginalis (Corynebacterium vaginale, Gardnerella vaginalis)* and associated microorganisms in patients with vaginal discharge has yet to be defined. Nonetheless, in the following sections a description of the epidemiology, diagnosis, and therapy of the condition called nonspecific vaginitis, nonspecific vaginosis, bacterial vaginosis, *Gardnerella vaginitis, Haemophilus vaginitis,* and *Corynebacterium vaginitis* will be discussed.

Epidemiology

Interest in the microbiology of abnormal vaginal discharges is not a new phenomenon. In 1913 Curtis[7] read a paper before the Chicago Gynecological Society in which he described microorganisms that were found in the vagina at the time of leukorrhea. In this report, he described many bacillary forms, including a "curved rod" as well as a short pleomorphic anaerobic bacillary form. Whether the organisms that Dr. Curtis described included *Gardnerella* is unclear from the writings. He does, however, point out the complex nature of the microbial flora in patients with an abnormal vaginal discharge. Many authors have done both qualitative and quantitative evaluations of the microbial flora of the female genital tract.[8-10] Additionally, serial sampling in patients has also been conducted.[11] The results of all of these studies indicate that *Gardnerella vaginalis* is a common organism isolated from the genital tract, and, although it has been associated with patients in whom there is an abnormal vaginal discharge, it is frequently found in the asymptomatic host. Osborne and associates[12] were able to demonstrate that the organism was isolated in 23% of symptomatic women, whereas it was only found in 5% of asymptomatic women in a series of patients that had multiple sexually transmitted agents. McCormack and colleagues,[13] however, found that there was no association between the colonization with this organism and an abnormal vaginal discharge, either as reported by the patient or as noted by the examiner. He also noted the association of isolation with the patient being of nonwhite race, using oral contraceptives, being unmarried, and having had a previous pregnancy. Previous sexual experience did not appear to influence the rate of colonization. The organism was isolated in 29% of sexually inexperienced women and in 41% of those who had had previous intercourse with six or more men. Similar findings were described by Levinson and his associates[14] when they performed a quantitative study of the microflora of the reproductive tract. He noted that 40% of patients with no evidence of inflammatory vaginal disease were harboring the organism. These findings are similar to that of McCormack. McCormack and associates[13] alluded to the association between oral contraceptive use and the isolation of *Gardnerella vaginalis*. A similar finding was obtained by Josey and Lambe[15] in 184 patients infected with the organism. They compared these patients to 140 women in a control group. It was noted that 51% of the study patients were taking oral contraceptives, as compared with 35% of their controls. Additionally, another sexually transmitted agent was concomitantly harbored, or had previously been isolated, in 52% of the women in the study group, compared with 38% of controls. Another interesting finding was the rate of cervical neoplasia in their population. They found that 13.6% of the study patients had this finding, compared with 5.7% of the control group. In view of these findings, it was their interpretation that *Gardnerella vaginalis* is a sexually transmitted organism.

The prevalence of *Gardnerella* in the aforementioned studies varies between 12 and approximately 50%. These data are obtained from a one-time culture on a specific patient and may not reflect the overall harboring of the organisms. Sautter and Brown[11] did serial sampling two to three times per week for one month in seven patients. They collected a total of 65 specimens, and noted that 58% of the cultures were positive for *Gardnerella*. It was the predominant organism in 40% of cases, and persisted throughout the entire cycle in more than 50% of the serial cultures in 60% of patients evaluated. In one subject, it was found in all samples, and in another, it was only found in 1 off 11 samples. It should be noted that all patients had the organism isolated at one time or another during the course of their cycle. Because of the small number of subjects, no attempts were made to correlate the finding of the organism with sexual activity and/or contraceptive employment. It is of note, however, that with this high frequency of finding none of the patients were symptomatic. This allowed the authors to postulate that it appears to be normal flora in a high percentage of women, and may cause infection only when proper circumstances of irritation, increased secretions, or other conditions are met. This view was likewise reported by Tashjian and his colleagues,[16] upon their evaluation of the vaginal flora in asymptomatic women. They noted in four groups of patients—pregnant women, premenopausal patients on oral contraceptives, premenopausal patients not using oral contraceptives and postmenopausal patients—that the organism was isolated, although their patients were asymptomatic. Hence they supported the idea that this organism is asymptomatically harbored and may constitute part of the normal flora of the reproductive tract.

Complications

Although *Gardnerella vaginalis* is considered part of the normal flora of the female reproductive tract and is associated with abnormal vaginal discharge, on occasion it has also been associated with severe illness. Edmunds,[17] Regamey and Schoenknecht,[18] and Venkataramani and Rathbun[19] have reported purpural fever, purpural sepsis, and bacteremia associated with this organism. The data presented by Edmunds are not as convincing as those of the other authors, who were able to demonstrate isolation of the organism from the blood. Recent work by Gravett and Eshenbach[20] have demonstrated similar phenomena. The role of this organism in the pathogenesis of significant infection needs to be further delineated. Platt[21] presents

two cases in which there is apparent transfer from the mother to the neonate. One case demonstrated potential ascending endometritis and amniotic infection syndrome, resulting in congenital sepsis and death; and the other was a superficial infection that may have been acquired during passage through the birth canal. The adverse outcomes that were associated with both of these cases were determined microbiologically to be associated with *Gardnerella*. Rotheram and Schick,[22] in describing sepsis associated with abortion, demonstrated one patient to have a pure culture of *Gardnerella* in this condition.

The aforementioned cases suggest that the organism, which is basically ubiquitous, can be associated with significant serious illness. Fortunately, the very low frequency of this particular event is encouraging and supports the lack of need to diagnose and then treat prophylactically patients who might be harboring the organism. However, when patients with significant infection are encountered, the potential of *Gardnerella* as being causative must not be underestimated.

Diagnosis

CLINICAL DIAGNOSIS

The syndrome, first described by Gardner and Dukes, included women who complained of an abnormal vaginal discharge. It was pointed out by these authors that not all patients presented with a complaint of an abnormal vaginal discharge, but they did verify the problem once they were specifically asked. Additionally, many gave histories of having to use douching and other hygienic measures because of an odor or discharge. Although it is unclear from studies, both past and present, what the absolute prevalence of abnormal vaginal discharge is in the condition, it certainly appears to exist in over 50% of the patients.

Once the symptom of abnormal vaginal discharge, frequently associated with a disagreeable odor, is elicited, then further clinical steps can be utilized to make the diagnosis. The findings include the presence of an abnormal, increased discharge in the vagina, which is usually grayish-white, adherent to the vaginal walls, and homogeneous in quality. When the pH of the discharge is measured, it is usually above 4.5, and commonly is between 5.0 and 6.0. When a specimen of a discharge is mixed with normal saline, placed on a microscope slide and then covered with a coverslip, and then is viewed microscopically, the characteristic clue cell, as first described by Gardner and Dukes, is visualized. This is an epithelial cell that appears to be stippled or granular. The stippling or granularity is thought to be secondary to the close adherence of the organism *Gardnerella* to the surface of the cell. Additionally, when one looks in the background, one sees large numbers of the microorganism in the vaginal fluid. The paucity of white blood cells has raised the question as to whether this is a true vaginitis. However, this is one more feature that aids in the diagnosis. Recently the so-called "whiff test" has been described.[23] This test is conducted by placing a small amount of the vaginal discharge on a microscope slide, and mixing it with 10% potassium hydroxide. The production of aromatic and aliphatic amines results in a fishy odor. It is thought that the diamines, putrescine and cadaverine, are most responsible for this particular phenomenon.[24]

LABORATORY DIAGNOSIS

The most readily available and easily usable laboratory tool to assist in the diagnosis is the microscope. This is employed, as is described above in the Clinical Diagnosis section, in identifying the presence of the clue cell. Additionally, specimens from the vaginal discharge can be placed on a microscope slide, dried, heat-fixed, and then stained with Gram's reagents. This results in the ready identification of a gram-negative, small bacillary form. When epithelial cells are noted in the preparation, the clue cell can be identified as being an epithelial cell that is almost in its totality covered with these small microorganisms. Additionally, they are seen in the background. Frequently the organism stains gram-variable and appears as a coccobacillus.[25] The utility of the diagnosis by Gram's stain was recently supported by Spiegel and her associates.[26]

Lewis and O'Brien[27] evaluated 441 patients by Papanicolaou smear and compared this with the culture diagnosis. They demonstrated that they could correctly interpret the presence of *Gardnerella* on Pap smear in 87.4% cases. However, they had a false positive rate of 10.4%. In a smaller study, Smith and associates[28] compared Gram-stained vaginal smears with cervical Papanicolaou smears isolation. They likewise reported a high rate of false positives when Papanicolaou smear was compared with culture. In view of these findings, one should be cautioned to not place high reliance on the Papanicolaou smear for making the diagnosis. This is specifically true in the asymptomatic patient.

Immunofluorescent procedures have also been utilized in the identification of *Gardnerella*.[29] These authors compared immunofluorescent techniques to culture, microscopic evaluation of clue cells, ang Gram stains in 132 patients derived from three separate sources. They found a very strong correlation between the fluorescent antibody method and culture methods. They also noted that the fluorescent antibody techniques picked up five other patients that had been missed by culture. To rule out nonspecific fluorescence, they did in vitro interspecies testing with all bacteria isolated and demonstrated the specificity of their reaction. They also noted that, although "clue cells" on wet preparation as well as positive Gram stains were common, they were unable to either culture the organism or demonstrate specific fluorescence in many of those patients. The implication being that the clue cell and the Gram stain are less specific and may be derived from organisms other than *Gardnerella*.

The absolute standard for identification using laboratory techniques is culture. In his initial investigations, Leopold[2] employed Casman's blood agar for the isolation of the organism. Although there have been many other variations of blood agars and broths employed for the identification of *Gardnerella,* this has been the primary standard.[30-32] Because of the colonization of the genital tract with a multitude of microorganisms the addition of colistin, nalidixic acid, and amphotericin to the isolation media to preclude growth by concomitant organisms has been popular. The organisms being facultative anaerobes also have their isolation enhanced by incubation in either a candle extinction jar or a gas pack system.[33] Identification is by colony morphology and specific growth characteristics as well as sugar fermentation. Further confirmation is the demonstration of catalase positivity. Recently, there has been an interest in further substantiating the identity of the organism by gas-liquid partition chromatography, measuring the volatile fatty acids produced by sugar fermentation.s;3[4]

Although culture diagnosis as well as various types of chromatography are helpful in research endeavors, it is not needed in evaluating the individual patient. The diagnosis of a patient is based on the presence of an abnormal discharge and the symptom complex that hallmarks the syndrome. One can further substantiate the diagnosis employing various laboratory methods. The single most simple and reliable technique for supporting the diagnosis is identification of the "clue cell" on wet preparation. Because of the high number of positive cultures in the normal population, routine employment of culture is probably not cost-effective.

Therapy

The recommendations for therapy for *Gardnerella vaginalis* vaginitis are difficult to support on a scientific basis. Since the pathogenesis of this particular phenomenon is not well-understood and the microbiology associated with it is even less well-understood, it is difficult to appreciate how a specific recommendation for therapy can be made. It is thought that the nonspecific vaginitis associated with *Gardnerella vaginalis* is a synergistic infection between that organism and vaginal anaerobes. This hypothesis is consistent with using metronidazole for therapy. However, the high carriage rate of *Gardnerella* and anaerobes in asymptomatic, normal healthy women is also well-established. Hence, the syndrome has to have other, yet to be defined, components.

Therapy of the *Gardnerella vaginalis* vaginitis syndrome with topical agents has been popular.[35,36] Jones and coworkers[37] recently reported that in vitro tests demonstrated both Bacteroides strains found in the vagina as well as *Gardnerella vaginalis* were susceptible to at least two of three sulfonamides at high concentration. This corresponds to previous observations where these agents have been demonstrated to be effective in from one third to one half of the patients that have been treated.[35-38] Because of the high failure rate (approximately 50%) with the topical agents, and lower failure rates encountered when systemic agents are used, the majority of clinicians have opted for the more successful forms of therapy.

Although immediate relief may result upon instillation of a cream with this agent in the vagina, it is difficult to determine if an abnormal discharge was present or not. Additionally, cure rates may have been the result of decreasing the total vaginal flora. Follow-up studies to determine the frequency of recurrence of symptoms are not readily available. It is possible that the topical agents that have been employed suppressed the growth of the microorganisms in the vagina to the point where the patient became asymptomatic. However, upon the discontinuation of the cream, the flora could be reestablished and, within a time period, could result in recurrence of symptoms.

Ampicillin and tetracycline have been employed for this condition, with varying degrees of success. Gardner and Kaufman[39] reported that ampicillin 500 mg every six hours for five days was the most effective therapy, and this was substantiated in a subsequent report by Lee and Schmale.[40] Ampicillin has become standard therapy for this condition.

In 1978 Pheifer and associates[23] evaluated topical sulfonamides, oral doxycycline, oral ampicillin, and oral metronidazole in the therapy of the nonspecific vaginitis thought to be associated with *Gardnerella vaginalis*. Their results with the first three agents were poor. However, they noted that 80 or 81 patients given oral metronidazole were cured, with a regimen of 500 mg twice daily for seven days. This result was surprising because of the differences in activity between ampicillin and metronidazole in the in vitro situation.[41] The response they noted may have been due to the nonspecific activity that metronidazole has against many of the anaerobes found in the reproductive tract. Another explanation is based on the metabolism of metronidazole.[42] One of the metabolic by-products of the breakdown of metronidazole is a 2-hydroxy-methyl compound. This metabolite has been demonstrated by Balsdon and Jackson[43] to be more active than metronidazole against *Gardnerella*. It is possible that the activity of this metabolite against *Gardnerella* as well as the activity of unchanged metronidazole and its metabolites against anaerobic flora caused the response noted.

The dose of metronidazole that was chosen by Pheifer and his associates[23] was strictly empiric and does not appear to have a scientific foundation. Although this agent is effective in this dosage, one has to question whether the side effects of nausea as well as the risk of mutagenic potential of this agent should not be taken into consideration and a lower dose sought. In a large study of imprisoned women, a single 2-g oral dose of metronidazole was employed to treat this condition.[44] The authors found that, although they did not reach the high levels of cure demonstrated by Pheifer, their cure rate was quite good. In view of this report, it seems reasonable that an approach to the treatment of this particular phenomenon would be a single course employing 2 g of the agent orally. If failure was encountered with this regimen, then one might want to go to a more prolonged course of therapy.

The treatment of sexual partners always becomes a question. In the original report by Leopold,[2] the organism was found in the urethras of men and also in their sexual partners. Additionally, the concomitant occurrence with other sexually transmitted pathogens, as well as the epidemiologic characteristics of the population that are infected, would imply that the agent is sexually transmitted. Gardner and Dukes[3] encouraged their patients to have condom intercourse because of the risk of sexual transmission. Dawson and associates[45] found that up to 14% of males attending a sexually transmitted diseases clinic were harboring this organism asymptomatically. In view of these findings one must question whether the male partner should be treated at the time of diagnosis. If, however, the organism is normal flora of the female reproductive tract, it seems only reasonable that the flora found in the male urethra would be reflective of what was in his sexual partner. For that reason, it may be construed that *Gardnerella vaginalis* is also normal flora of the male urethra. Hence there would not be a need to treat men who are asymptomatic. Additionally, this syndrome appears to be multifactorial and have more than the simple component of just the presence of *Gardnerella* as being causative. This is demonstrated in the high incidence of carriage of this microorganism in perfectly normal patients. This reasoning has led us to not treat the male sexual partner of a woman with *Gardnerella vaginalis* vaginitis during her first epidsode. The patient is usually treated with a single oral 2-g dose of metronidazole at first occurrence, and then requested to return for follow-up one week later. She is asked to refrain from sexual intercourse in the intervening period of time. If at the time of return for follow-up the patient has not had sexual intercourse and is still symptomatic, she is given the more prolonged course of therapy as recommended by Pheifer. The patient is again requested not to engage in sexual intercourse. She is then returned one week after the completion of that therapy and reevaluated. If she has no evidence of any active disease, then she is allowed to resume activity as normal. If she is still symptomatic or has a recurrence of her condition within the subsequent four weeks, both she and her partner are treated. The dose employed for the two of them is a single 2-g oral dose initially, and then as outlined above based on response.

Summary

Nonspecific vaginitis has probably come full circle. The term nonspecific vaginitis was employed for years until Gardner and Dukes[3] published their data. This drew attention to previous reports of the microorganism and resulted in the subsequent investigation of what appears to be an extremely common problem in women. Prevalence figures for the percentage of vaginitis caused by *Gardnerella* and other nonspecific agents is difficult to ascertain because there are no nationally kept data such as we have for gonorrhea and syphilis

infections. However, rough estimates suggest that approximately one half of patients that present for complaints of an abnormal vaginal discharge have neither evidence of a fungal infection nor trichomoniasis.[46]

The role of *Gardnerella vaginalis* as a pathogen is unclear. Although the organism has been associated with extragenital disease in the form of puerperal sepsis and bacteremia, the high frequency with which it is found in the genital tracts of normal, healthy women makes its significance very controversial. It is possible that the organism has certain strains or types that are more virulent than others as has been demonstrated in the streptococcus. It may be a phenomenon that is dependent upon the absolute numbers of the organism present. Another explanation is that the organism is a biologic marker that grows in large numbers when adverse conditions are present in the vagina, and it has nothing to do with the pathologic process. Whatever the relationship *Gardnerella vaginalis* has with abnormal vaginal discharge, it is clear that a syndrome associated with this organism does exist. The diagnosis of this syndrome is based on patient symptoms and clinical findings, and the therapy that has been proposed appears to be effective. This therapy is strictly empiric and at the current time, does not have a strong scientific basis. Only through continued efforts to better understand the microecology of the female reproductive tract and the pathogenesis of the syndromes that affect it, are we going to gain the understanding that we need to put *Gardnerella vaginalis* in proper perspective.

TRICHOMONAS VAGINALIS VAGINITIS

History and Background

There are three trichomonads that infect man: *Trichomonas vaginalis*, *Trichomonas tenax*, and *Pentatrichomonas hominis*. *Tri-*

chomonas vaginalis is the only one of the three that infects the urogenital tract. The other two infect the oral cavity and the gastrointestinal tract, respectively. Although each of the three organisms can interchange sites for brief periods of time, the environments are such as to preclude colonization and/or infection.

In 1836 Donne[47] described a motile, flagellated organism in secretions coming from the urogenital tracts of both men and women. He named this organism *Tricomonas vaginale*. He did not relate the presence of this organism to any symptoms from the patients that were harboring it. Two years later, Ehrenberg[48] renamed the organism *Trichomonas vaginalis*.

In 1894 Marchand[49] described a male patient with a urethral infection from whom he isolated *Trichomonas vaginalis*. In the same year in Japan, Miura[50] likewise described an infectious urethritis in a male patient harboring this organism. Miura also described a prostatitis in his patient. These represent the first documentation of *T. vaginalis* causing disease in men.

The first United States report of a *Trichomonas* infection was made by Dock[51] in 1896. Subsequent to that there were innumerable reports in the literature. At the turn of the century, Curtis[52] described the microbial inhabitants of leukorrhea and made mention of this protozoan parasite. Although innumerable authors made contributions over the subsequent 30 years, the first major review of this subject was in the form of a monograph by Trussel[53] in 1947.

Early therapy for *T. vaginalis* infections was a problem. Although symptomatic therapy was available, cures were uncommon. Additionally, the sexually transmitted nature of the infection resulted in not only two patients being involved, but also multiple recurrences. French investigators evaluated an oral drug for *T. vaginalis* infections, which proved to be effective. Durel and associates[54] published their report in 1960, demonstrating the efficacy of metronida-

zole for the treatment of *T. vaginalis* vaginitis. This was the first drug that was truly curative. The agent became very popular and its use soon was widely disseminated. However, one year later it was noted that drug resistance might be a problem.[55] It was questioned at this time, however, whether the failure of therapy was based on true drug resistance of the organism, an inability to absorb the agent, or an alteration in its metabolism. Meingassner and Thurner,[56] Forsgren and Forssman,[57] and Muller and colleagues,[58] in a series of papers that appeared in 1979 and 1980, demonstrated that metronidazole resistance due to decreased susceptibility of the organism to the drug in vitro was a problem.

In the subsequent sections the association between *T. vaginalis* and human disease will be discussed. The epidemiology of this organism and its associated conditions will be presented. The diagnostic methods from both the clinical and laboratory point of view will be described. Current aspects with regard to the forms of available therapy will also be discussed.

Epidemiology

The prevalence of *Trichomonas vaginalis* infections varies between 3 and 88%, depending upon the populations studied and the means by which the diagnosis is made. It is estimated that approximately $2\frac{1}{2}$ million cases of *T. vaginalis* infections occur in the United States on an annual basis in women.[59] This may be a significant underestimation, in that public health statistics for this condition are not kept and these estimates are only crude and based on anecdotal reports and small surveys. In a report to the National Institute of Allergy and Infectious Diseases in 1980, Wiesner[60] estimated that almost a million office visits were made by women for sexually transmitted diseases. One of the more common reasons that a woman seeks health care for sexually transmitted disease is because of an abnormal vaginal discharge.

The patient that is infected with *Trichomonas* can present with an abnormal vaginal discharge or she can be completely asymptomatic, as will be described subsequently. However, the male sexual partners of women that are infected with *Trichomonas* are more often asymptomatic. Cornell and Riba[61] noted that two of three patients that were infected with *T. vaginalis* at the time of urologic evaulation were asymptomatic. *T. vaginalis* also has a role in nonspecific urethritis in male patients. Feo[62] in his evaluation of inductees into the Army found that 121 of these patients (16.5%) had *T. vaginalis* in their urethras. All of these patients that Feo evaluated were complaining of a urethral discharge. Catterall[63] likewise noted a relationship between urethritis and the ability to isolate *T. vaginalis*. However, he noted that 30% of his patients that were harboring this organism in their urethra were asymptomatic at the time of examination, and only complained of either a morning discharge or dysuria.

The natural history of *Trichomonas vaginalis* infections is not well-understood. It is unequivocally a sexually transmitted disease. Catterall and Nicol,[64] in evaluating 56 male patients with urethritis and their partners, found that 100% of the female consorts of these men were infected with the organism. That the organism can be transferred from one person to another by other means is always a question in evaluating patients with sexually transmitted diseases. Kessel and Thompson[65] were able to demonstrate that they could inoculate enameled blocks of wood with the organism. They allowed the discharge to dry and were able to recover it at subsequent times. Burch and coworkers[66] likewise evaluated inanimate materials. They were able to demonstrate the ability to recover *Trichomonas* from wet bath towels 23 hours after they had been inoculated. This would imply the potential of transfer of this organism from the soiled linens to others in a sharing situation. However, suffice it to say, that the overwhelming majority of *T. vaginalis* infections that are transferred from one patient to another are through sexual contact.

The patient with a *Trichomonas* infection will usually present in one of three ways.[67,68] She will be completely and totally asymptomatic, she might have mild symptoms such as slightly increased discharge, some dyspareunia, or an odor, or she may have the "classical findings" that are often described in the textbook. It is unclear how long a person can harbor the organism asymptomatically, but it is distinctly possible that one person could be harboring the organism asymptomatically and transfer it to a second individual, who would become severely symptomatic. Likewise, it is possible that the patient, having the florid discharge that is so frequently described in textbooks, may have a self-limiting condition that disappears spontaneously in time. Usually, however, the patient, because of the degree of discomfort, will seek medical attention and have the condition treated. Less is understood about the disease in men; however, in this gender the condition appears to be self-limiting.

The epidemiology of *Trichomonas* infections and the risk factors involved have been well-delineated by Willcox.[69] He noted that the infection is found predominantly in the sexually active age group, and occurs most often in patients between the ages of 16 and 35. It is a sexually transmitted condition and the isolation of the organism from one individual will often lead to the ready identification of the organism in their sexual partner. Male sexual partners, however, because the infection can be self-limiting, may be negative in the face of having a positive female partner. On the other hand, it is not the case that the infected male usually has an infected sexual partner. The frequency of intercourse and the time from the last intercourse to the time that the infection is diagnosed do not appear to be important.[68] There is also an increased risk of infection in oral contraceptive users. The socioeconomic status and race of the patient were thought to be important. However, this probably represents a skewing of the data since the poor and nonwhite groups usually seek health care from providers where there will be an increased likelihood of their infection being documented.

The major complications that have been associated with *Trichomonas vaginalis* infections have been reviewed by Jirovec and Petru.[70] These authors described endometritis and salpingitis in patients with this infection as well as an increased risk of postpartum fever in patients that are infected and go on to deliver. Patients that have *Trichomonas vaginalis* infections might likewise also be at an increased risk of being infertile.[71] However, this is very difficult to sort out because of the high frequency of these patients having other sexually transmitted infections. It is possible that one of the other agents such as *Neisseria gonorrhoeae* or *Chlamydia trachomatis,* which is known to be common of patients with *Trichomonas* infections, may be the underlying cause for the infertility.

Prostatovesiculitis was reported in male patients with *Trichomonas* infections. Unfortunately the authors did not attempt to isolate other organisms such as *Neisseria gonorrhoeae* and *Chlamydia trachomatis* which are also associated with these conditions. Although the trichomonad was isolated, it is possible that it was not the causative agent for these conditions.

Another important aspect of *Trichomonas* infections is the presence of resistant forms. These have been alluded to previously. Mattern and Spence[72] have collected a large number of patients that are infected with metronidazole-resistant *Trichomonas* and have extensively studied the organism. Other than the metronidazole resistance, there does not appear to be any difference between these organisms and those that are sensitive to this particular drug. The organism appears to be ubiquitous and has been isolated from a large geographic area of the United States as well as from Canada and continental Europe. Thus far, all cases that have been reported have been sporadic and no distinct epidemiologic pattern has been defined.

The association between *T. vaginalis* and abnormal Papanicolaou smears has led some investigators to question a cause-effect role.[73–77] Kulda and associates[73] demonstrated a relationship between the pathogenicity of the *Trichomonas* organism in a laboratory system and an associated increased risk of an abnormal Pap smear. This work was subsequently substantiated by Honigberg and his associates[74] in a more extensive evaluation. These authors found that as the virulence of the organism in an animal model increased, the patient harboring the organism was more likely to have a severe dysplastic change on her Pap smear. This phenomenon is not new and was reported by Papanicolaou and Wolinska[75] in the 1950s. Pahen and coworkers[76] in a mouse model inoculated trichomonad intravaginally and were able to demonstrate dysplastic changes in the mouse vaginal epithelium. These changes regressed when the offending agent (*T. vaginalis*) was removed. Borten and Friedman[77] colposcopically evaluated patients infected with *Trichomonas.* They found that once the *Trichomonas* infection had been cured, the colposcopic changes regressed over the next subsequent few weeks. The findings described by Papanicolaou and Wolinska[75] as well as the experimental results of Pahen and associates[76] and the findings of Borten and Friedman would lead one to believe that a cause-effect relationship between precancerous lesions of the cervix and *Trichomonas* probably do not exist. The epidemiology for the two conditions should be similar in that both are probably sexually transmitted, but the observations of Kulda and then subsequently Honigberg and associates must be placed in proper perspective. The findings described by Papanicolaou and Wolinska were not malignant transformations. They were atypical changes found in the nucleus, but did not appear to be precancerous. Additionally, the development of carcinoma of the cervix is something that takes place over several years and it is highly unlikely that the finding of an organism in someone's vagina at a specific point in time is going to be related to a longstanding condition that evolved over years. Therefore, although it is very interesting that patients harboring virulent trichomonads have abnormal Pap smears, a cause-effect relationship probably does not exist.

Al-Salihi and coworkers[78] describe neonatal infections of *T. vaginalis* and reviewed the literature. These authors proposed that the infection could be transmitted to the neonate as it passed through an infected birth canal. This undoubtedly can happen; however, when one encounters a *Trichomonas vaginalis* infection in a young child, especially outside the neonatal period, the question of child abuse must be entertained. Although *T. vaginalis* can be transmitted to the offspring by passage through the infected birth canal and possibly the transmission of the organism can occur through soiled bath linens, the most common means of transmission is sexual contact.

Diagnosis

CLINICAL DIAGNOSIS

The clinical diagnosis has received a great deal of attention because it appears to be the most important aspect with regard to the management of patients with trichomoniasis.[53,67,68] The symptom complex that afflicts the patient is quite variable. Approximately one-half of the patients that have trichomoniasis have absolutely no symptoms at all. Their infection is discovered serendipitously when a wet preparation or other diagnostic test is done either as a routine procedure or for some other reason. Patients will also present complaining of a bad body odor. They will state that they have used numerous feminine hygiene sprays, deodorants, douches, and other hygienic devices to no avail. Upon evaluation, the source of their odor is determined to be secondary to their infection. Dyspareunia is not an uncommon complaint of a woman with *Trichomonas* infection. It is usually not a complaint where she has discomfort with initial insertion, nor is it pain on deep penetration. Rather the dyspareunia associated with trichomoniasis is a generalized discomfort with the sex act as well as an aching discomfort afterward. Dans and Klaus[79] evaluated patients presenting with the complaint of dysuria. They found that a very common reason that a woman would come in with a complaint of dysuria was the presence of a *Trichomonas* infection. This organism does inhabit the bladder and urethra as well as cause irritation to the external genitalia. It could be any of the three aforementioned, or some combination thereof, mechanisms that cause the patient discomfort. The patients upon examination were found not to have urinary tract infections. Pruritis is another complaint that afflicts the patient with a *T. vaginalis* infection. The itching is usually right at the introitus, but also can be on the external genitalia involving the labia majora. It does not appear to vary with the time of day, nor does it appear to be as intense as that found with fungal infection. However, occasionally a patient will have evidence of external genital excoriation secondary to her scratching from her pruritis. The discharge associated with this condition is irritating and patients, in addition to pruritis, will also complain of a burning irritation of their external genitalia and of their vagina. This appears to be an irritative discomfort that is difficult to alleviate. The abnormal vaginal discharge that is thought to hallmark the condition is only a complaint of approximately 25% of patients that have the diagnosis substantiated. It can vary in nature from very slight, to a moderate, to a copious quantity. One must remember that vaginal discharges are normal for women and must be placed in context of the patient that has it and how she perceives it. The symptoms that are found in the male sexual partner of the woman with *Trichomonas* are usually none. The overwhelming majority of these individuals are totally and completely asymptomatic and only seek attention when directed by the woman. Occasionally however, the male that does have an infection with *Trichomonas* will complain of a urethral discharge. The discharge quite frequently is described as a "morning drip" and is often associated with mild dysuria. Some patients can have a clear, urethral discharge secondary to *T. vaginalis*. Patients with nongonococcal urethritis that do not respond to firstline therapy must be considered as potentially having a *Trichomonas* infection.

Signs that are found on physical examination of a patient with Trichomoniasis, much like the symptoms, are quite variable. Approximately 50% of the patients that have this infection have no evidence of any active disease process whatsoever. They have no complaints, nor do they have physical findings consistent with an infection. Occasionally only minimal evidences of excoriations or scratchings are found on the external genitalia, and the patient may give a vague history of pruritis. However, one can also see a very marked and severe involvement of the genital tract with this microorganism. The mucous membranes can be mildly erythematous to violaceous with significant edema and the so-called "strawberry cervix." The vaginal discharge like the rest of the examination is quite variable and should be evaluated with regard to its quantity, character, color, and effect on the patient. The quantity can be normal, to slightly increased, to copious. The character is usually that of a thin, homogeneous discharge that does not have the commonly seen lumps of epithelial cells. The odor also is usually offensive. This can be mild or quite significant. There is frequently a bubbly or frothy character of the discharge. The color of the discharge can be white, slate gray, yellow, or yellow-green. Occasionally, because of the irritation of the vaginal tissues and the attendant bleeding, it will have a bloody appearance. Because of the chronic moisture that is engendered by the presence of the discharge, the tissues can be quite irritated, erythematous, edematous, and friable.

Patients that have a severe *Trichomonas* infection are often extremely tender. The tenderness is more than just to touch on the external genitalia where the moistness has caused an irritation of the mucous membranes and surrounding tissues. It can be quite significant on examination whereby the vagina is so tender that the introduction of the speculum results in vaginismus. Cervical involvement can result in cervical motion tenderness as well as the complaint of low back pain with manipulation of the cervix. Additionally, significant involvement of the fornices of the vagina can result in the patient having what appears to be adnexal or uterine tenderness on bimanual examination. This tenderness on bimanual examination has misled many examiners because of its severity. Patients with this sign can occasionally be interpreted as having early pelvic inflammatory disease and inappropriate therapy initiated.

LABORATORY DIAGNOSIS

Laboratory modalities available to supplement the clinical diagnosis are extensive.[80–86] One of the most frequently used methods for making the diagnosis of trichomoniasis is the "hanging-drop" or "wet preparation." This technique requires a microscope. A specimen of the patient's discharge is mixed with normal saline and then evaluated microscopically. There are two ways to obtain the discharge. One is to take a nonabsorbent instrument, such as a spatula, and obtain some of the discharge from the posterior fornix and mix it with a drop of normal saline that has been placed on a glass microscope slide. The two are stirred together to make the mixture homogeneous and then it is covered with a 22-mm coverslip. Another means by which the discharge can be obtained is to take a cotton-tipped applicator or some other absorbent applicator and place it in the discharge and then mix it with approximately 1 to 2 cc of normal saline that has been placed in a clean test tube. A drop of this solution can then be placed on a microscope slide and covered with a coverslip. The specimens should be visualized under low power (10×). The occulars of most microscopes are 10× magnification and using the 10× objective, the fields are magnified 100 times. To use the higher magnification will usually result in failure to evaluate the entire specimen. One looks for the presence of the motile organism that is about the same size as a pus cell (white blood cell). The organism's movement is usually spinning and jerky. Upon its identification, a higher power can be utilized to have a closer look at the organism. Dark field microscopy can also be used for this purpose. However, dark field microscopy requires a high power magnification and is best used to confirm the presence of the organism rather than make the initial diagnosis. This technique allows one to quite often see the four anterior flagella and the undulating membrane.

Occasionally, on reading progress notes, one will see the interpretation of "dead trich." The microscopic diagnosis of *Trichomonas vaginalis* on wet preparation is dependent upon seeing the motile organisms. One cannot make the diagnosis of dead trichomonads using this technique.

Even expert microscopists are loathed to differentiate a trichomonad from a white blood cell without seeing motility or using special stains. Hence, the diagnosis of "dead trich" must be viewed with suspicion.

Obtaining films of the discharge, placing them on a microscope slide, allowing them to dry, heat-fixing them, and then staining them with various stains is another mechanism that may be employed. The stains described by Giemsa, Gram, and Wright have all been utilized in the aforementioned studies. All of these appear to have a lower sensitivity than the wet preparation. Papanicolaou's stain, however, has been demonstrated to be quite effective in identifying the presence of the organism. This stain, however, is not readily available and usually requires an extended period of time with preparation of the slide. Another technique that has been employed is the use of acridine-orange. This stain results in the organism fluorescing a red color and the nuclei having an apple-green color. Fripp and associates[82] found this to be a very valuable technique in making the laboratory diagnosis of *Trichomonas vaginalis*. The sensitivity and specificity of this particular stain was similar to culture.

Papanicolaou smears, as mentioned earlier, can be very sensitive.[85] Additionally, the routine obtainment of the Papanicolaou smear in a patient coming in for an annual pelvic examination will often lead to this diagnosis. Because this technique is not 100% accurate, one should always confirm the diagnosis before initiating therapy. It is a poor medical practice, unless you know your cytologist very well, to initiate therapy on the basis of the Papanicolaou smear indicating that *Trichomonas vaginalis* is present without further evaluating the patient.

The most sensitive method of making the diagnosis of *Trichomonas vaginalis* is through culture. In 1957 Feinberg and Whittington[87] reviewed the literature with regard to the various culture techniques that were available and described a method of their own. In that same year, Diamond[88] described his media. There are many media that are available for the isolation and identification of *T. vaginalis,* and several of these have subsequently undergone significant modification. All of these media require the additon of serum or other complex ingredients. To date no chemically defined medium has been described for the isolation and identification of *Trichomonas vaginalis.* The organism is a facultative anaerobe and grows well under aerobic conditions. A reducing agent is frequently employed in the media. Hollander and Frost[89] described a variation in reducing agents and presented a semisolid media that could be employed. Likewise it has been demonstrated that the growth of the organism can be altered by altering the iron and ascorbate levels (two reducing agents) in the media.[90]

A good serologic test to evaluate patients with trichomoniasis would be helpful. Although much work has been done in the area, two recent reports have directed attention to the indirect hemagglutination technique and the ELISA.[91,92] Although these authors found their respective tests satisfactory, they encountered the problem that continues to plague all that want a serologic test for the diagnosis of trichomoniasis. A good serologic test has to be both sensitive and specific. Neither of these properties seem to be met with the tests that have been developed thus far. Although the tests may be sensitive and identify the individual who has had *Trichomonas* infection, it does not allow one to identify the patient who is infected at a specific point in time. After the infection has been cleared, the patient quite often remains with a positive serologic test. Because of the immune response, the patient could be harboring the infection and not be positive until after symptoms had developed. The tool might be useful in epidemiologic studies of populations of low-risk groups in whom other diagnostic tests cannot be employed. However, as a general screening tool or to be employed in wide-scale use in a sexually transmitted disease clinic, these tests will probably have little utility.

Hence, the diagnosis of *Trichomonas vaginalis* depends upon either a patient presenting with a symptom complex and having signs of disease, or its serendipitously being determined at the time of routine examination. Fouts and Kraus[67] as well as McLellan and coworkers[68] have demonstrated that the clinical impression for clinical diagnosis of *Trichomonas* is not reliable. One must have a high index of suspicion and in appropriate populations, employ good screening methods. Once a tentative diagnosis is made, there are innumerable laboratory techniques to support and substantiate the diagnosis.

Therapy

Treatment of patients with *Trichomonas vaginalis* infections was highly unsuccessful until the late 1950s. In the "premetronidazole era," most of the therapy was local, palliative, and, unfortunately, frequently associated with recurrence. In 1960 Durel and his associates[58] published their report on the use of metronidazole in the treatment of trichomoniasis. They employed both the systemic form as well as a local suppository of this medication. The duration of therapy that they employed in the early studies was up to 10 days. Familiarization with the drug resulted in the decrease in the dosage employed for therapy. In 1971 Csonka[93] demonstrated that a single gram oral dose of metronidazole was equally effective as the medication given in a regimen of 200 mg three times a day for seven days. This work was subsequently substantiated in this country by Hager and associates.[94]

There are now an increasing number of metronidazole-resistant strains of *Trichomonas vaginalis* being discovered. Lossick,[95] in collaboration with Muller, has isolated, identified, and done sensitivity testing on over 40 such isolates. Similar work has been conducted by Mattern and Spence.[96] These organisms are not absolutely resistant to metronidazole, but require dosages far in excess of what are considered standard therapy in order to effect a cure. Meingassner and Mieth[97] have demonstrated that if metronidazole resistance is present, these organisms are also resistant to other 5-nitroimidazoles. In order to counteract this problem, other forms of therapy have been sought. Recently, Rein and his associates[98] have conducted a randomized prospective study employing clotrimazole as a therapeutic agent for *Trichomonas vaginalis* infections. Unfortunately their work does not support that this agent will be effective in treating trichomoniasis.

Metronidazole has been demonstrated in bacterial systems as well as in experimental animals to be mutagenic.[99–101] For this reason, it is not recommended that this drug be prescribed and given to pregnant patients. However, there have never been reports that have demonstrated that the drug can result in oncogenesis in the human host.[102] Studies evaluating this phenomenon, however, may not have a large enough population from which they are derived and they may not have followed their patients for a long enough period of time. Because of this potential adverse effect from this drug, many question whether asymptomatic patients should be treated. It must be pointed out, however, that since *Trichomonas vaginalis* is a sexually transmitted pathogen that can result in a significant degree of morbidity in patients, in order to break the chain of infection it is probably in the best interest to treat the infection when it is encountered.

Recently the role of zinc in the treatment of trichomoniasis has attracted attention.[103] It is unclear at this time what, if any, effect zinc ion has on this organism and how it might affect its growth and/or spread of infection. It has been demonstrated, however, that concentrations of zinc as low as those found in prostatic fluid have been inhibitory to the growth of the microorganism. Hence, this might be one mechanism by which the male has a self-limiting condition. Ejaculation of a fluid that is inhibitory to the organism could result in spontaneous cure of this infection out of therapy that seems relatively attractive. It might be further demonstrated that individuals in whom the prostatitis or prostatovesiculitis occurs have low levels of zinc in their prostatic fluid. Only further studies will help to delineate these phenomena.

Summary

Trichomonas vaginalis infections have probably been around since antiquity. However, their description is relatively young (less than 150 years). The agent is widespread and is probably one of the more common, if not the most common, sexually transmitted diseases. Its spread will continue at a rapid rate because of the large number of patients with the infestation or infection that are asymptomatic. This makes it difficult to diagnose, not only in the infected male patient, but also in the majority of female patients. The laboratory methods that are available for diagnosing the condition are simple and safe. However, they are time-consuming and not usually employed on a routine basis. The simplest and most sensitive laboratory technique, culture, is probably not cost-effective.

The therapy for the condition is specific, but unfortunately there is only one agent. There is now evidence of a growing resistance to metronidazole and hence, in the past 25 years, it appears as if we have come full circle. That is, having an effective agent that is gradually losing its potency.

The future for *Trichomonas vaginalis* infections is quite bright. We need to develop better, more cost-effective, more efficient methods by which we can make the diagnosis. We must also search for alternate medications for therapy. It appears that we are living on borrowed time with regard to the usefulness of metronidazole. It is highly unlikely that a vaccine will be developed that will be effective against this agent because of the well-established phenomenon that the natural infection does not confer immunity on the host. There is much to be learned about this organism. Only through continued efforts to gain a better understanding of the pathogenesis and natural history of this infection as well as effective means of therapy will our control of trichomoniasis become successful.

REFERENCES

1. Amsel R, Totten P, Spiegel C, et al: Nonspecific vaginitis. Am J Med 74:14, 1983
2. Leopold S: Heretofore undescribed organism isolated from the genitourinary system. US Armed Forces Med J 4:263, 1953
3. Gardner H, Dukes C: Haemophilus vaginalis vaginitis—A newly defined specific infection previously classified "nonspecific" vaginitis. Am J Obstet Gynecol 69:962, 1955
4. Criswell BS, Ladwig CL, et al: *Haemophilus vaginalis:* Vaginitis by inoculatiion from culture. Obstet Gynecol 33:195, 1969
5. Zinnemann K, Turner G: The taxonomic position of "Haemophilus vaginalis [Corynebacterium vaginale]." J Pathol Bacteriol, 85:213, 1963
6. Greenwood JR, Pickett MJ: Transfer of Hemophilus vaginalis Gardner and Dukes to a new genus Gardnerella: G. vaginalis (Gardner and Dukes) comb. nov. Int J Syst Bacteriol 30:170, 1980
7. Curtis AH: On the etiology and bacteriology of leucorrhea. Surg Gynecol Obstet 18:299, 1914
8. Bartlett JG, Moon NE, Goldstein PR, et al: Cervical and vaginal bacterial flora: Ecologic niches in the female lower genital tract. Am J Obstet Gynecol 130:658, 1978
9. Bartlett JG, Onderdonk AB, Drude E, et al: Quantitative bacteriology of the vaginal flora. J Infect Dis 136:271, 1977
10. Levison ME, Trestman I, Quach R, et al: Quantitative bacteriology of the vaginal flora in vaginitis. Am J Obstet Gynecol 133:139, 1979
11. Sautter RL, Brown WJ: Sequential vaginal cultures from normal young women. J Clin Microbiol 11:479, 1980
12. Osborne NG, Grubin L, Pratson L: Vaginitis in sexually active women: Relationship to nine sexually transmitted organisms. 142:962, 1982
13. McCormack WM, Hayes CH, Rosner B, et al: Vaginal colonization with Corynebacterium vaginale (Haemophilus vaginalis). J Infect Dis 136:740, 1977
14. Levison ME, Corman LC, Carrinton ER, et al: Quantitative microflora of the vagina. Am J Obstet Gynecol 127:80, 1977
15. Josey WE, Lambe DW: Epidemiologic characteristics of women infected with Corynebacterium vaginale (Haemophilus vaginalis). J Am Vener Dis Assoc 3:9, 1976
16. Tashjiam JH, Coulam CB, Washington JA: Vaginal flora in asymptomatic women. Mayo Clin Proc 51:557, 1976
17. Edmunds PN: *Haemophilus vaginalis:* Its association with puerperal pyrexia and leucorrhoea. J Obstet Gynecol 66:917, 1959
18. Regamey C, Schoenknecht FD: Puerperal fever with Haemophilus vaginalis septicemia. JAMA 225:1621, 1973
19. Venkataramani TK, Rathbun HK: Corynebacterium vaginale (Hemophilus vaginalis) bacteremia: Clinical study of 29 cases. Johns Hopkins Med J 139:93, 1976
20. Gravett M, Eschenbach DE: Personal communication
21. Platt MS: Neonatal Hemophilus vaginalis (Corynebacterium vaginalis) infection. Clin Pediatr (Phila) 10:513, 1971
22. Rotheram EB, Schick SF, Nonclostridial anaerobic bacteria in septic abortion. Am J Med 46:80, 1969
23. Pheifer TA, Forsyth PS, Durfee MA, et al: Nonspecific vaginitis: Role of Haemophilus vaginalis and treatment with metronidazole. N Engl J Med 298:1429, 1978
24. Chen KC, Forsyth PS, Buchanan TM, et al: Amine content of vaginal fluid from untreated and treated patients with nonspecific vaginitis. J Clin Invest 63:828, 1979

25. Brewer JI, Halpern B, Thomas G: Hemophilus vaginalis vaginitis. Am J Obstet Gynecol 74:834, 1957
26. Spiegel CA, et al: Diagnosis of bacterial vaginosis by direct Gram stain of vaginal fluid. J Clin Microbiol 18:170, 1983
27. Lewis JF, O'Brien S: Diagnosis of Haemophilus vaginalis by Papanicolaou smears. Tech Bull Registry Med Tech 39:34, 1969
28. Smith RF, Rodgers HA, Hines PA, et al: Comparisons between direct microscopic and cultural methods for recognition of Corynebacterium vaginale in women with vaginitis. J Clin Microbiol 5:268, 1977
29. Redmond DL, Kotcher E: Comparison of cultural and immunofluorescent procedures in the identification of Haemophilus vaginalis. J Gen Microbiol 33:89, 1963
30. Dunkelberg WE: Corynebacterium vaginale. Sex Transm Dis 4:69, 1976
31. Totten PA, Amsel R, Hale J, et al: Selective differential human blood bilayer media for isolation of Gardnerella (Haemophilus) vaginalis. J Clin Microbiol 15:141, 1982
32. Wells JI, Goei SH: Rapid identification of Corynebacterium vaginale in nonpurulent vaginitis. J Clin Pathol 34:917, 1981
33. Malone BH, Schreiber M, Schneider NJ, et al: Obligately anaerobic strains of Corynebacterium vaginale (Haemophilus vaginalis). J Clin Microbiol 2:272, 1975
34. Csango PA, Hagen N, Jagars G: Method for isolation of Gardnerella vaginalis (Haemophilus vaginalis). Acta Pathol Microbiol Immunol Scand [B] 90:89, 1982
35. Malouf M, Fortier M, Morin G, et al: Treatment of Haemophilus vaginalis vaginitis. Obstet Gynecol 57:711, 1981
36. Heltai A, Taleghany P: Nonspecific vaginal infections. Am J Obstet Gynecol 77: 144, 1959
37. Jones BM, Kinghorn GR, Geary I: In vitro susceptibility of Gardnerella vaginalis and Bacteroides organisms, associated with nonspecific vaginitis, to sulfonamide preparations. Antimicrob Agents Chemother 21:870, 1982
38. Rein MF: Current therapy of vulvovaginitis. Sex Transm Dis 8:316, 1981
39. Gardner HL, Kaufman RH: Benign Diseases of the Vulva and Vagina. p 191. Mosby, St. Louis, 1969
40. Lee L, Schmale JD: Ampicillin therapy for Corynebacterium vaginale (Haemophilus vaginalis) vaginitis. Am J Obstet Gynecol 115:786, 1973
41. Ralph ED, Austin TW, Pattison FLM, et al: Inhibition of Haemophilus vaginalis (Corynebacterium vaginale) by metronidazole, tetracycline and ampicillin. J Sex Transm Dis 6:199, 1979
42. Easmon CS, Ison CA, Kaye CM, et al: Pharmacokinetics of metronidazole and its principal metabolites and their activity against Gardnerella vaginalis. Br J Vener Dis 58:246, 1982
43. Balsdon J, Jackson D: Metronidazole metabolite and Gardnerella vaginalis (Corynebacterium vaginale) Lancet *1*:1112, 1981
44. Minkowski WL, Baker CJ, Alleyne D, et al: Single oral dose metronidazole therapy for Gardnerella vaginalis vaginitis in adolescent females. J Adolesc Health Care 4:113, 1983
45. Dawson SG, Ison CA, Csonka G, et al: Male carriage of Gardnerella vaginalis. Br J Vener Dis 58:243, 1982
46. Baldson MJ, Taylor GE, Pead L, et al: Corynebacterium vaginale and vaginitis: A controlled trial of treatment. Lancet 1:501, 1980
47. Donné MA: Animalcules observés dans les matières purulentes et le produit des secretions des organes genitaux de l'homme et de la femme extrait d'une lettre. Acad Sci (Paris) 3:385, 1836
48. Ehrenberg CG: Die Infusion-thierchen als volkommene Organismen: Ein Blick in das tiefere organische, Leben der Natur. p 331. L. Voss, Leipzig, 1838
49. Marchand F: Uber das Vorkommen von Trichomonas im Harne eines Mannes, nebst Bermerkungen uber Trichomonas vaginalis. Zentralbl Bakteriol 15:709, 1894
50. Miura K: Trichomonas vaginalis in the freshly voided urine of man. Zentrabl Bakteriol 16:67, 1894
51. Dock G: Trichomonas as a parasite of man. Am J Med Sci 3:1, 1896
52. Curtis AH: On the etiology and bacteriology of leukorrhea. Surg Gynecol Obstet 18:299, 1914
53. Trussell RE: Trichomonas vaginalis and trichomoniasis. Charles C Thomas, Springfield, IL, 1947

54. Durel P, Roiron V, Siboulet A, et al: Systemic treatment of human trichomoniasis with a derivative of nitro-imidazole, 8823 R.P. Br J Vener Dis 36:21, 1960

55. Kane PO, McFadzean JA, Squires S: Absorption and excretion of metronidazole II. Studies on primary failures. Br J Vener Dis 37:276, 1961

56. Meingassner JG, Thurner J: Strain of Trichomonas vaginalis resistant to metronidazole and other 5-nitroimidazoles. Antimicrob Agents Chemother 15:254, 1979

57. Forsgren A, Forssman L: Metronidazole-resistant Trichomonas vaginalis. Br J Vener Dis 55:351, 1979

58. Muller M, Meingassner J, Miller WA, et al: Three metronidazole-resistant strains of Trichomonas vaginalis from the United States. Am J Obstet Gynecol 138:808, 1980

59. Rein MF, Chapel TA: Trichomoniasis, candidiasis, and the minor venereal diseases. Clin Obstet Gynecol 18:73, 1975

60. Wiesner PJ: Magnitude of the problem of sexually transmitted diseases in the United States. p 21. In NIAID Study Group: Sexually Transmitted Diseases, 1980 Status Report. U.S. Government Printing Office, Washington, DC, 1981

61. Cornell EL, Riba LW: Treatment of Trichomonas vaginalis and Trichomonas in the male. Surg Gynecol Obstet 63:511, 1936

62. Feo LG: The incidence and significance of Trichomonas vaginalis infestation in the male. Am J Trop Med 24:195, 1944

63. Catterall RD: Diagnosis and treatment of trichomonal urethritis in men. Br Med J 1:113, 1960

64. Catterall RD, Nicol CS: Is trichomonal infestation a venereal disease? Br Med J 1:1177, 1960

65. Kessel JF, Thompson CF: Survival of Trichomonas vaginalis in vaginal discharge. Proc Soc Exper Biol Med 74:755, 1950

66. Burch TA, Rees CW, Reardon LV: Epidemiological studies on human trichomoniasis. Am J Trop Med Hyg 8:167, 1959

67. Fouts AC, Kraus SJ: Trichomonas vaginalis; reevaluation of its clinical presentation and laboratory diagnosis. J Infect Dis 141:137, 1980

68. McLellan R, Spence MR, Smith JL: The clinical diagnosis of trichomoniasis. Obstet Gynecol 60:30, 1982

69. Willcox RR: Epidemiological aspects of human trichomoniasis. Br J Vener Dis 36:167, 1960

70. Jirovec O, Petru M: Trichomonas vaginalis and trichomoniasis. Adv Parasitol 6:117, 1968

71. Hume JC: Trichomoniasis, candidiasis and Gardnerella vaginalis vaginitis as sexually transmitted diseases. Dermatol Clin 1:137, 1983

72. Mattern CFT, Spence MR: Unpublished observation

73. Kulda J, Honigberg BM, Frost JK: Pathogenicity of Trichomonas vaginalis. A clinical and biologic study. Am J Obstet Gynecol 108:908, 1970

74. Honigberg BM, Gupta PK, Spence MR, et al: Pathogenicity of Trichomonas vaginalis: Cytopathologic and histopathologic changes of the cervical epithelium. Obstet Gynecol 64:179, 1984

75. Papanicolaou GN, Wolinska WH: Symposium on trichomoniasis. Part I. Vaginal cytology in Trichomonas infestation. Intern Med 168:55, 1955

76. Pahen SF, Hughes CP, Reagan JW: An experimental study of the relationship between Trichomonas vaginalis and dysplasia in the uterine cervix. Acta Cytol 7:187, 1963

77. Borten M, Friedman EA: Duration of colposcopic changes associated with Trichomonas vaginalis. Obstet Gynecol 51:111, 1978

78. Al-Salihi FL, Curran JP, Wang J: Neonatal Trichomonas vaginalis: Report of three cases and review of the literature. Pediatrics 53:196, 1974

79. Dans PE, Klaus B: Dysuria in women. Johns Hopkins Med J 138:13, 1976

80. Burch TA, Rees CW, Kayhole DE: Laboratory and clinical studies on vaginal trichomoniasis. Am J Obstet Gynecol 76:658, 1958

81. McLennan MT, Smith JM, McLennan CE: Diagnosis of vaginal mycosis and trichomoniasis: Reliability of cytologic smear, wet smear and culture. Obstet Gynecol 40:231, 1972

82. Fripp PJ, Mason PR, Super H: A method for the diagnosis of Trichomonas vaginalis using acridine orange. J Parasitol 61:966, 1975

83. Mason PR, Super H, Fripp PJ: Comparison of four techniques for the routine diagnosis of Trichomonas vaginalis infection. J Clin Pathol 29:154, 1976

84. McCann JS: Comparison of direct microscopy and culture in the diagnosis of trichomoniasis. Br J Vener Dis 50:450, 1974

85. Spence MR, Hollander DH, Smith JL, et al: The clinical and laboratory diagnosis of Trichomonas vaginalis infection. Sex Transm Dis 7:168, 1980

86. Perl G: Errors in the Diagnosis of Trichomonas vaginalis infection as observed among 1199 patients. Obstet Gynecol 39:709, 1972

87. Feinberg JG, Whittington MJ: A culture medium for Trichomonas vaginalis Donné and species of Candida. J Clin Pathol 10:327, 1957

88. Diamond LS: The establishment of various trichomonads of animals and humans in axenic cultures. J Parasitol 43:488, 1957

89. Hollander DH, Frost JK: Demonstration of a minimum oxidation-reduction potential requirement for Trichomonas vaginalis. J Bacteriol 80:1610, 1965

90. Meingassner JG, Heyworth PG: Sensitivity of Trichomonas vaginalis to metronidazole in medium with different concentrations of iron and ascorbate. J Parasitol 68:1163, 1982

91. Kuberski T: Evaluation of the indirect hemagglutination technique for study of Trichomonas vaginalis infections, particularly in men. Sex Transm Dis 5:92, 1978

92. Street DA, Taylor-Robinson D, Ackers JP, et al: Evaluation of an enzyme-linked immunosorbent assay for the detection of antibody to Trichomonas vaginalis in sera and vaginal secretions. Br J Vener Dis 58:330, 1982

93. Csonka GW: Trichomonal vaginitis treated with one dose of metronidazole. Br J Vener Dis 47:456, 1971

94. Hager WD, Brown ST, Kraus S, et al: Metronidazole for vaginal trichomoniasis: Seven days versus single dose regimen. JAMA 244:1219, 1980

95. Lossick JG: Personal communication

96. Spence MR, Mattern CFT: Unpublished observations

97. Meingassner JG, Mieth H: Cross-resistance of trichomonads to 5-nitroimidazole derivatives. Experientia 15:183, 1976

98. Rein MF: Personal communication

99. Legator MS, Connor TH, Stoeckel M: Detection of mutagenic activity of metronidazole and niridazole in body fluids of humans and mice. Science 118:1118, 1975

100. Rustia M, Shubik P: Induction of lung tumors and malignant lymphomas in mice by metronidazole. J Natl Cancer Inst 48:721, 1972

101. Roe JFC: A critical appraisal of the toxicology of metronidazole. p 215. In Phillips I, Collier J (eds): Metronidazole. (Royal Society of Medicine International Congress and Symposium Series No. 18). Academic Press, London, 1979

102. Beard CM, Noller KL, O'Fallon WM, et al: Lack of evidence for cancer due to use of metronidazole. N Engl J Med 301:519, 1979

103. Krieger JN, Rein MF: Zinc sensitivity of Trichomonas vaginalis: In vitro studies and clinical implications. J Infect Dis 141:137, 1980

Index

Note: Page numbers followed by t denote tables; those followed by f denote figures.